Onco-Neurogastroenterology

George Triadafilopoulos
Editor

David M. Richards
Lavanya Viswanathan
Mehnaz A. Shafi
Associate Editors

Onco-Neurogastroenterology

Gastrointestinal Motility and Sensation Across the Cancer Spectrum

Springer

Editor
George Triadafilopoulos
Department of Gastroenterology
Hepatology and Nutrition
UT MD Anderson Cancer Center
Houston, TX, USA

Associate Editors
David M. Richards
Department of Gastroenterology
Hepatology and Nutrition
UT MD Anderson Cancer Center
Houston, TX, USA

Lavanya Viswanathan
Department of Gastroenterology
Hepatology and Nutrition
UT MD Anderson Cancer Center
Houston, TX, USA

Mehnaz A. Shafi
Department of Gastroenterology
Hepatology and Nutrition
UT MD Anderson Cancer Center
Houston, TX, USA

ISBN 978-3-031-98847-9 ISBN 978-3-031-98848-6 (eBook)
https://doi.org/10.1007/978-3-031-98848-6

This Springer imprint is published by the registered company Springer Nature Switzerland AG
The registered company address is: Gewerbestrasse 11, 6330 Cham, Switzerland

Competing Interests

The authors have no competing interests to declare that are relevant to the content of this manuscript.

About This Book

Onco-gastroenterology is a subspecialty that is not just about gastrointestinal and liver cancer; it is about any cancer and cancer-related treatments and their effects on the gut and liver. Medical and surgical oncologists and gastroenterologists have been treating gastrointestinal cancer for decades by endoscopically or surgically removing the tumor, and by implementing chemotherapy and/or radiation. But recently, onco-gastroenterology has taken an additional focus: the management of gut health in the presence of aggressive therapies for treating cancer in the digestive tract and other organs and understanding how chemotherapy, novel targeted therapies, and immunotherapies used to treat cancer impact the gut. Conceptually, onco-gastroenterology involves an interdisciplinary cooperation in managing complex cases of patients suffering from both digestive and liver disease and cancer, regardless the origin (Fig. 1).

Within this construct, Onco-Neurogastroenterology (ONG) addresses any gastrointestinal dysmotility and altered sensation in patients with cancer that may occur at different phases in cancer evolution, during the pre-cancer state (i.e., Barrett's esophagus or esophageal achalasia), during the active cancer phase, and particularly during its treatment (i.e., chemotherapy, immunotherapy, radiation therapy, or surgery), or months or years later, during the cancer survivorship phase, often as a result of prior cancer treatment (i.e., radiation), and focusing on the diagnosis, and management of such patients to optimize their clinical care while maximizing their

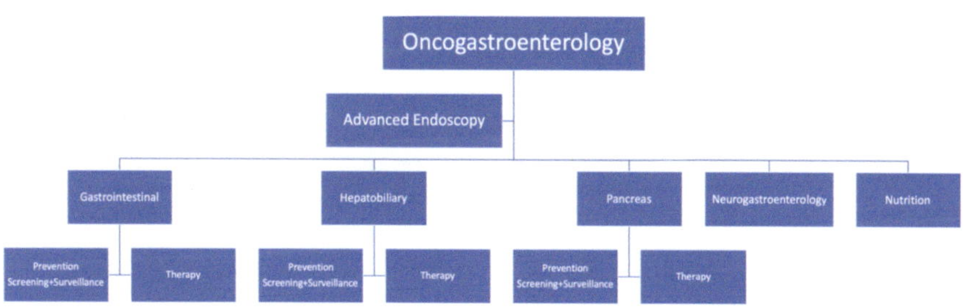

Fig. 1 Organizational structure of the Oncogastroenterology Department at MD Anderson Cancer Center, in Houston, TX, USA

quality of life. Onco-Neurogastroenterology involves an interdisciplinary cooperation in managing complex cases of patients suffering from functional digestive issues and cancer, regardless of origin.

Hence, this book was designed to help general gastroenterologists, medical and surgical oncologists, and radiation therapists take care of their patients with gastrointestinal problems that are not straightforward to master. The text is written from the standpoint of four expert gastroenterologists practicing at MD Anderson Cancer Center, the leading Oncology Institution in the USA, who frequently deal with gastrointestinal dysmotility and altered sensation in patients across the cancer spectrum.

The main objective of this book is to practically compile and present the most clinically important issues in Onco-Neurogastroenterology to help anyone taking care of patients with cancer-related gastrointestinal problems. This is not an exhaustive textbook, but more of a practical manual in Onco-neurogastroenterology as it stands in 2026, as a new subspecialty of Gastroenterology. As such, it is bound to change dramatically in the next few years, as the field grows and more focused research is conducted and new diagnostic and therapeutic tools are developed and validated. While the text may be targeted particularly toward practicing general gastroenterologists, it certainly can be of benefit to Gastroenterology fellows in training, medical, radiation, and surgical oncologists, and general internists and surgeons with a strong interest in cancer, as well as advanced practice providers involved in the care of cancer patients.

Contents

Introduction to Cancer and Gastrointestinal Motility and Sensation

1

George Triadafilopoulos

Alterations in gastric, intestinal, and colonic motor and sensory functions affect a large proportion of the population worldwide, impair quality of life (QoL), and cause considerable health-care costs. Assessment of gastrointestinal motility in these patients can serve to establish diagnosis and to guide therapy [1]. Through basic and translational research, there have been significant advances in understanding the mechanisms of disorders of gastrointestinal motility and sensation, and in targeting the receptors or mediators involved, through clinical trials involving biomarkers and patient outcomes. These advances have led to relief of patients' symptoms and improved QoL although there are still significant unmet needs [2]. Gastrointestinal dysmotility and altered sensation in patients with cancer may occur at different phases in cancer evolution, during the precancer state (i.e., Barrett's esophagus or esophageal achalasia), during the active cancer phase, and particularly during its treatment (i.e., chemotherapy or surgery), or months or years later, during the cancer survivorship phase, often a result of prior cancer treatment (i.e., radiation. XRT) (Fig. 1.1). Within such construct, we highlight the essential elements of pathophysiology, diagnosis, and its relation to cancer, as well as the management of such patients to optimize their clinical care and maximize their quality of life.

Cancer survivors are living longer, and their gastrointestinal needs are changing and wide-ranging, from postoperative sequela to long-term chemotherapy, such as chemotherapy-induced constipation or radiation-induced symptoms that require complex and often multidisciplinary approach and expert perspective. We frequently do not fully understand the pathophysiology of how these interactions work or have large-scale trials to guide our management. The neuroscience of cancers arising outside of the CNS is complex and multifactorial, ranging from altered synaptic miscommunication in somatic and autonomic peripheral

G. Triadafilopoulos (✉)
Department of Gastroenterology, Hepatology and Nutrition, UT MD Anderson Cancer Center, Houston, TX, USA
e-mail: gtriadafilopoulo@mdanderson.org

G. Triadafilopoulos (ed.), *Onco-Neurogastroenterology*,
https://doi.org/10.1007/978-3-031-98848-6_1

nervous system of the gut, metabolic and trophic support of cancer cells, the role of glial cells, and the influence of innervation on cancer treatment efficacy (Fig. 1.2) [3].

Onco-neurogastroenterology addresses primary or secondary motor and sensory dysfunction, gut immunology, and alterations of the gut microbiome before, during, or after cancer development and/or therapy, which require further study and precision-driven clinical management and objectives that are summarized in Fig. 1.3. An essential element before a neurogastroenterological evaluation is an in-depth understanding of the background history, with precise timing and chronology, prior surgeries for both benign and malignant disease, radiation therapy

Fig. 1.1 The three phases of cancer evolution that may be affecting gastrointestinal motility and sensation

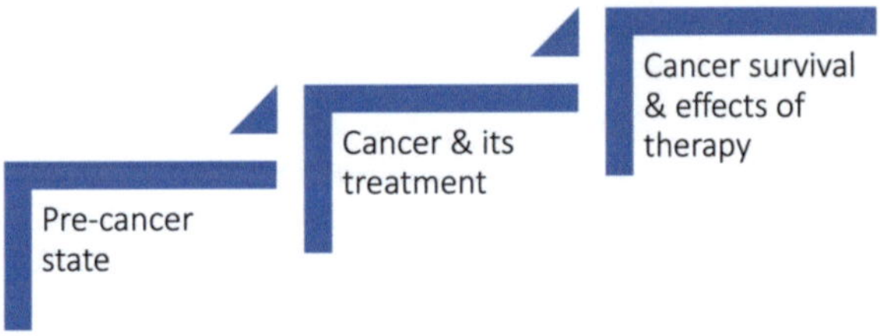
Pre-cancer state
Cancer & its treatment
Cancer survival & effects of therapy

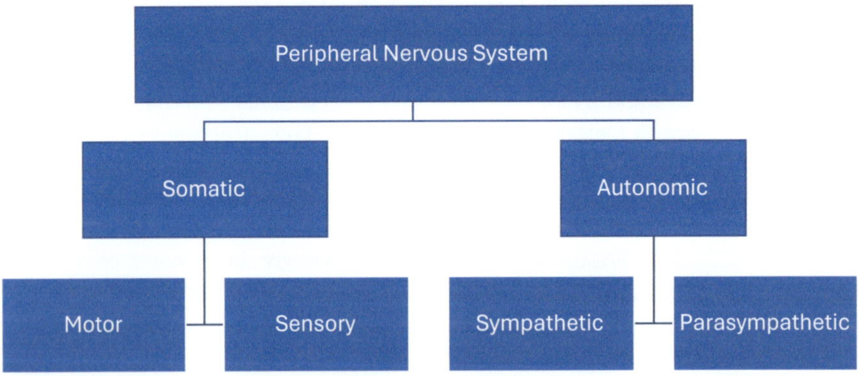

Fig. 1.2 Peripheral neuroscience of cancer

Fig. 1.3 Highlights of the sequential examination and ultimate management in onco-neurogastroenterology. Beyond altered motility and sensation, gut immunology, and alterations of the gut microbiome may play a role

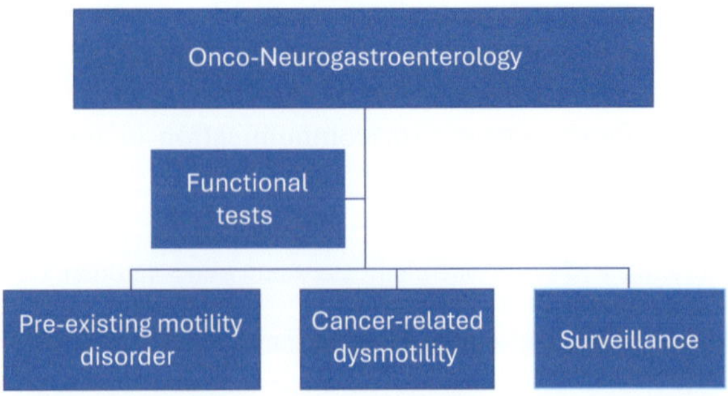

with its location, timing, and dosage as well as timing, nature, and side effects encountered using chemotherapy and/or immunotherapy. The next step is a fresh assessment of the structural integrity of the gastrointestinal tract to rule out mucosal pathology that could explain the patient's symptom presentation, typically using endoscopy, colonoscopy, video capsule endoscopy, and endoscopic ultrasound, as needed. If the assessment of the mucosa is negative, an evaluation of the wall of the gastrointestinal tract using imaging (i.e., CT, MRI) will importantly highlight any structural abnormalities, such as wall thickening, mass, or stricture, or even fluid in the chest, abdomen, or pelvis. If no answer is found, functional studies, such as high-resolution manometry and nuclear scintigraphy, will inform about gastrointestinal motility. Finally, assessment of the luminal contents (pH by ambulatory pH monitoring, enzymes, such fecal elastase, or markers of inflammation, such as fecal calprotectin, and examination of the microbiome using glucose, or lactulose breath testing should be considered. Although typically causing acute symptoms, specific GI infections are often examined by stool PCR testing. This approach may identify a preexisting motility abnormality, a cancer-related dysmotility, a sensory abnormality, or luminal alterations and guide relevant therapy. Ultimately, to establish restoration of quality of life based on therapeutic intervention, periodic surveillance is needed, to modify and optimize therapy, as needed.

In complex cases, which are frequently encountered in onco-neurogastroenterology, it is helpful to identify key features in the background, middle ground, and foreground that will form the clinical landscape (Fig. 1.4). Assessing the chronology and acuity of various and at times overlapping symptoms will allow a synthetic approach and diagnosis. A thorough clinical and neurological examination matched by neuroimaging assists the clinician in the neuroanatomical localization of the problem in the brain, spinal cord, nerve roots and peripheral nerves, the neuromuscular junction or the muscle, as well as the involvement of the enteric nervous system. Metabolic derangements, primary or secondary, as well as therapy-related neurotoxicity, also need to be entertained.

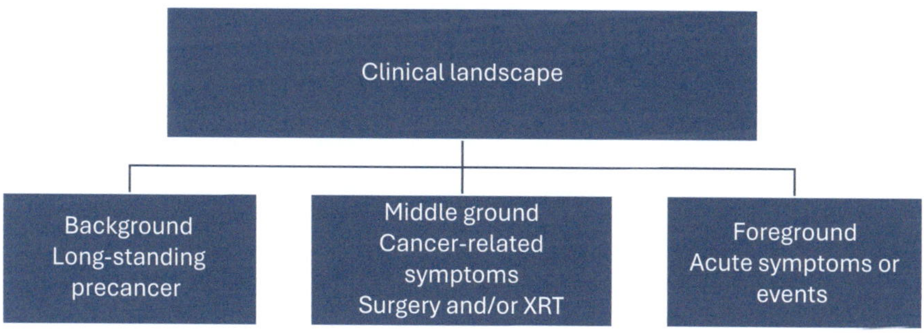

Fig. 1.4 Assessing the clinical landscape in onco-neurogastroenterology

1.1 Essentials of GI Sensory-Motor Function

The gastrointestinal sensory-motor system works continuously to process the intake of nutrients that supply the body with energy and promote tissue growth and repair. Its complex neurohormonal and muscular functions allow for the seamless delivery of 1.5–3 kcal per day from the diet, while simultaneously absorbing 2 L of dietary fluids and 7 L of salivary, gastric, pancreaticobiliary, and intestinal secretions. The GI tract also is an integral portal for eliminating waste. The functions require multiple complex processes including chewing, swallowing, gastrointestinal motility passing the contents through the tract and sweeping away debris, secretion, absorption, and sensation. All of this is coordinated by the brain-gut axis that includes both the central (CNS) and enteric nervous systems (ENS) and various enteroendocrine cells that coordinate nutrient processing and transport [4].

The placement of food in the mouth starts the mastication reflexes. Oral mechanoreceptors relay sensory input to the brain stem that in turn coordinates alternating contractions and relaxations of the jaw muscles, mostly through trigeminal innervation. Chewing breaks down food boluses while mixing and lubricating them with saliva and salivary amylase. Deglutition starts with the mostly involuntary transport of the food bolus from the pharynx into the esophagus. The soft palate is pulled upward, closing the posterior nares and preventing food from being refluxed into the nose. The larynx moves upward and forward due to suprahyoid and thyrohyoid muscle contraction. The epiglottis blocks food from entering the trachea driven by hypolaryngeal elevation, pharyngeal constriction, and bolus transit. Movement of the hypolaryngeal complex allows the larynx to be covered by the tongue base. Respiration is transiently inhibited. As the food bolus exits the pharynx, the swallowing reflex coordinates upper esophageal sphincter (UES) relaxation. UES opening also involves traction from the superior and anterior movement of the hyolaryngeal complex and mechanical pressure from the advancing bolus into the esophagus [5]. The UES then closes, preventing laryngopharyngeal reflux (LPR). A primary esophageal peristaltic wave is initiated, resulting in a sequence of aboral contractions, propelling the bolus toward the stomach. If the bolus is not cleared, a secondary peristaltic wave, triggered by esophageal distention and mediated by the ENS, arises and repeats until the bolus is cleared. As the bolus approaches the esophago-gastric junction (EGJ), the lower esophageal sphincter (LES) opens through activation of myenteric inhibitory neurons that release VIP. As the food bolus moves from the esophagus into the stomach, distention in the lower esophagus triggers fundic receptive relaxation and gastric accommodation through a vagovagal reflex, in turn decreasing the gastric pressure and increasing gastric volume. A wave of distal relaxation, due to VIP-releasing myenteric neurons, then allows the peristaltic contraction to move the bolus toward the distal stomach and duodenum [6].

Contractions of the gastric muscular wall propel the food forward, often against the contracted pylorus, decreasing the size of the food bolus particles and mixing them with gastric secretions. This produces a semifluid mixture under the command of the gastric pacemaker located in the greater curvature of the stomach and composed of the interstitial cells of Cajal (ICC). These mesenchymal cells are critical components of gastrointestinal motility by transducing nitrergic and cholinergic signals to smooth muscle cells. ICC generate spontaneous electrical slow (3–5 cpm) waves and transmit these waves to the smooth muscle cells in the gut to generate phasic contractions and peristalsis [7, 8].

Such gastric slow wave depolarizes the gastric smooth muscle cells, causing contractions of increasing intensity toward the antrum, propelling some of the gastric contents through the pylorus into the duodenum when the particle size has been optimized, followed by closure of the pylorus that forces most gastric contents back into the stomach for more mixing and particle size reduction. Vagal stimulation, gastrin release, and local distention increase gastric contractility. Sympathetic stimulation, secretin, and gastric inhibitory peptide (GIP) release eventually result in a decrease in the force of gastric contractions and slow emptying into the duodenum, usually within 3 h, that ultimately allows for proper digestion and absorption in the small intestine. Practically, liquids empty faster than solids, carbohydrates faster than proteins, and proteins faster than fats. Concomitantly, enterogastric reflexes may suppress gastric emptying, mostly driven by duodenal distention, low pH, or altered osmolarity of the duodenal contents regulated by cholecystokinin (CCK), GIP, and secretin counteracting gastrin [9].

The small intestinal motility and secretions facilitate the timely digestion and absorption of nutrients by mixing luminal contents with digestive enzymes through distention-triggered, segmenting contractions. Under ENS influence, distention triggers regularly spaced concentric contractions along the entire length of the small intestine causing segmentations, typically at 12 cpm. Acetylcholine and substance P trigger contractions, while VIP and nitric oxide facilitate distal relaxation. Other hormones (e.g., thyroxine, gastrin, CCK, and insulin) increase small bowel peristalsis; in contrast, secretin and glucagon decrease peristalsis. Somatostatin inhibits the secretion of growth hormone (GH), insulin, glucagon, and other gut hormones that are generally inhibitory to gastrointestinal motility. Increased distention and exposure of intestinal contents in the terminal ileum increase peristalsis and relax the ileocecal valve, allowing for cecal access. Conversely, increased cecal pressure decreases ileal peristalsis and increases contraction of the ileocecal valve, preventing backflow of colonic contents into the small intestine [10].

The main function of the right colon is the absorption of water and electrolytes from the lumen, while the left colon desiccates and stores the feces. Segmental contractions mix the large bowel contents, facilitating exposure of feces to the colonic mucosal absorptive surface. Triggered by meals, the gastrocolic or gastroduodenal reflexes, or simply colonic distention or irritation, mass colonic movements propel the contents from the hepatic flexure to the sigmoid colon usually 1–3 times per day [11].

Defecation is both involuntary and voluntary. As the rectum fills with feces, the recto-sphincteric reflex causes the rectum to contract and the internal anal sphincter (IAS) to relax, creating an urge to evacuate. However, this urge is thwarted by the tonically contracted external anal sphincter (EAS). When it is opportune to defecate, the abdominal wall muscles voluntarily contract increasing the intra-abdominal pressure, the external anal sphincter relaxes, and the rectal smooth muscle contracts, expelling the feces from the rectum [12].

1.2 Essential Concepts in Gastrointestinal Cancer Neuroscience

Cancer cells reciprocally interact with many other cell types in their surrounding tumor microenvironment (TME) to influence cancer initiation, growth, progression, and response to various antitumor therapies, such as immunotherapy (Fig. 1.5) [13]. The autonomic, sensory, and enteric nerves are major cancer drivers despite being often overlooked in the TME, in part because their cell bodies reside outside of the primary tumor (usually within ganglia or central nuclei), but also because of inadequate resolution for detection through spatial transcriptomics, or the use of multiplex immunofluorescence.

Cancer cell interactions with nerves promote axonogenesis (i.e., neurite outgrowth) into the TME [14]. In contrast to the preexisting "normal" neuronal networks, these tumor-associated nerves carry novel functions capable of mitigating tumor growth. The autonomic nervous system, with its sympathetic and parasympathetic components, is a major player in cancer development and progression, by releasing norepinephrine and acetylcholine, respectively. Typically, the sympathetic nerves mediate involuntary "stress-related" biological processes, often enhancing the first stages of tumor development, while the parasympathetic ones mostly mediate physiologic functions at rest and control tumor progression [15]. However, their specific effects usually differ across various tumors, differentially influencing both the tumor cells and stromal elements within the TME. Sympathetic innervation mainly regulates tumor vasculature and induces immune suppression, while the parasympathetic contributions to components of the TME are likely due to site-specific receptor expression and innervation patterns. Developing novel tools to monitor and manipulate select populations of tumor-associated nerves will allow for site- and neuron-specific mapping and tracing within solid tumors. Many tumors also contain sensory nerves, including nociceptor neurons that may promote cancer-associated pain and cancer progression through neuropeptide release. Manipulation of the crosstalk between the

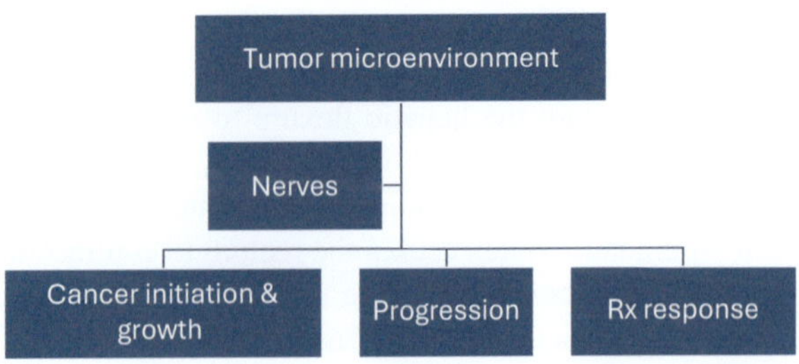

Fig. 1.5 Role of nerves in affecting the tumor microenvironment, in turn altering cancer initiation, progression, and response to oncologic therapy

sensory and immune systems could in turn lead to durable antitumor immunity [16]. Studies on sensory nerves within tumors may help us understand how pain signals are centrally relayed and processed before the brain subsequently sends signals back to the tumor to further affect its neuronal function, excitability, and growth [17]. Given the heterogeneous nature of tissue innervation and the diverse immune landscape of peripheral organs, sensory neurons may in turn regulate site-specific antitumor immunity.

The peripheral nervous system is directly controlled by "top-down" signals that originate in the brain and spinal cord, like the experience of stress, which activates the brain to elicit diverse "system-wide" effects, including heart rate increases, cortisol release, and immune alterations throughout the body. Such "top-down" signaling may also regulate cancer progression through connections between tumor-infiltrating nerves embedded in the tumor bed and the brain [18]. Newly formed sympathetic neurites within the TME develop long-range connections to the brain, triggering sympathetic output to the primary tumor, increasing local norepinephrine release, enhancing tumor growth, and promoting changes in the intra-tumor immune activity that could be modified by anxiolytic treatment. Using state-of-the-art neuroscience tools, we can interrogate specific neural circuits and cell types involved in cancer initiation, development, progression, and therapeutic resistance.

Furthermore, the nervous system often receives "collateral" damage throughout cancer therapy, exemplified by chemotherapy-induced peripheral neuropathy, which causes numbness and pain, particularly in response to platinum-based drugs, and requires dose limitation or early termination of chemotherapy, compromising the therapeutic response and patient survival [19].

1.3 Pathophysiology of Gastrointestinal Dysmotility and Altered Sensation

Multiple pathophysiological mechanisms are involved in the development of gut motility disorders and guide the use of relevant pharmacologic agents, as outlined in Table 1.1. Many of these mechanisms cross-interact within the gut, such as lumen-to-mucosa microbiota effects, mucosa-to-intestinal wall immune, and ENS-driven neuromuscular alterations, or may involve other organs, such as the secretory apparatus of the pancreatic-biliary system, or, more remotely, the brain, leading to a multitude of disorders of brain gut interactions (DGBI) [20].

Altered Gut Motility Propulsion of food and digestive fluids through the gut is driven by well-orchestrated peristaltic movements under the control of the interstitial nerves of Cajal (ICCs), enterochromaffin (EC) cells, the enteric nervous system (ENS), and the smooth muscle cells (SMC) cells of both the longitudinal and circular muscle layers. Any defects of ICCs, SMCs, EC cells, enteric neurons, and immune cells can compromise gut peristalsis.

Table 1.1 Potential pathophysiological mechanisms and relevant pharmacologic agents available for clinical use in onco-neurogastroenterology

Pathophysiological mechanism	Pharmacologic agent(s)
Altered gut motility	5-HT4R agonists, 5-HT3R antagonists, 5-HT1AR agonists, ghrelin receptor agonists, dopamine-2 receptor antagonists, and muscarinic receptor antagonists
Gut microbial dysbiosis	Probiotics, antibiotics, and fecal microbiota transplantation (FMT)
Gut immune dysfunction	Ketotifen, proton pump inhibitors (PPI)
Intestinal barrier dysfunction	Probiotics, diet, amino acids, vitamin D
Visceral hypersensitivity	Capsaicin, ebastine, CB2R agonists, oliceridine, neuromodulators, TCAs
Altered gut-brain interaction	Neuromodulators (TCA, TeCA, SSRIs, SNRIs)
Gastrointestinal secretion	Linaclotide, lubiprostone
Bile secretion	Elobixibat, obeticholic acid

Gut Microbial Dysbiosis Alteration of the gut microbial composition (dysbiosis) leads to gut barrier dysfunction (leaky gut), which in turn causes gut dysmotility and visceral hypersensitivity. Metabolites generated by the gut microbiota, particularly short-chain fatty acids (SCFAs), signal and regulate normal digestion and altered gut motility. Further, microbial dysbiosis-induced alterations in bile acids (BA) may also lead to gut dysmotility and visceral pain [21].

Gut Immune Dysfunction An increase in the number of immune cells in the gut (such as mast cells, T cells, macrophages, and eosinophils) have been found in functional gastrointestinal disorders (FGIDs). Activated mast cells release cytokines, histamines, prostaglandins, and tryptase and are in turn associated with intestinal barrier dysfunction and altered nociception. Intestinal barrier dysfunction leads to the permeation of pathogens and food antigens, which further enhance the gut immune response and contributes to symptom severity [22].

Intestinal Barrier Dysfunction Through special tight junction proteins, the gut epithelium is an important barrier that prevents harmful toxins, metabolites, and pathogens from penetrating the gut epithelium while allowing for the normal crossing of essential nutrients. Decreased expression of tight junction proteins leads to intestinal barrier dysfunction. Diet, dietary supplements, probiotics, and drugs that alter intestinal permeability are under investigation [23].

Visceral Hypersensitivity Due to the proximity of intestinal neurons to immune cells and the degree of inflammatory reaction, an increased perception of gut mechanochemical stimulation ensues, manifesting in pain and burning. Activation of transient receptor potential vanilloid subtype 1 (TRPV1) is triggered by nerve growth factor (NGF), thermal stimulus, capsaicin, prostaglandins, acidic pH, and inflammatory mediators, which further release neuropeptides that aid in visceral pain sensation.

Altered Gut-Brain Interactions Gut function is strongly influenced by the coordinated bidirectional interaction between the gut and the brain that is essential for normal gut motility, visceral sensation, intestinal barrier integrity, gastric secretion, and various immune responses. The gut-brain axis also aids in indirect signaling between the host and gut microbiota. Alterations to the gut microbiota may regulate neurotransmitter synthesis or consumption, leading to behavior alterations. Many patients with FGIDs also experience psychological conditions, such as stress, anxiety, and depression, which in turn lead to altered gut physiology, such as gut dysmotility and enhanced visceral sensitivity.

1.4 Nature and Location of Precancer, Cancer, and Post-cancer

Structural and/or neurological sensory-motor dysfunction can be direct, from the gastrointestinal (GI) tract (i.e., esophageal, gastric, small intestinal, colonic, or multiregional), or indirect (primary or secondary), from an extra-intestinal origin (Fig. 1.6).

Gastrointestinal tract cancers can be primary sources of sensory-motor GI disorders and so can non-GI tract cancers and hematologic malignancies (i.e., lymphoma, multiple myeloma). Cancer treatments may lead to functional symptoms, either acutely or chronically. Radiation therapy is an example of treatment that exhibits delayed onset effects, often starting years after the treatment (Table 1.2).

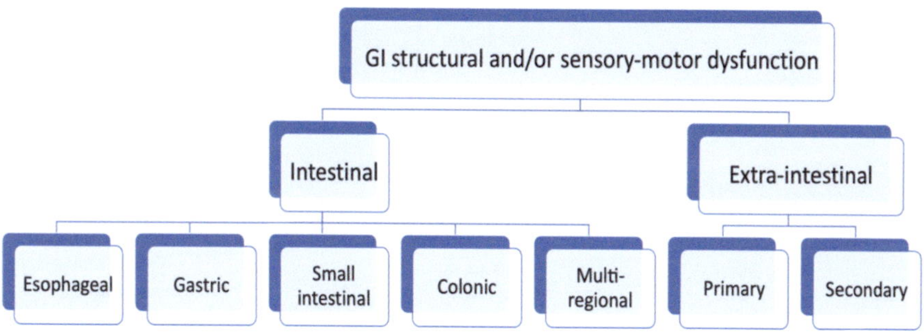

Fig. 1.6 Location of structural and/or neurological sensory-motor dysfunction. Overlapping syndromes simultaneously affecting multiple GI organs may occur and should always be clinically considered

Table 1.2 Various gastrointestinal sensory-motor abnormalities in patients with precancer, cancer, and cancer survivorship reviewed according to GI organ involvement

Organ	Gastrointestinal sensory-motor abnormalities
Hypopharynx and upper esophageal sphincter	Myasthenia gravis Lambert-Eaton syndrome Dermatomyositis Radiation-induced oro-hypopharyngeal injury Post-laryngectomy Upper esophageal sphincter (UES) dysfunction Surgical defects Laryngopharyngeal reflux (LPR)
Esophagus	Gastroesophageal reflux (GERD) Barrett's esophagus (BE) Esophageal stricture Immune checkpoint inhibitor (ICI) esophagitis Achalasia and cancer-associated achalasia (CAA) Ineffective esophageal motility (IEM) Dysmotility following endoscopic submucosal dissection (ESD) Medication-induced esophageal dysfunction Esophageal dysmotility after total laryngectomy Radiation-induced esophageal injury Post-esophagectomy syndrome (PES) Emetogenic esophagitis Eosinophilic Esophagitis (EoE)
Stomach	*H. pylori* infection Autoimmune gastritis Gastric intestinal metaplasia Postoperative gastroparesis GERD-related gastroparesis Glucagon-like peptide-1 receptor agonists-gastroparesis Malignancy-associated gastroparesis Gastric emptying after ESD for gastric cancer Postsurgical conditions (gastrectomy, RYGB) Immunotherapy-associated gastroparesis Duodenogastric bile reflux
Biliary-pancreas	Pancreatic neuroendocrine tumors (NETs) Sphincter of Oddi dysfunction Pancreatic insufficiency

(continued)

Table 1.2 (continued)

Organ	Gastrointestinal sensory-motor abnormalities
Small intestine	Neuroendocrine tumors (NETs) Zollinger Ellison syndrome (ZES) Dumping syndrome Celiac disease Non-celiac gluten sensitivity Small intestinal intussusception Small intestinal bacterial overgrowth (SIBO) Intestinal methanogen overgrowth (IMO) Small intestinal fungal overgrowth (SIFO) Carbohydrate malabsorption Bile acid malabsorption (BAM) Roux-en-Y limb motility after total gastrectomy Chronic intestinal pseudo-obstruction (CIPO) Radiation-induced enteritis Afferent loop syndrome Blind loop syndrome ICI toxicity Postoperative ileus Paraneoplastic chronic watery diarrhea Narcotic bowel syndrome Systemic mastocytosis Short bowel syndrome (SBS)
Colon	Irritable bowel syndrome (IBS) Ulcerative colitis (UC) Crohn's disease (CD) *C. difficile* infection Chronic colonic pseudo-obstruction (CCPO) Opioid-induced constipation (OIC) Structural anorectal disorders (hemorrhoids, anal fissure) Pelvic floor dysfunction and prolapse Low anterior resection (LAR) syndrome Dyssynergic defecation Radiation proctopathy Chemotherapy-induced constipation Postoperative (loss of IC break, bile salt diarrhea) Diverticulosis Segmental colitis associated with diverticulosis
Multiregional	Disorders of brain-gut interaction (DBGI) Radiation injury Intra-abdominal adhesions Endometriosis Postural orthostatic tachycardia syndrome (POTS) Cancer therapy-induced gastrointestinal dysfunction Opioid-induced bowel dysfunction (OIBD) Paraneoplastic MEN2B and ganglioneuromas Neurofibromatosis Cannabinoid gut Amyloidosis Adrenal insufficiency Thyroid disorders

References

1. Keller J, Bassotti G, Clarke J, Dinning P, Fox M, Grover M, Hellström PM, Ke M, Layer P, Malagelada C, Parkman HP, Scott SM, Tack J, Simren M, Törnblom H, Camilleri M. International Working Group for Disorders of Gastrointestinal Motility and Function. Expert consensus document: advances in the diagnosis and classification of gastric and intestinal motility disorders. Nat Rev Gastroenterol Hepatol. 2018;15(5):291–308. https://doi.org/10.1038/nrgastro.2018.7. Epub 2018 Apr 6. PMID: 29622808; PMCID: PMC6646879.
2. Camilleri M. Pharmacological agents currently in clinical trials for disorders in neurogastroenterology. J Clin Invest. 2013;123(10):4111–20. https://doi.org/10.1172/JCI70837. Epub 2013 Oct 1. PMID: 24084743; PMCID: PMC3784550.
3. Amit M, Anastasaki C, Dantzer R, Demir IE, Deneen B, Dixon KO, Egeblad M, Gibson EM, Hervey-Jumper SL, Hondermarck H, Magnon C, Monje M, Na'ara S, Pan Y, Repasky EA, Scheff NN, Sloan EK, Talbot S, Tracey KJ, Trotman LC, Valiente M, Van Aelst L, Venkataramani V, Venkatesh HS, Vermeer PD, Winkler F, Wong RJ, Gutmann DH, Borniger JC. Next directions in the neuroscience of cancers arising outside the CNS. Cancer Discov. 2024;14(4):669–73.
4. Sanders KM, Kito Y, Hwang SJ, Ward SM. Regulation of gastrointestinal smooth muscle function by interstitial cells. Physiology (Bethesda). 2016;31(5):316–26. https://doi.org/10.1152/physiol.00006.2016. PMID: 27488743; PMCID: PMC5504460.
5. Mankekar G, Chavan K. Physiology of swallowing and esophageal function tests. In: Swallowing – physiology, disorders, diagnosis and therapy. Springer (India) Private Limited; 2015. p. 21–38. https://doi.org/10.1007/978-81-322-2419-8_2.
6. Lottrup C, Khan A, Rangan V, Clarke JO. Esophageal physiology-an overview of esophageal disorders from a pathophysiological point of view. Ann N Y Acad Sci. 2020;1481(1):182–97. https://doi.org/10.1111/nyas.14417. Epub 2020 Jul 10. PMID: 32648992.
7. Camilleri M, Sanders KM. Gastroparesis. Gastroenterology. 2022;162(1):68–87.e1. https://doi.org/10.1053/j.gastro.2021.10.028. Epub 2021 Oct 27. PMID: 34717924; PMCID: PMC8678360.
8. O'Grady G, Carbone F, Tack J. Gastric sensorimotor function and its clinical measurement. Neurogastroenterol Motil. 2022;34(12):e14489. https://doi.org/10.1111/nmo.14489. Epub 2022 Nov 13. PMID: 36371709.
9. Ramsay PT, Carr A. Gastric acid and digestive physiology. Surg Clin North Am. 2011;91(5):977–82. https://doi.org/10.1016/j.suc.2011.06.010. PMID: 21889024
10. Patel YA, Pasricha PJ. Enteric neuromodulation for the gut and beyond. Cold Spring Harb Perspect Med. 2020;10(1):a034355. https://doi.org/10.1101/cshperspect.a034355. PMID: 30858329; PMCID: PMC6938660.
11. Dinning PG. A new understanding of the physiology and pathophysiology of colonic motility? Neurogastroenterol Motil. 2018;30(11):e13395. https://doi.org/10.1111/nmo.13395. Epub 2018 Jul 4. PMID: 29971850.
12. Bharucha AE, Lacy BE. Mechanisms, evaluation, and management of chronic constipation. Gastroenterology. 2020;158(5):1232–1249.e3. https://doi.org/10.1053/j.gastro.2019.12.034. Epub 2020 Jan 13. PMID: 31945360; PMCID: PMC7573977.
13. Hanahan D, Monje M. Cancer hallmarks intersect with neuroscience in the tumor microenvironment. Cancer Cell. 2023;41(3):573–80.
14. Amit M, Takahashi H, Dragomir MP, Lindemann A, Gleber-Netto FO, Pickering CR, Anfossi S, Osman AA, Cai Y, Wang R, Knutsen E, Shimizu M, Ivan C, Rao X, Wang J, Silverman DA, Tam S, Zhao M, Caulin C, Zinger A, Tasciotti E, Dougherty PM, El-Naggar A, Calin GA, Myers JN. Loss of p53 drives neuron reprogramming in head and neck cancer. Nature. 2020;578(7795):449–54.
15. Kamiya A, Hayama Y, Kato S, Shimomura A, Shimomura T, Irie K, Kaneko R, Yanagawa Y, Kobayashi K, Ochiya T. Genetic manipulation of autonomic nerve fiber innervation and activity and its effect on breast cancer progression. Nat Neurosci. 2019;22(8):1289–305.

16. Balood M, Ahmadi M, Eichwald T, Ahmadi A, Majdoubi A, Roversi K, Roversi K, Lucido CT, Restaino AC, Huang S, Ji L, Huang KC, Semerena E, Thomas SC, Trevino AE, Merrison H, Parrin A, Doyle B, Vermeer DW, Spanos WC, Williamson CS, Seehus CR, Foster SL, Dai H, Shu CJ, Rangachari M, Thibodeau J, V Del Rincon S, Drapkin R, Rafei M, Ghasemlou N, Vermeer PD, Woolf CJ, Talbot S. Nociceptor neurons affect cancer immunosurveillance. Nature. 2022;611(7935):405–12.
17. Magnon C, Hondermarck H. The neural addiction of cancer. Nat Rev Cancer. 2023;23(5):317–34.
18. Zhang Z, Li Y, Lv X, Zhao L, Wang X. VLM catecholaminergic neurons control tumor growth by regulating CD8+ T cells. Proc Natl Acad Sci USA. 2021;118(28):e2103505118.
19. Zajączkowska R, Kocot-Kępska M, Leppert W, Wrzosek A, Mika J, Wordliczek J. Mechanisms of chemotherapy-induced peripheral neuropathy. Int J Mol Sci. 2019;20(6):1451.
20. Furness JB. The enteric nervous system and neurogastroenterology. Nat Rev Gastroentero. 2012;9:286–94.
21. Jacobson A, Yang D, Vella M, Chiu IM. The intestinal neuro-immune axis: crosstalk between neurons, immune cells, and microbes. Mucosal Immunol. 2021;14(3):555–65. https://doi.org/10.1038/s41385-020-00368-1. Epub 2021 Feb 4. PMID: 33542493; PMCID: PMC8075967.
22. Pace LA, Kong N, Itani MI, Hemp J. The neuroimmune axis in gastrointestinal disorders - an underrecognized problem. Curr Gastroenterol Rep. 2025;27(1):28. https://doi.org/10.1007/s11894-025-00973-9. PMID: 40232527.
23. Twardowska A, Makaro A, Binienda A, Fichna J, Salaga M. Preventing bacterial translocation in patients with leaky gut syndrome: nutrition and pharmacological treatment options. Int J Mol Sci. 2022;23(6):3204. https://doi.org/10.3390/ijms23063204. PMID: 35328624; PMCID: PMC8949204.

Symptom Etiology

2

George Triadafilopoulos

2.1 Symptom Etiology

The approach to gastrointestinal (GI) symptoms starts with three questions: Are the symptoms [1] related to an underlying structural process; [2] the result of a functional process; and [3] due to a combination of structural and functional disturbances. Structural processes can be obstructive (like a malignant luminal obstruction), or non-obstructive, like the physical destruction of nerves, mucosal absorptive surfaces (including loss of brush border enzymes), direct drug effects (i.e., ICI toxicity), alterations in blood and lymphatic flow, or muscle tissue. Functional processes can cause changes in movement leading to changes in transit (both too fast, or too slow), or they can result in disordered sensation (Fig. 2.1).

G. Triadafilopoulos (✉)
Department of Gastroenterology, Hepatology and Nutrition,
UT MD Anderson Cancer Center, Houston, TX, USA
e-mail: gtriadafilopoulo@mdanderson.org

G. Triadafilopoulos (ed.), *Onco-Neurogastroenterology*,
https://doi.org/10.1007/978-3-031-98848-6_2

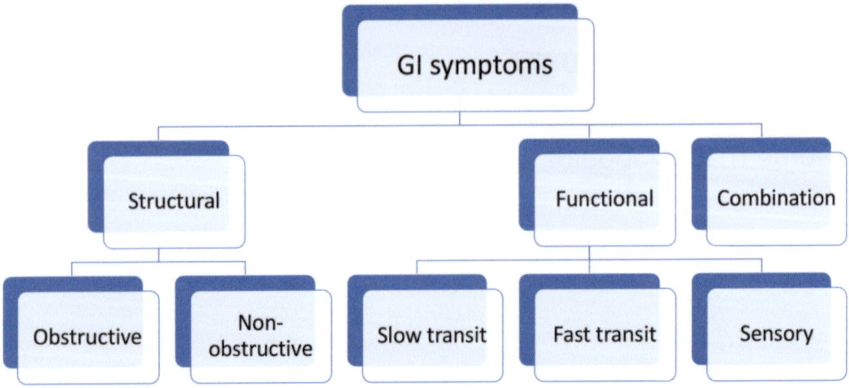

Fig. 2.1 Differentiating the diagnostic exploratory process of symptoms in onco-neurogastroenterology. Before investigating gastrointestinal motor or sensory function, mucosal or structural diseases, such as inflammatory or malignancy should be excluded

2.2 Gastrointestinal Symptom Questionnaire

The use of a simple and practical gastrointestinal symptom questionnaire is highly recommended before every visit to the physician, regardless of their specialty. The patient has the time to examine if they have any symptoms and to what degree such symptoms affect their quality of life by grading their frequency and severity. Relaying this information to the physician will then initiate a conversation and decision-making. The physician will be alerted to the problem and will decide about its management, specifically by an intervention or a referral. The questionnaire can also be used by the patient, week after week, month after month, to assess how they are doing overall, with or without any intervention. Changes in the nature, frequency, and severity of symptoms will in turn allow the recognition of a new problem or the improvement or worsening of an existing problem. Importantly, the questionnaire focuses the discussion with the patient and sets goals to be met by a particular intervention. The questionnaire also facilitates the communication between the primary physician and the gastroenterologist so they can coordinate care, adjust medical therapy, or ensure ongoing monitoring.

The questionnaire (Table 2.1) has been particularly easy to fill out by the patient and their caretakers and provides very useful information to their physicians in a time-efficient manner. At the time of the visit, and with a brief glance, the physician can quickly decide how significant the gastrointestinal symptoms are, if they are focal or general in nature, and to what degree they are linked to the patient's presentation, or they potentially reflect side effects of therapy. If an intervention is decided upon, the questionnaire can be used as an assessment tool in judging its success or failure, the need for further testing, or advancement of therapy [1].

Although the symptoms of neurological dysfunction can often be attributed to an abnormality of a specific organ along the length of the gut, mixed presentations are not uncommon, and coexistent issues need to be kept in mind, particularly when

Table 2.1 Gastrointestinal symptom questionnaire

Symptom	Score			
Difficulty swallowing (dysphagia)	0	1	2	3
Chest pain with swallowing (odynophagia)	0	1	2	3
Fluid (acid or bile) regurgitation	0	1	2	3
Pain in upper stomach (above belly button)	0	1	2	3
Is this pain relieved with food or acid blockers	0	1	2	3
Is this pain worse with greasy foods	0	1	2	3
Is this pain waking you up at night	0	1	2	3
Pain in lower stomach (below belly button)	0	1	2	3
Is this pain waking you up at night?	0	1	2	3
Is this pain better with passing stool or gas?	0	1	2	3
Burping (belching)	0	1	2	3
Loss of appetite	0	1	2	3
Nausea (stomach sickness)	0	1	2	3
Early satiety (fullness after meals)	0	1	2	3
Bloating	0	1	2	3
Abdominal distention	0	1	2	3
Constipation (hard and infrequent) stool	0	1	2	3
Straining at stool evacuation	0	1	2	3
Unable to complete bowel movement	0	1	2	3
Urgency to pass stool	0	1	2	3
Stool (fecal) incontinence, or loss of bowel control	0	1	2	3
Diarrhea (loose and frequent) stool	0	1	2	3
Bleeding through the rectum	0	1	2	3
Unintentional weight loss (>10 lbs)	0	1	2	3

Please *circle* your response to the questions below. Use the following *scale* to score your symptoms:

0 No problem
1 Problem of *mild* intensity (<3/10) and/or frequency (<50% of the time)
2 Problem of *moderate* intensity (3–6/10) and/or frequency (50–75% of the time)
3 Problem of *severe* intensity (>7/10) and/or frequency (>75% of the time)

patients do not respond to an empirically prescribed therapy, such as acid suppression (Table 2.2). Because there is a possibility of such overlap, radical therapies (such as surgery) need to be avoided, unless necessitated for specific diagnosis. The preexisting magnitude of the neurological dysfunction will also need to be considered prior to any further oncologic therapies being implemented, to minimize any further QoL impairment.

2.3 Symptom Localization and Assessment

2.3.1 Mouth and Tongue

Dental Problems Because of their face dexterity, poor jaw opening, and coordination difficulties, patients with head and neck cancer who undergo radiation therapy, surgery, or both brush their teeth and seek dental care less frequently than healthy adults. This leads to an increased risk for gum problems, caries, and the need for teeth extractions prior to radiation therapy, making them vulnerable to osteoradionecrosis, infectious complications, reconstructions with dental and jaw resections,

Table 2.2 Symptoms originating from various organs of the gut; overlap may occur

Motor and sensory symptoms resulting from specific organ involvement
Mouth
Dental problems
Xerostomia (dry mouth)
Altered taste (dysgeusia)
Pharynx and esophagus
Lump in throat (Globus)
Dysphagia
Odynophagia (painful swallowing)
Chest pain
Heartburn and regurgitation
Belching
Laryngo-pharyngeal reflux (LPR)
Stomach
Fullness and early satiety
Nausea and vomiting
Bloating
Abdominal pain
Biliary-pancreas
Abdominal pain
Diarrhea
Small intestine
Bloating
Abdominal pain
Weight loss and malnutrition
Small intestinal bacterial overgrowth (SIBO)
Colon and anus
Bloating and abdominal distention
Diarrhea
Constipation
Fecal urgency and incontinence
Rectal bleeding

or mouth opening due to loss of oral structures. Such patients can have palatal defects that require obturators, limiting their ability to chew and impacting swallowing and nutrition.

Xerostomia A dry mouth might impair the self-cleaning mechanism of the mouth, causing bad breath, altered taste, and poor food intake. Hyposalivation and subjective experience (xerostomia) are common in patients with cancer. Dry mouth is often a result of medication use, specifically anticholinergics. The complexity of these salivary problems necessitates a multidisciplinary approach to avoid mutually counteracting treatments from different healthcare professionals. Dry mouth from damage to salivary structures leads to dysphagia, dental issues, Candida esophagitis, oral thrush, globus, and a persistent sensation of thick mucus in the mouth with the need for throat clearing [2]. In a quality-of-life study of head and neck cancer survivors, xerostomia was the most frequently reported symptom and the symptom with the highest mean severity across all patients, followed by dysphagia [3].

Altered Taste (Dysgeusia) Chemotherapy is often accompanied by taste alterations, due to different mechanisms. Although clinicians usually underestimate dysgeusia, it is considered very worrying and disturbing by cancer patients, because it induces changes in dietary choices and social habits, affecting their physical and psychological health, with a profound impact on their quality of life. Several strategies and therapies have been proposed to prevent or alleviate dysgeusia. A feeling of burning in the mouth without any obvious abnormalities on examination may be reported and clinically noted [4].

2.3.2 Pharynx, Hypopharynx, Larynx, and Esophagus

Lump in the Throat Globus is the near constant sensation of a foreign body in the throat. History is key in identifying any possible pathology and in directing further investigations and management. Typically, investigations yield negative results. Treatment of globus mainly centers on patient reassurance and counselling, but it may include reflux management, neuromodulation, or speech therapy in selected cases and treatment of any identified cause [5]. When performed, esophageal manometry is abnormal in 63% of patients, and esophageal pH monitoring identifies underlying acid reflux in approximately 20%. Barium esophagram identifies abnormalities in 24% of patients, and endoscopy identifies abnormalities in 22% [6].

Dysphagia Dysphagia, or difficulty swallowing, can be seen in many patients across the cancer spectrum and may be related to precancerous conditions, such as esophageal achalasia, cancer itself and its therapies, or late in its course. It can originate in the mouth and the pharynx because of poor coordination, and rigidity of the swallowing muscles in patients with head and neck cancer, or, more distally, from the esophagus. This tube-like muscle carries the food into the stomach. The first kind is called *oropharyngeal*, or *transfer* dysphagia, while the other is called *esophageal* dysphagia. Both types can be subjectively reported, but sometimes they are found only upon testing, predisposing patients to aspiration pneumonia. Clinical signs of laryngeal penetration or aspiration include coughing, throat clearing, and voice changes. Patients suffering from silent aspiration demonstrate no clinical symptoms or present with recurrent lower respiratory tract infections and respiratory failure. Patients may unknowingly reduce their oral intake and lose weight. Aspiration may be found in 30% of patients with head and neck cancer and it may be silent in 20% of patients. Dysphagia is typically seen in more advanced or end-stage disease. Clinical examination of swallowing can miss up to 50% of cases of silent aspiration [7].

Abnormal swallowing may also be found in patients when tested by videofluoroscopy, barium swallow, or high-resolution esophageal manometry and a high index of suspicion is needed, since nocturnal poor clearance and stagnation of oropharyngeal and esophageal secretions may lead to silent aspiration pneumonia. There are several factors contributing to dysphagia, making its management challenging. Patients with head and neck cancer may have either oropharyngeal (OD), or esophageal dysphagia (ED), or both. Dysphagia can be a large detriment to the quality of life and likely contributes to the weight loss. When oropharyngeal dysphagia is present together with dysarthria (also known as bulbar symptoms), weakness of the oropharyngeal muscles resulting from myasthenia or Lambert-Eaton syndrome should be suspected. Other cranial nerve palsies may be found in patients with head and neck cancers after surgery or chemoradiation.

The steps to be taken when evaluating a cancer patient who presents with dysphagia are highlighted in Fig. 2.2. It is always essential to exclude a structural abnormality, such as a benign esophageal stricture or cancer, by endoscopy, before proceeding with other (functional) studies. Radiologic assessment of esophageal transit using fluoroscopic imaging and barium radiography [8] and the assessment of esophageal pressures, peristaltic coordination, and esophagogastric junction (EGJ) relaxation by high-resolution esophageal manometry (HREM) and esophageal pressure topography (EPT) are important clinical tools for the diagnosis of dysphagia and other esophageal symptoms (i.e. heartburn or regurgitation) in such patients [9]. HREM provides greater resolution, minimizes artifacts, and generates three-dimensional topographical plots of intraluminal pressure profiles, increasing the diagnostic accuracy of esophageal dysfunction and clearance in patients with ED [10].

Esophageal motility disorders should be suspected in patients with a history of cervical or thoracic radiotherapy in patients with dysphagia and other upper GI symptoms, such as need to clear the back of the throat from saliva and normal endoscopy, and they are under-diagnosed unless HREM is used. Breast cancer is the most common indication for radiation (40%), while lung, head, and neck tumors and Hodgkin's lymphoma should be considered either during therapy or many years thereafter. The most frequent motility disorder is ineffective esophageal motility in 40% patients; rarely (5%) patients may present with classic achalasia [11]. There is a significant decrease in the contractility of the striated esophagus in such patients and patients with oropharyngeal without neuromuscular disease. This is important for two key reasons: First, the striated esophagus is near the trachea, and its

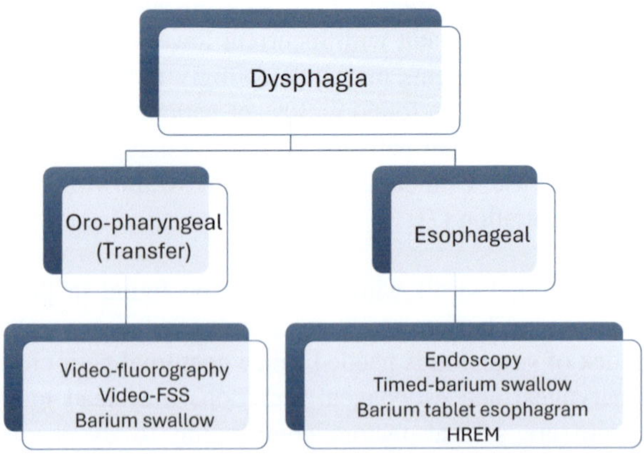

Fig. 2.2 Steps to be taken when evaluating a cancer patient who presents with dysphagia

dysfunction could place patients at increased risk of aspiration pneumonia. Second, the impaired contractility likely inhibits proper bolus propulsion, leading to retention and reflux into the hypopharynx, increasing the risk of laryngeal penetration. Unlike oropharyngeal dysphagia, which can improve with expiratory muscle strength training, there are currently good therapeutic options to strengthen the con tractility esophagus [12].

Odynophagia (Painful Swallowing) The most frequent reason for odynophagia in a patient with cancer is drug-induced esophagitis, which usually reflects improper administration of pills without adequate water intake, particularly at night. In the proper setting, acute onset of painful swallowing should also raise the suspicion of foreign body impaction, typically from a fish bone, or a foreign body (partial dentures) and will require extraction using endoscopy. This is in contrast to food bolus impaction that is mostly responsible for acute onset of dysphagia. Odynophagia should also raise the suspicion of chemotherapy or radiation therapy-induced oropharyngeal mucositis. More distally, *Candida* or viral (Herpes, CMV) esophagitis will require endoscopic and histologic confirmation and therapy [2].

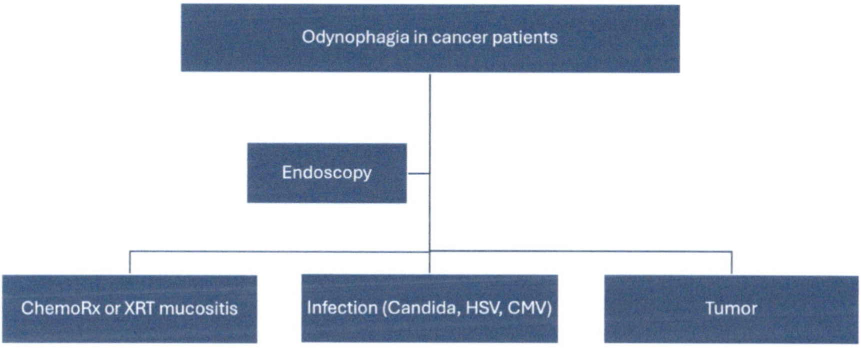

Laryngopharyngeal Reflux (LPR) Rather than a single disorder, laryngopharyngeal reflux (LPR) represents a varying spectrum of clinical subtypes with signs and symptoms that arise from the direct and/or indirect effects of refluxate, physical and molecular mucosal injury, as well as neurologic responses to esophageal events [13]. Specific elements of the refluxate exert distinct mucosal responses and immediate or delayed effects, resulting in transient or persistent symptoms and/or laryngeal hypersensitivity. Hypopharyngeal-esophageal multichannel intraluminal impedance-pH (HEMI-pH) monitoring provides detailed analysis of reflux events, in turn guiding individualized treatment planning. Figure 2.3 highlights the various tests used for LPR detection and quantification. Alginates offer temporary symptom relief and antireflux surgery may provide benefit for recalcitrant symptoms. Pepsin inhibitors hold promise. Laryngeal hypersensitivity during acidic/weakly acidic or nonacidic reflux may play a role [14].

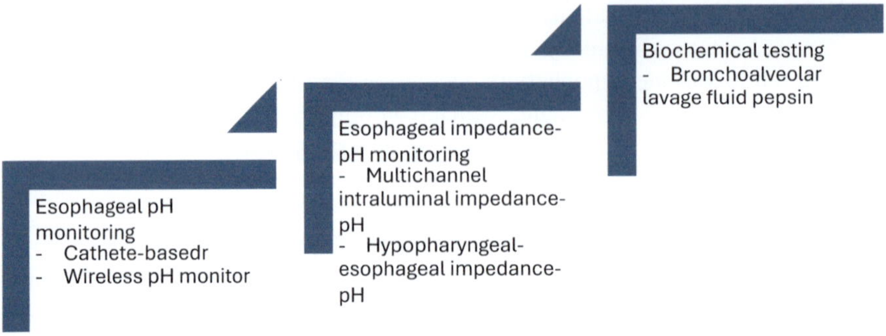

Fig. 2.3 LPR testing modalities

Chest Pain Like angina pectoris, chest pain may arise from an esophageal cause, such as GERD or motility disorder, such as esophageal spasm. Given that most patients with cancer are older and at risk for coronary artery disease, further cardiac evaluation is universally advised. The evaluation of esophageal causes of chest pain in patients across the cancer spectrum may involve complementary tests, such as barium swallow, but high-resolution esophageal manometry (HREM) is most often needed to clarify the diagnosis. Chest pain and dysphagia can be triggered by mechanical stimulation and then get conveyed to the central nervous system via the sensory vagal and spinal afferent nerve fibers. There are three main types of afferent nerve endings, mucosal afferent, intramuscular arrays (IMAs), and intra-ganglionic laminar endings (IGLEs). Calcitonin gene-related peptide (CGRP), a neurotransmitter expressed in the esophageal mucosa, may play a role in symptom induction [15]. In patients with cancer, chest pain may be related to musculoskeletal disorders (i.e., bone metastases), pericardial or pleural involvement, inflammatory, or neoplastic in origin. The characteristics of the pain should be carefully elicited to guide the physician toward the proper diagnosis.

Heartburn and Regurgitation Typical symptoms of GERD consist of heartburn, esophageal chest pain, and regurgitation. Although heartburn responds well to antacids and other acid blockers, regurgitation, the effortless presence of sour or bitter gastric content in the mouth, often does not fully improve with acid suppression alone. Chronic cough, hoarseness, globus, nausea, abdominal pain, and wheezing have a low but potential pathophysiological relationship to GERD. Regurgitation needs differentiation from rumination, a subconsciously learned postprandial behavior that is treated with behavioral therapy. Retrosternal burning, rising from the epigastrium toward the throat, is a type of dyspepsia due to reflux of acid and bile into the lower esophagus secondary to excessive relaxation of the lower esophageal sphincter (LES), or other times, resulting from a hiatal hernia. In select patients with cancer, coexisting esophageal dysmotility may further impair acid/bile clearance back into the stomach. Symptoms are typically aggravated by eating large or fatty meals, lying flat (particularly shortly after meals), or stooping. Endoscopic findings do not correlate with symptoms. Often the esophagus appears normal (non-erosive reflux disease; NERD). Other times, patients with only mild symptoms have significant reflux esophagitis with inflammation, erosions, or ulcers. Such patients typically have underlying ineffective esophageal motility (IEM) and poor acid clearance. Since many such patients are elderly, Barrett's esophagus, that is the replacement of the distal esophageal squamous mucosa with intestinal-type columnar epithelium, due to chronic acid and bile reflux into the distal esophagus, may be found. A diagnosis of acid and/or bile reflux and esophageal dysmotility is made by high-resolution esophageal manometry (HREM) and ambulatory esophageal pH studies [16]. Figure 2.4 diagrammatically depicts the key determinants of GERD, emphasizing the balance between defensive and offensive factors

Collectively, the constellation of heartburn, regurgitation, and intermittent or continuous nonprogressive dysphagia strongly suggest the diagnosis of GERD that will require endoscopic and histologic evaluation, followed by careful assessment of symptom severity that, in turn, will guide therapy, using acid suppressive therapies upon demand, or continuously (Fig. 2.5). This is particularly true in patients with cancer receiving chemotherapy who are at risk for opportunistic infections of the esophagus or those receiving radiation therapy with potential for damage to the esophageal mucosa and muscle. Risk stratification in these patients will require endoscopy to define the severity of esophagitis, HERM to assess the effectiveness of esophageal peristalsis and clearance, and ambulatory pH monitoring while on acid suppressive therapy, to validate its adequacy in controlling esophageal acidity. Further, the use of HREM and pH monitoring may help clinicians predict the disease course and the possible need for antireflux surgery, risk for neoplasia, and potentially the need for endoscopic eradication therapy (EET).

Based on the degree of abnormalities identified, the onco-neurogastroenterogist may apply primary and secondary prevention strategies and further identify and treat complications, as they arise (Fig. 2.6). As an example, early recognition and pharmacologic or surgical intervention may mitigate the evolution of reflux esophagitis toward cancer (Fig. 2.7).

Proton-pump inhibitors (PPI) are the best initial therapy for reflux, being superior to H2-receptor antagonists or antacids alone. Alginates are often useful as "as

Fig. 2.4 Key determinants of GERD

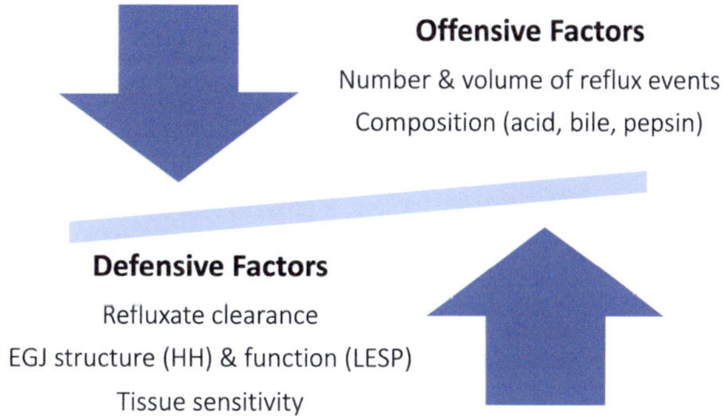

Fig. 2.5 Detailed GERD diagnosis allows severity assessment, course prediction, and refinement of cancer risk

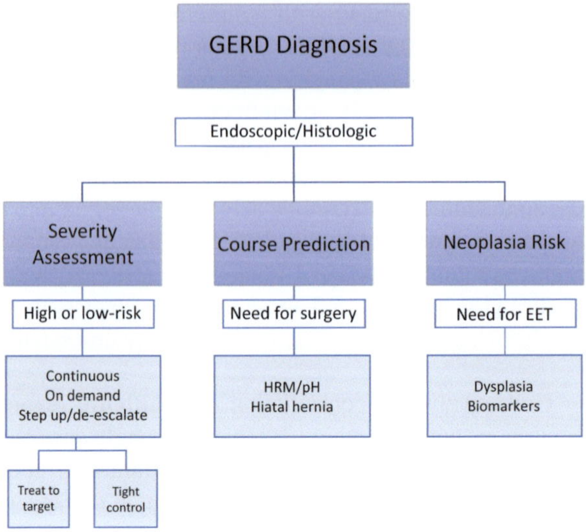

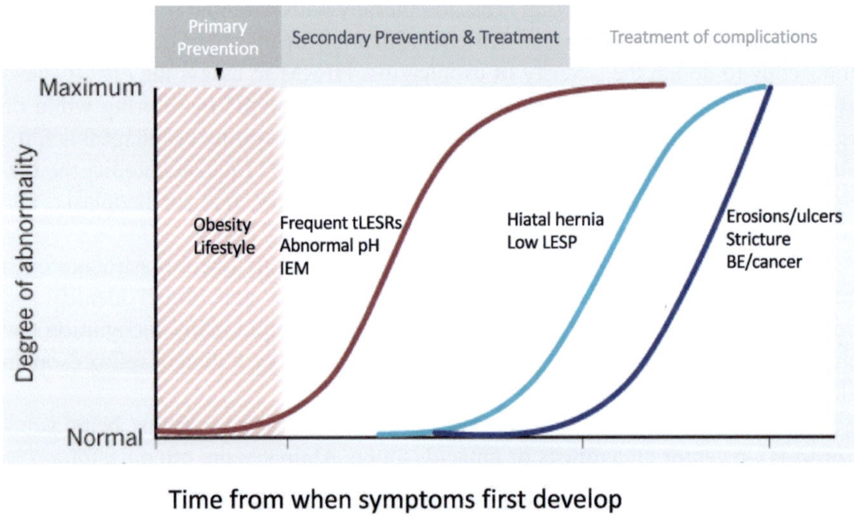

Fig. 2.6 GERD evolution and steps in management

needed" treatments. Lifestyle alterations, including weight reduction, avoidance of fatty foods, and raising the head of the bed, may help. In some patients with long-standing *Helicobacter pylori*, a gastric antrum-dwelling bacterium, may induce acid reflux. Endoscopic techniques for treating GERD include esophageal radiofrequency energy delivery (Stretta) procedure, transoral incisionless fundoplication (TIF), or endoscopic full-thickness plication. Other novel techniques include antireflux mucosectomy (ARMS), peroral endoscopic cardiac constriction, endoscopic submucosal dissection, and endoscopic band ligation. Concomitant hiatal hernia

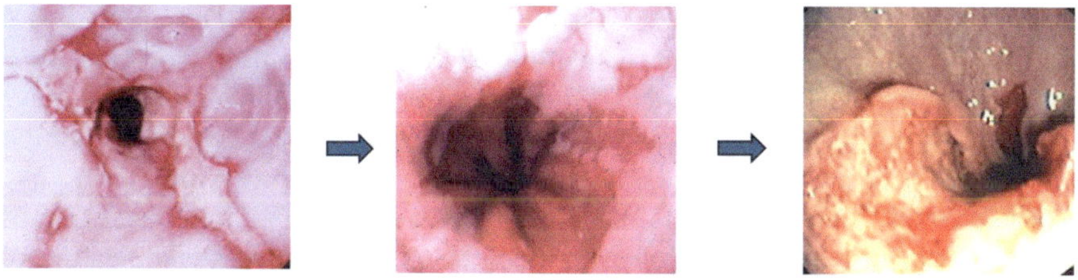

Fig. 2.7 Endoscopic images depicting the progression of erosive esophagitis to Barrett's esophagus and esophageal adenocarcinoma. The use of proton pump inhibitors has the potential of preventing and healing erosive esophagitis, the development of BE, and its progression to cancer

(HH) repair with TIF (cTIF) is often offered as an alternative to conventional antireflux surgery (ARS) [17–19].

In refractory patients with well-validated GERD, particularly those with significant hiatal hernia, surgical treatment is antireflux surgery (ARS) (typically, laparoscopic fundoplication) whereby the fundus is wrapped behind the esophagus and the hernia is reduced back into the abdomen (hernia repair). In those patients with compromised esophageal motility, complications may include dysphagia and bloating due to an inability to belch. Partial posterior fundoplication (Toupet fundoplication, TF) may provide equivalent outcomes in reflux symptom control with a lower risk of postoperative dysphagia compared with total (360°) fundoplication [20]. Long-term (>20 years) experience with laparoscopic fundoplication carries a success rate of ~80% among uncomplicated GERD patients and ~63% among patients with large hiatal hernias [21].

A clinical practice guideline from the American Society for Gastrointestinal Endoscopy (ASGE) recently addressed the indications for endoscopy in patients with GERD, as well as in those who develop GERD after sleeve gastrectomy or peroral endoscopic myotomy. The guideline also discusses how to endoscopically evaluate gastroesophageal junctional integrity and discusses management strategies for GERD, including the role of lifestyle interventions, PPI use, and endoscopic antireflux therapy [22].

Belching Eructation (belching or burping) is a common benign—yet distressing—symptom that is frequently encountered in patients across the cancer spectrum, but it is also reported by normal individuals as well as in patients with dyspepsia or gastroesophageal reflux disease (GERD). Belching is frequently a manifestation of drug-induced dyspepsia. In such cases, it is transient and resolves upon treatment discontinuation (i.e., chemotherapy). The belch reflex is a physiological mechanism to expel swallowed air (aerophagia) from the stomach and therefore may be more common after meals. The reflex consists of transient lower esophageal sphincter (LES) relaxation, gas reflux from the stomach to the esophagus to produce a "common cavity" event, upper esophageal sphincter (UES) relaxation, esophago-pharyngeal gas reflux, and restoration of esophageal pressure to baseline pressures through effective esophageal peristalsis [23]. Normally, physiological acid reflux may occur after meals in association with possible leakage of acid as gas is refluxed through the relaxed LES. Belching and acid reflux in normal adults often occur simultaneously. In addition, transient LES relaxations are observed during belching events. Studies with air insufflation have shown that transient LES relaxations are provoked by stomach distention similar to those seen before pathological acid reflux events in patients with GERD [24]. Chronic excessive belching has often been attributed to aerophagia and treated with behavior modification. However, since belching can be a manifestation of GERD, this diagnosis should be considered, and ambulatory pH monitoring can assess for symptom association and severity of esophageal acid exposure that would be amenable to medical, surgical, or endoscopic therapy [25]. A 24-h pH impedance testing can also visualize aerophagia and belching [26]. Further, underlying functional esophageal dysmotility, functional dyspepsia, and gastroparesis may all play a role and they will need further assessment, using HREM and gastric scintigraphy.

2.3.2.1 Stomach

Indigestion Dyspepsia (indigestion) is a vague term that describes a constellation of symptoms, such as upper abdominal discomfort or bloating, belching, retrosternal or epigastric pain, nausea, loss of appetite, and early satiety after a meal. Dyspepsia affects up to 40% of the population, and in only 25% of cases is a cause found. Alarm features, such as age over 50, new onset of symptoms, persistent dyspepsia despite empiric treatment, history of peptic ulcers or cancer, NSAID or aspirin use, associated dysphagia, weight loss, or vomiting, call for an upper endoscopy to rule out structural abnormalities, particularly cancer, and *Helicobacter pylori* infection. *H. pylori* infection may induce gastroparesis, resulting in a prolonged transit time for drugs to reach the small intestine for absorption. Non-ulcer, (functional) dyspepsia (FD), is a common and costly disease, currently defined by symptoms, using the Rome consensus on functional bowel disorders. Such symptoms include abdominal pain and are often meal-related and there are two major subtypes, postprandial distress syndrome and epigastric pain syndrome, both in the absence of an endoscopically identifiable pathology. Increasingly however, tangible pathologies occur in FD, for example, *Helicobacter pylori*, duodenal eosinophilia, permeability alterations, structural neuronal changes, and microbial duodenal dysbiosis, suggestive of a true disease entity due to allergy, immune disorder, or infection. Anxiety and depression may precede or follow FD [27]. An upper abdominal ultrasound may be justified to exclude gallstones. The optimal treatment for non-ulcer dyspepsia is unknown, but acid suppression is helpful for many. A key consideration in patients with refractory FD is to exclude the presence of gastroparesis that will require gastroenterology consultation and possibly more aggressive therapy [28].

Loss of Appetite (Anorexia) The etiology of the anorexia in aging adults, particularly those with cancer, is multifactorial, and it includes a combination of declining taste, reduced central and peripheral drive to eat, delayed gastric emptying, pathological conditions (such as depression, medications and iatrogenic interventions, oral-health status), and social factors (poverty, loneliness). Anorexia in the aging cancer patient is associated with protein-energy malnutrition, sarcopenia, frailty, functional deterioration, morbidity, and mortality. Since this symptom can lead to dramatic consequences, early identification, and effective, mostly nutritional interventions are needed [29].

Cancer-related anorexia-cachexia (CRAC), very common in advanced cancer patients, is associated with impaired QoL and shorter survival. To combat this, medications include branched-chain amino acids, eicosapentaenoic acid, thalidomide, cytokine inhibitors, steroids, anti-serotoninergic medications (mirtazapine), and megestrol acetate. Due to their low toxicity, anti-inflammatory effects, and catabolic pathway inhibitory qualities, nutraceuticals, such as green tea, fish oil, and curcumin, have been used [30].

Nausea and Vomiting Alterations in the upper GI function occur after gastric surgery for malignant gastric lesions. Gastric accommodation response is impaired after partial gastric resection. Vagotomy can result in loss of fundus and pyloric relaxation and reduced antral contractions resulting in gastric retention [31]. Symptoms suggestive of delayed gastric emptying include early satiety, nausea, vomiting, regurgitation, bloating, postprandial fullness, visible upper abdominal distention, abdominal pain, and weight loss. However, most patients with rapid gastric emptying present with similar abdominal symptoms. Hence, gastric emptying tests and intraluminal measurements of contractility are necessary to further delineate gastric motor dysfunction. Gastroparesis, or delayed emptying of food from the stomach after meals, may be noted in both early and advanced gastric neoplasia, or more often, opioid use, and it may cause no symptoms. When present, such symptoms include nausea, vomiting, early satiety, and excessive fullness after meals, bloating, and abdominal distension. Such symptoms are more likely to occur with solid meals, particularly greasy or fatty, high-fiber intake, and less so with soups or liquids. Gastroparesis is most likely a result of involvement of the gut nervous system, but it can also reflect brain involvement. Abnormal ghrelin function might be involved, since this so-called "hunger hormone" is normally secreted when the stomach is empty, thus increasing gastrointestinal motility in preparation for ingestion of food. Patients with gastroparesis may experience delayed delivery of an orally administered drug or complete loss of its benefit due to poor timing of absorption and leading to an unpredictable duration of action [32].

Early Satiety (Fullness after Meals) Early satiety is the inability to eat a full meal or feeling full after only a small amount of food. This is most likely due to gastroparesis, a condition in which the stomach is slow to empty and is typically seen in opioid users [33]. The patient feels full soon, less than 30 min after initiating a meal, and is unable to complete a normal portion. This eventually, but not always, leads to weight loss, nutrient deficiency, and malnutrition. Since early satiety may also be a sign of serious medical conditions, such as stomach cancer, ulcers, or diabetes, an endoscopy is imperative to rule out structural etiologies.

Bloating and Abdominal Distention This is a hard to define symptom complex, particularly in cancer patients who have undergone previous abdominal surgery. Patients may describe their abdomen feeling full (bloating) more than usual, abdominal pressure, either soon after meals (early satiety), or hours thereafter. Distention is the physical enlargement of the abdomen/abdominal girth [34]. Upper abdominal pain or discomfort, abdominal rumbling (borborygmi), or even excessive belching and passing of gas are frequently associated with bloating and distention. It is essential to rule out structural causes (i.e., peritoneal carcinomatosis) for these symptoms, preferably using abdominal and pelvic CT or MRI using oral contrast.

In the absence of obstruction, and, depending on the timing after meals (early v. late) and the dominant location of the discomfort, clinicians should entertain several scenarios to be evaluated by further testing or empiric therapy. When bloating occurs soon after meals and is not associated with significant distention, but, instead with a sensation of early satiety that limits the completion of a meal, one should consider the stomach as the primary source of the problem. Gastroparesis should be explored by performing wireless motility capsule testing, gastric scintigraphy, or electrogastrography. Figure 2.8 provides a simplistic approach to understanding the reasons behind dysmotility-related bloating and abdominal distention, based on the symptom onset after a meal and its possible relationship to an underlying organ dysfunction. However, overlap may frequently occur.

When bloating happens soon after meals and is not associated with significant distention, but, instead with a sensation of early satiety that limits the completion of a meal, one should consider the stomach as the primary source of the problem. Gastroparesis should be explored by performing wireless motility capsule testing, gastric scintigraphy, or electrogastrography. Bloating and abdominal distention that is not clearly related to meals is usually long-lasting and not alleviated with belching or passing gas is most likely due to abnormal gut-brain interaction [35] or small bowel dysmotility, often associated with small intestinal bacterial overgrowth (SIBO) or intestinal methanogen overgrowth (IMO). In the latter scenario, lactulose breath testing (LBT), wireless motility capsule (WMC) testing, or antroduodenal

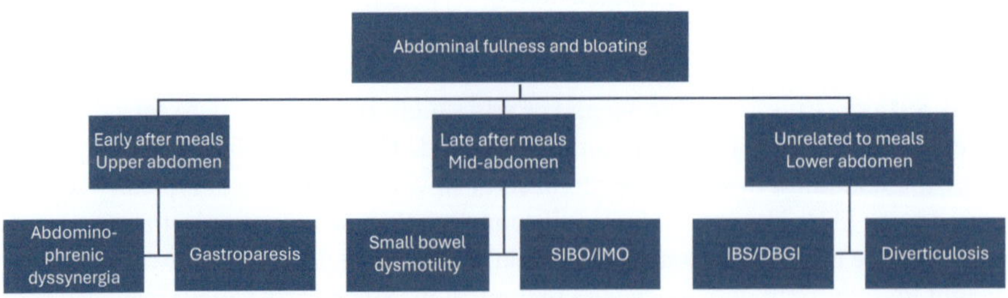

Fig. 2.8 Key considerations in patients who present with abdominal fullness and bloating

manometry (ADM) should be considered. Small intestinal manometry is useful in distinguishing gastrointestinal neuropathy, myopathy, or both, from partial small bowel obstruction, each revealing characteristic tracings and denoting different prognosis and management. If these studies are not available, alternate options could be the use of video capsule endoscopy (VCE) or MR enterography (MRE) to indirectly assess small bowel transit and rule out structural issues at the level of the small bowel. When bloating and abdominal distention are not readily related to meals, and they transiently improve by passing of stool or gas, a colonic origin should be sought (Fig. 2.9). After excluding a structural etiology (diverticulosis, stricture, or colon cancer) by colonoscopy, measuring colon transit time using WMC, or sitzmarks testing, should be considered, since slow transit constipation (STC), due to generalized colonic inertia, is a possibility. High-resolution anorectal manometry, balloon expulsion testing, and rectal sensory testing assess the sphincter competence and neuromuscular coordination during defecation. These tests are generally more readily available and could be used early in the evaluation of patients with abdominal bloating and distention. Except for lower rates of anal hypertonicity in patients with slow colon transit time, disorders of recto-anal coordination, and rectal sensation are commonly seen [36]. MR defecography is reserved for patients with possible defecatory dysfunction, typically elicited by a careful history.

Visible abdominal distension may reflect distorted perception, true intestinal gas accumulation, or abdomino-phrenic dyssynergia (diaphragmatic push and anterior wall relaxation). Objective evidence of abdominal distension may be obtained using a tape measure, by CT imaging in most patients, or by abdominal EMG (a research tool that shows reduced activity, i.e., relaxation) or increased activity (diaphragmatic contraction) by EMG [35]. Abdominal distention can result from abdomino-phrenic dyssynergia (i.e., diaphragmatic contraction and abdominal wall relaxation) in patients with disorders of gut-brain interaction. Abdominothoracic wall movements serve as an effective biofeedback signal for correcting abdomino-phrenic dyssynergia and abdominal distention [37].

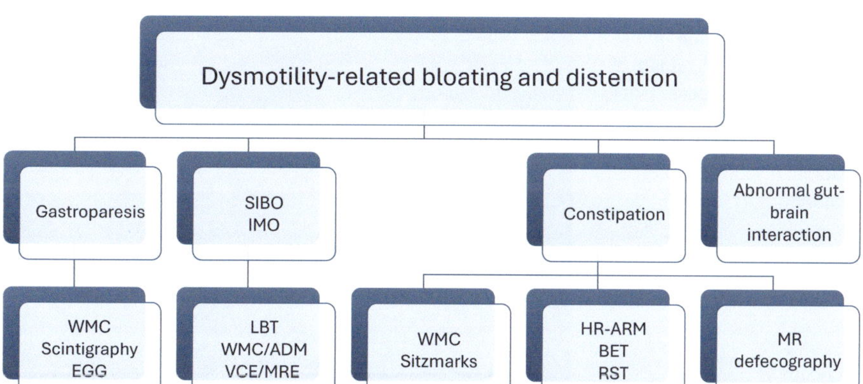

Fig. 2.9 Diagnostic considerations and tools to further examine the origin and nature of dysmotility-related bloating and distention

2.3.2.2 Biliary-Pancreas

Abdominal Pain Biliary dyskinesia is a condition where the gallbladder does not contract properly, leading to episodic right upper quadrant pain, at times radiating to the right shoulder, with sharp, cramping, or dull quality, typically provoked by eating fatty foods. Nausea and vomiting, bloating, indigestion, heartburn, and regurgitation may coexist. The diagnosis is often made in patients with biliary-type pain, a sonographically normal gallbladder, and a reduced gallbladder ejection fraction on cholecystokinin-cholescintigraphy (CCK-HIDA) scan and requires exclusion of other diagnoses, such as gallstones or gallbladder cancer, which is frequently made by abdominal imaging using abdominal ultrasound, CT, or MRI (Fig. 2.10) [38].

The sphincter of Oddi (SO) is a neuromuscular structure located at the junction of the biliary-pancreatic system and the duodenum. Sphincter of Oddi dysfunction (SOD) can result in various clinical manifestations, including biliary-type pain and recurrent idiopathic pancreatitis. Type I SOD is defined as biliary-type pain with both elevated liver enzymes and a dilated bile duct. Type II SOD presents with biliary-type pain with either elevated liver enzymes or a dilated bile duct. Type III SOD patients have biliary-type pain only without biochemical or imaging abnormalities. Type III SOD may reflect central sensitization and visceral hyperalgesia, and it can be found in cancer patients using narcotics regularly [39]. Because ERCP and sphincterotomy may not be effective [40], and a leading cause of pancreatitis, antidepressants are occasionally prescribed [41].

Many patients with intraductal papillary mucinous neoplasm of the pancreas (IPMN) have no symptoms, and they are detected incidentally when imaging studies are performed for unrelated indications. Other patients may have nausea, vomiting, abdominal pain, back pain, weight loss, or anorexia. Because the main

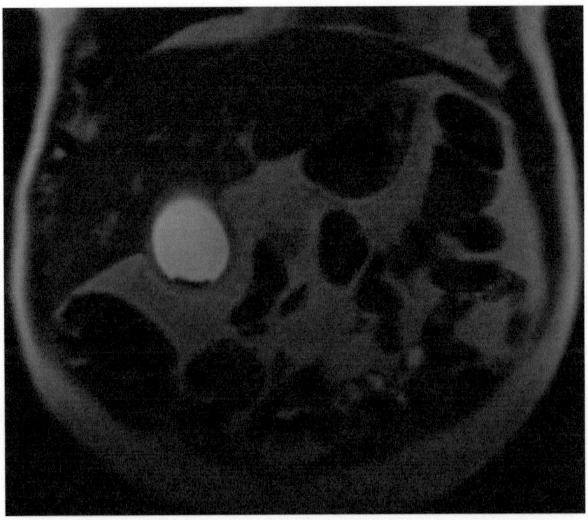

Fig. 2.10 Abdominal MRI imaging of the gallbladder depicting layering sludge and small gallstones in a patient presenting with intermittent right upper quadrant discomfort and bloating

pancreatic duct may be obstructed by mucin, some patients have pancreatitis-like symptoms and may develop exocrine and endocrine pancreatic insufficiency and maldigestion. Often there is a delay in diagnosis of up to several months due to the insidious nature of this disease. Patients with IPMN are at risk for both pancreatic and extrapancreatic malignancies [42].

Diarrhea and Steatorrhea Diarrhea and steatorrhea are distinct from each other, but they may coexist. Steatorrhea occurs because of impaired fat digestion in patients with pancreatic enzyme deficiency or as a result of impaired fat absorption. Steatorrhea is a manifestation of severe exocrine deficiency and implies loss of over 90% of pancreatic function before it becomes clinically evident. Both bile salt deficiency and small intestinal disease can lead to fat malabsorption (Fig. 2.11). Idiopathic recurrent pancreatitis and, over time, chronic idiopathic pancreatitis may result from pancreatic sphincter stenosis or dyskinesia and marked by pancreatic-type pain, often radiating to the back, and associated with altered bowels, mostly diarrhea, steatorrhea, and weight loss [43]. In contrast to those with pancreatic cancer who report significant anorexia, patients with pancreatitis have a good appetite and consume larger meals, more frequently.

The incidence of Immune checkpoint inhibitors (ICI)-induced pancreatitis is 1–2%, clinically ranging from asymptomatic enzyme elevations to severe pancreatitis. The diagnosis is based on clinical symptoms, elevated pancreatic enzymes, and imaging findings, on MRI or endoscopic ultrasound (EUS). Management involves IV fluid administration, pain control, and nutritional support. The efficacy of corticosteroids is controversial. Long-term monitoring is crucial due to the risk of chronic pancreatitis and pancreatic insufficiency [44].

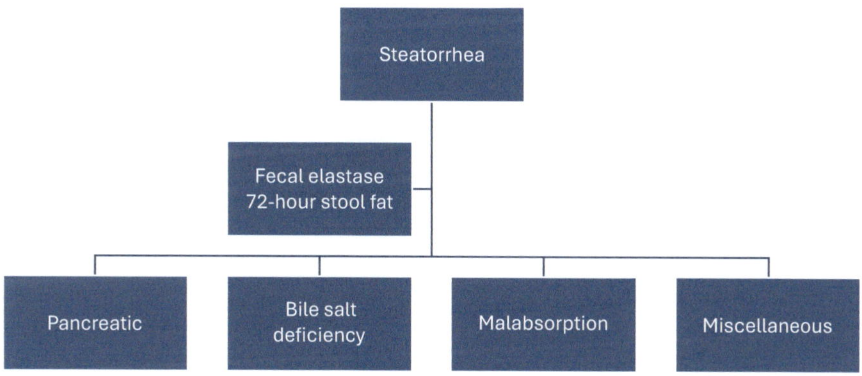

Fig. 2.11 Approach to a patient with steatorrhea

2.3.2.3 Small Intestine

Abdominal Distention and Bloating Abdominal bloating and distention can occur independently of one another, and they can be acute or chronic. These symptoms frequently coexist, although they can occur separately. Bloating is a symptom, while abdominal distension is a sign that should be quantified using a measuring tape. Bloating may be due to gas or accumulated fluid or digestive contents. Bacteria are the sole producers of intestinal hydrogen, and the glucose breath test (GBT) or lactulose breath test (LBT) are based on bacterial metabolism of the ingested sugar into hydrogen or methane [45]. Normally, the small bowel contains only small numbers of bacteria and ingested lactulose is metabolized when it reaches the dense population of bacteria in the colon, giving rise to a late peak in breath hydrogen and/or methane content. In patients with small intestinal bacterial overgrowth (SIBO), the glucose or lactulose metabolism by bacteria produces an early rise of breath hydrogen, while in a similar fashion, methane production suggests the presence of methanogens. Methanogens are achaea, prokaryotic organisms that are neither bacteria nor eukaryotes that produce methane. Methanobrevibacter smithii is the predominant methanogen in the human gut [45]. SIBO may cause nonspecific abdominal distention and bloating, irregular bowel evacuation pattern, and foul-smelling stool and is at times associated with worse motor function. By convention, an increase of greater or equal to 20 parts per million (ppm) from baseline in hydrogen by 90 min is considered a positive test to diagnose SIBO. A level of greater than or equal to 10 ppm in methane at any point in the study is considered positive for methanogenic overgrowth. Thus, instead of SIBO, the term intestinal methanogen overgrowth (IMO) is used for a positive methane breath test, which has been associated with constipation because methane blocks intestinal transit. Both hydrogen (for SIBO) and methane (for IMO) should be measured during breath testing. Before the breath test is performed, antibiotics should be avoided for 4 weeks and laxatives should be avoided for 1 week. Diet, smoking, and physical activity may also need to be altered [46].

Diarrhea Diarrhea is defined as the passage of three of more loose stools per day. Based on the duration of symptoms, diarrhea is further classified as acute (<14 days), persistent (14–29 days), or chronic (>30 days) (Fig. 2.12). The origin of diarrhea may be a challenge to localize; it may be related to gastric hyperacidity (i.e., Zollinger-Ellison syndrome), small intestinal malabsorption, mucosal hypersecretion or inflammation, or colonic etiologies (see below). Typically, diarrhea originating from the small intestine is larger in volume and more fluid; in contrast, small volume diarrhea is colonic in origin. Placing the patient on 24-h fasting challenge significantly curtails or eliminates osmotic diarrhea, while secretory diarrhea continues unabated. Mixed diarrhea that is intermittent, small volume, and non-bloody is due to colonic motor dysfunction. If associated with blood, pus, or mucus, it could be related to inflammatory bowel disease or immunotherapy-induced enterocolitis (ICI).

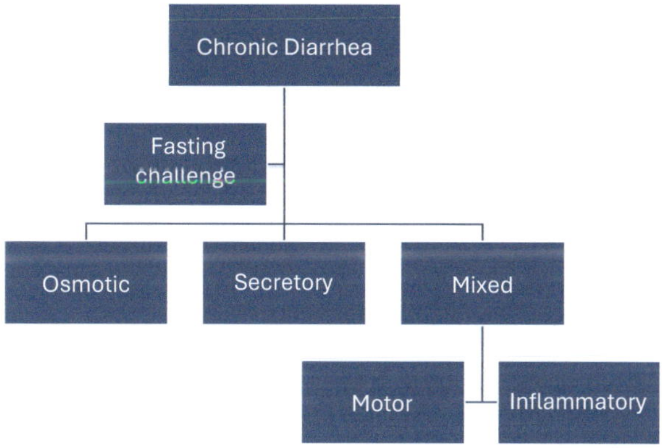

Fig. 2.12 Practical algorithm for evaluation of chronic diarrhea

The commonest causes of acute diarrhea are bacterial, such as *Salmonella, Campylobacter*, Shiga-toxin producing *E. coli*, *Vibrio*, and *Yersinia*. *Clostridium difficile* infection is an important cause of diarrhea following antibiotic or immunosuppressant treatment and in hospitalized patients. Antibiotic-associated diarrhea occurs in the absence of *Clostridium difficile* infection and is probably due to small intestinal bacterial overgrowth (SIBO). During the treatment of cancer, diarrhea may reflect the administration of chemotherapy or immunotherapy.

When assessing a cancer patient with chronic intermittent diarrhea, it is essential to clearly distinguish it from fecal incontinence associated with fecal impaction and overflow, a much more common issue. In turn, if true diarrhea is suspected, it is practical to classify it as "osmotic" (due to impaired fluid absorption, resulting from malabsorption, which improves with fasting) and "secretory" (excessive liquid stools >1 l/day, usually due to infection or hypersecretory state, which persists with fasting). Frequent, small-volume stools suggest a colonic origin, whereas less frequent, but large volume, often watery stools indicate a possible small bowel source.

Because cancer is a disease of older adults, the presence of frequent, small, usually formed, stools should suggest colonic source, such as colorectal cancer, diverticulosis, or solitary rectal ulcer and a colonoscopy should always be considered. In contrast, frequent, watery bowel movements should raise the suspicion of small bowel bacterial overgrowth (SIBO), usually associated with pale, large-volume, foul-smelling stools with bloating, borborygmi and weight loss, or microscopic (lymphocytic or collagenous) colitis, particularly in women. In such instances, hydrogen/methane breath testing and colonoscopy with multiple random biopsies should be considered.

In acute persistent diarrhea, stool samples should be analyzed for parasites and bacteria. In chronic cases, stool should also be tested for elastase (low in pancreatic insufficiency) and calprotectin (elevated in any inflammatory condition and thereby useful to distinguish inflammatory from functional causes). Elastase measurements are limited in the setting of profuse watery diarrhea in which dilution alone can cause low values. Pancreatic insufficiency is more likely in steatorrhea or soft but relatively formed stools. Imaging studies (particularly MRI enterography) can

Table 2.3 Common agents that may cause diarrhea

Medications or supplements potentially causing diarrhea
5-aminosalicylates
Selective serotonin reuptake inhibitors (SSRIs)
Serotonin and norepinephrine reuptake inhibitors (SNRIs)
Proton pump inhibitors
Magnesium containing antacids
Metformin

Table 2.4 Classes of agents that may cause diarrhea in cancer patients undergoing treatment

Agents potentially causing diarrhea in cancer patients
Conventional cytotoxic agents
Molecularly targeted agents
Tyrosine kinase inhibitors (TKI)
Anti-epidermal growth factor receptor (EGFR) monoclonal antibodies
Immune checkpoint inhibitors (ICI)
Antibody-drug conjugates

provide additional useful information on small-bowel anatomy and transit time, which may be affected in late stages of cancer involving the bowel wall and peritoneum. Table 2.3 lists common agents that may cause diarrhea that need consideration and at least a 2-week-long discontinuation to define an etiologic role, prior to embarking in complex and potentially invasive diagnostic studies. Chemotherapy-related diarrhea (CRD) is a common side effect of chemotherapy treatments. It occurs when chemotherapy drugs damage the cells lining the gastrointestinal (GI) tract, leading to inflammation and increased fluid secretion. Diarrhea may also occur in the context of immunotherapy and radiation therapy (Table 2.4).

2.3.2.4 Colon

Bloating, Belching, and Flatulence Normally, the volume of gas in the gut (200 ml) is relatively constant, both during fasting and after meals. Yet, abdominal bloating, feeling of distention, and excessive passing of flatus are common complaints. This is often due to involuntary poorly coordinated activity of the diaphragmatic and anterior abdominal wall muscles, rather than excessive amounts of intestinal gas [47]. Intermittent belching is commonly caused by swallowing air (aerophagia), typically while eating fast and talking, or eating certain foods, such as onions, cabbage, or fatty foods, that delay stomach emptying. If aerophagia is suspected, drinking through a straw helps. Further, placing a pencil in between the jaws inhibits subconscious air swallowing, in turn improving bloating. Excessive bloating may also be a symptom of lactose intolerance, gluten sensitivity, small intestinal bacterial overgrowth (SIBO), or delayed gastric emptying without mechanical obstruction (gastroparesis). Generalized feeling of abdominal bloating is mostly due to irritable bowel syndrome (IBS) and/or diverticulosis and is often associated with altered bowel habits, such as alternating constipation and diarrhea. Some foods contain high amounts of simple, poorly digested carbohydrates that are fermented by colonic bacteria leading to excess gas production and the formation of osmotically active substances. Reducing wheat, onions, broccoli, beans, and insoluble fiber may be useful [48]. Table 2.5 lists medications or supplements that frequently cause bloating, belching, flatulence, and feeling of abdominal distention, thereby requiring careful consideration. At least a 2-week-long drug discontinuation to define an etiologic role is useful prior to embarking in complex and potentially diagnostic studies. Table 2.6 lists various considerations in patients with bloating, belching, flatulence, and feeling of abdominal distention that clinicians need to entertain.

Chronic Constipation (CC) Chronic constipation is defined as stool evacuation frequency of <3 per week, usually described as "too infrequent, too little, too hard," usually for more than 3 months. Mostly related to opioid use for pain control, constipation is the most common gastrointestinal symptom in cancer patients. The underlying mechanisms are unknown, but reduced density or even absence of the gut nerves has been seen in patients with severe chronic constipation. Constipation is a common side effect of many drugs used in cancer, particularly chemotherapeutic agents, antiemetics, and anticholinergics. More frequently, particularly after pelvic surgery or radiation, patients might also have poorly coordinated or dyssynergic bowel evacuation, which is characterized by the inability, or paradoxical increase, of the pelvic floor and anal canal muscles to relax during attempted defecation. Dysfunction of the sacral and pelvic ganglia is suspected to be an underlying reason for such evacuation disorder.

Table 2.5 Medications or supplements that cause bloating, flatulence, and feeling of abdominal distention

Medications or supplements potentially causing bloating, flatulence, and abdominal distention
Probiotics and prebiotics
Excessive fiber intake
Cholestyramine
Glucagon peptide-1 agonists
Lactulose
Excessive use of carbonated agents

Table 2.6 Considerations in patients with bloating, belching, flatulence, and feeling of abdominal distention

Causes of bloating, flatulence, and abdominal distention
Aerophagia
Abdominophrenic dyssynergia
Gastroparesis
Constipation
IBS and diverticulosis

Figure 2.13 highlights the various forms of constipation, based on their clinical characteristics. Lack of urge to defecate suggests slow transit constipation (STC). Defecatory straining, a sense of incomplete stool evacuation, and the need to use digital maneuvers (through the anal canal into the rectum or through external pressure through the vagina) suggest evacuation disorder (ED). These two conditions may coexist in many patients (mixed constipation, MC). Obstructive constipation (OC) is a late form of fecal impaction (FI), due to hardened stool trapped in the rectum. FI may go unnoticed, typically confused as worsening constipation, or it may manifest as acute intestinal obstruction (bowel blockage), or colonic volvulus (twisting of the colon), causing severe abdominal bloating, distention, and pain, and it may lead to death if left untreated [49]. Under these circumstances an emergency evaluation, clinical examination (that includes a digital rectal examination by a physician), as well as the use of blood tests, abdominal radiographs and CT imaging are needed. Depending on the preliminary results, urgent attention by a gastroenterologist to perform a decompressing colonoscopy and release (untwisting) of volvulus or a surgeon to perform abdominal surgery are needed. Many such patients get hospitalized.

There are many causes of constipation in adults, as well as patients with cancer, and they always need to be considered. Mostly, constipation is functional, not related to significant underlying disease. In such cases, which can be acute, intermittent, or chronic, no abnormalities are found upon testing. Relief can be spontaneous or result from changes in the diet, fluid intake, or the transient use of laxatives. In patients with chronic or recurrent constipation, secondary causes need to be considered. In patients with cancer, constipation may result from drugs (i.e., narcotics, etc.), from the disease itself, from other metabolic causes (postoperative diabetes or hypothyroidism, electrolyte disturbances, etc.), or a combination. Mechanical obstruction by postoperative adhesions, a colon tumor, or twisted bowel (volvulus) needs to be always considered and properly treated, mostly surgically. Because constipation in patients across the cancer spectrum cancer is so common and driven by multiple factors, it requires a thorough initial evaluation as

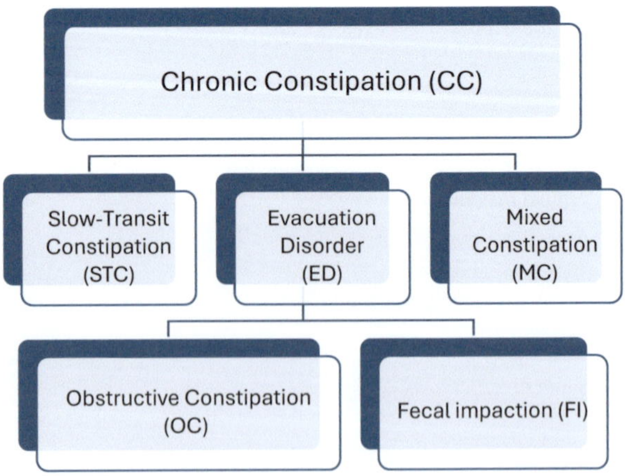

Fig. 2.13 Types of chronic constipation, based on their clinical characteristics

well as frequent assessments to ensure improvement, stability, or deterioration. Periodic evaluations, using ingestible radio-opaque markers (Sitzmarks) and abdominal radiographs, are recommended to monitor patients with chronic constipation, even those who report no issues. Re-evaluation is also recommended if there is change in the efficacy of prior therapy, new diagnosis of cancer, or any other progressive change or alarm symptoms. Based on such surveillance assessments and testing, preventive measures can be implemented to avoid progressive dilation, atony, and loss of the propulsive activity of the colon. Similar steps may need to be taken in patients who report bowel urgency, seepage, or stool incontinence, since that may be a hidden manifestation of stagnation of stool in the rectum, rectal distention, and intermittent release of mucus and fluid through the anal canal at unpredictable times, simulating diarrhea (overflow incontinence) (Fig. 2.14).

Table 2.7 lists common agents that may cause constipation and will require consideration and at least a 2-week-long agent discontinuation, to define an etiologic role, prior to embarking in complex and potentially invasive diagnostic studies.

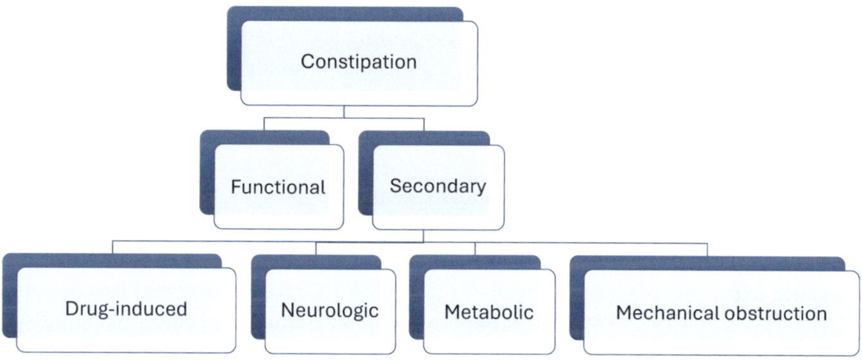

Fig. 2.14 Types of chronic constipation, based on their key etiology. Overlaps may occur

Table 2.7 Common agents that may cause constipation

Medications or supplements potentially causing constipation
Iron
Calcium
Antispasmodics
Opiates
Tricyclics
Serotonin and norepinephrine reuptake inhibitors
Antipsychotics
5-HT3 receptor antagonists
Calcium channel blockers
Aluminum containing antacids
Glucagon peptide-1 agonists

Fecal Incontinence (FInc) Anorectal control (continence) is normally maintained by a combination of several factors: [1] the internal (involuntary, smooth muscle) anal sphincter, [2] the external (voluntary, striated muscle) anal sphincter, [3] the puborectalis muscle (voluntary, striated muscle), and [4] anorectal sensation. Weakness of internal anal (involuntary) sphincter leads to incontinence of flatus and soiling, if the patient has diarrhea. A patient who is affected by the inadvertent fecal voiding through the anal canal (fecal incontinence) lives a life of social alienation and personal isolation. In general, looser and watery stools are more difficult to maintain control over than solid stools in the patient with urge incontinence. "Urge" incontinence is defined as the unwanted loss of stool despite active attempts to inhibit stool evacuation. "Passive" incontinence is defined as the unwanted loss of stool without the person being aware. Based on these definitions, there are three FInc subtypes (urge, passive, mixed). The various terms used to quantify the impact of fecal incontinence are listed in Table 2.8. Patients who report that they are almost exclusively incontinent because they have "urgency and cannot reach the toilet on time" are considered to have "urge" incontinence, whereas patients who are almost exclusively "unaware when the leakage is actually happening" are considered to have "passive" incontinence. Patients who report both are considered to have "mixed" incontinence [50]. It is essential to establish the degree of disability, since the management of the patient with partial soiling secondary to anal pathology will be very different from that of a patient with frequent incontinence of formed stool. Even profound anal sphincter deficits do not necessarily lead to incontinence if stool consistency is solid, while minor deficits may easily lead to gas incontinence.

Assessment of all three pelvic compartments, the anterior, with urinary incontinence, the middle with uterine and/or vaginal prolapse, and the posterior, with fecal incontinence, should be undertaken by a careful anal and pelvic examination and dynamic MR defecography. Cancer- or radiation-related rectovaginal fistulae also need to be considered in such patients. In the assessment of FInc, its duration, details of stool consistency using the Bristol stool form scale [51], and the presence of transit disorders, using the Rome IV criteria [52], should be collected, using standard questionnaires at baseline and during follow-up. FInc severity is assessed using the Cleveland Clinic Incontinence Score (CCIS) [53], or the Vaizey score, which incorporates the use of constipating medications and the lack of ability to defer defecation for 15 min [54]. Quality of life (QOL) is usually measured using the American Society of Colon and Rectal Surgeons QOL auto questionnaire for

Table 2.8 Various terms used to quantify the impact of fecal incontinence

Bowel urgency	Sudden and immediate need to have a bowel movement
Fecal incontinence	Involuntary loss of solid or liquid stool
Fecal seepage	Leakage of liquid stool after a normal bowel movement
Gas-bowel uncertainty	Inability to distinguish need to pass stool or gas
Passive incontinence	Involuntary passing of stool without awareness
Stool frequency	Visits to the toilet to pass stool, mucus, or gas
Urge incontinence	Involuntary passing of stool due to inability to reach the toilet in time

FInc (FIQL) [55]. One of the items of the embarrassment domain of the FIQL questionnaire is related to passive FInc, when patient reports "I leak stool without even knowing it."

The external anal sphincter can vigorously contract upon volition for approximately 60 s to prevent soiling in case of the presence of loose stool in the rectum. Most of the anorectal control is provided by the contraction of the puborectalis muscle, which creates an angle between the lower rectum and upper anal canal (the anorectal angle). Sharp angulation creates a flap-valve mechanism to operate, such that increases in intra-abdominal pressure cause the anterior rectal wall to close over the top of the anal canal, preventing rectal contents entering it. The sensation of a full rectum is probably caused by tension on pressure receptors in the pelvic floor musculature. The discrimination of the nature of rectal contents is accomplished by a locally mediated reflex whereby rectal distension (from flatus or stool) initiates internal anal sphincter relaxation. A sample of rectal contents thereby intrudes into the anal canal where it is perceived.

In all patients, a full clinical examination, perianal inspection, and dynamic digital rectal examination (at rest, upon squeeze and push maneuvers) should be enhanced by colonoscopy and high-resolution anorectal manometry, to further validate both the structural and functional integrity of the anorectum. In special cases, electromyography of the external anal sphincter and puborectalis muscles, anorectal ultrasound, and endo-FLIP measurements may be needed. Endo-FLIP utilizes high-resolution impedance planimetry during volume-controlled distention to measure luminal cross-sectional area (CSA) along an axial plane. This is synchronized to a singular pressure measure within a fluid-filled bag and thus allows for an assessment of luminal geometry and pressure akin to compliance measurement [56]. Dynamic MR defecography frequently provides valuable information on the integrity of the pelvic floor and the assessment of pelvic (uterine and bladder) and rectal prolapse. FInc does not necessarily imply deficiency of the anal sphincters or the pelvic floor musculature, because variable degrees of soiling may occur normally, if a person experiences acute or chronic diarrhea. This is why it is important to structurally examine the rectum because patients with inflammatory bowel disease or radiation proctopathy frequently state that the urgency and FInc is the most distressing element of their disease. Older patients may also have poor awareness of rectal filling, resulting in fecal impaction. In these patients the internal sphincter relaxes in response to rectal distension by impacted feces, facilitating leakage of loose stool fluid and mucus. Minor inadvertent loss of flatus or liquid stool through the anus typically results from a weak internal anal sphincter and it may be associated with intermittently prolapsing hemorrhoids or rectal prolapse. Major inadvertent and/or frequent loss of fully formed stool through the rectum suggests a more severe functional impairment of the anorectal structure and function and may result from surgical trauma of the external anal sphincter and the puborectalis muscle. Most of these patients have denervation of the striated (external) anal sphincter resulting from local nerve (i.e., pudendal) damage due to compression and stretching forces or from straining excessively with defecation. In some patients, partly because of sensory loss, fecal impaction ensues. This is typically encountered when tumors

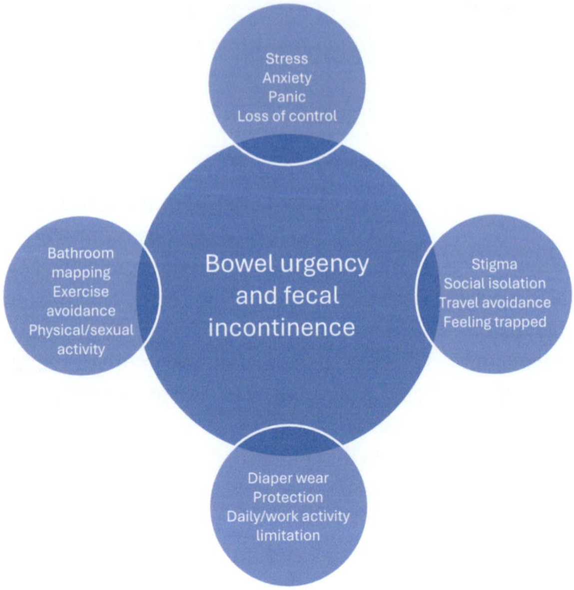

Fig. 2.15 Impact of bowel urgency on quality of life and social function

(primary or metastatic) impact the spinal cord and are associated with loss of perineal sensation. The impact of bowel urgency on quality of life and social function is shown in Fig. 2.15.

Rectal Bleeding Typically, rectal bleeding occurs in the context of distal colonic pathology and associated constipation, but other, more ominous conditions, such as colorectal cancer, need to be carefully considered. Because of the longstanding gut symptoms, such as fullness and nausea associated with gastroparesis or constipation, patients may not be adequately prepared for a colonoscopy and malignancy may be missed. A good-quality colonoscopy is imperative in all cases and will provide an explanation as to the origin and significance of the bleeding. Typically, bleeding is related to anal fissure, anal cancer, stercoral ulceration, diverticulosis, radiation proctopathy, or internal hemorrhoids. Unlikely etiologies include colonic ischemia and inflammatory bowel disease or infectious colitis. An important lesion, often overlooked at colonoscopy, is anal dysplasia or cancer. If concern is raised, a high-resolution anoscopy should be performed [57].

References

1. Rosa-E-Silva L, Gerson L, Davila M, et al. Clinical, radiologic, and manometric characteristics of chronic intestinal dysmotility: the Stanford experience. Clin Gastroenterol Hepatol. 2006;4:866–73. https://doi.org/10.1016/j.cgh.2006.05.001.
2. Stoopler ET, Villa A, Bindakhil M, Díaz DLO, Sollecito TP. Common oral conditions: a review. JAMA. 2024;331(12):1045–54. https://doi.org/10.1001/jama.2024.0953. PMID: 38530258

3. Townes TG, et al. Assessing patient-reported symptom burden of long-term head and neck cancer survivors at annual surveillance in survivorship clinic. Head Neck. 2020;42(8):1919–27.
4. Pellegrini M, Merlo FD, Agnello E, Monge T, Devecchi A, Casalone V, Montemurro F, Ghigo E, Sapino A, Bo S. Dysgeusia in patients with breast cancer treated with chemotherapy – a narrative review. Nutrients. 2023;15(1):226. https://doi.org/10.3390/nu15010226. PMID: 36615883; PMCID: PMC9823517
5. Siau R, Kinshuck A, Houghton L. The assessment and management of globus pharyngeus. Br J Hosp Med (Lond). 2021;82(3):1–8. https://doi.org/10.12968/hmed.2021.0038. Epub 2021 Mar 31. PMID: 33792382
6. Van Daele DJ. Esophageal manometry, pH testing, endoscopy, and videofluoroscopy in patients with globus sensation. Laryngoscope. 2020;130(9):2120–5. https://doi.org/10.1002/lary.28289. Epub 2019 Sep 9. PMID: 31498462
7. Jamróz B, Sobol M, Chmielewska-Walczak J, Milewska M, Niemczyk K. The risk factors for silent aspiration: a retrospective case series and literature review. Int J Lang Commun Disord. 2024;59(4):1538–52. https://doi.org/10.1111/1460-6984.13013. Epub 2024 Feb 1. PMID: 38301043
8. Lin Z, Nicodème F, Lin CY, Mogni B, Friesen L, Kahrilas PJ, Pandolfino JE. Parameters for quantifying bolus retention with high-resolution impedance manometry. Neurogastroenterol Motil 2014 Jul;26(7):929–936. doi: https://doi.org/10.1111/nmo.12346. Epub 2014 Apr 22. PMID: 24750336; PMCID: PMC4120956.
9. Bulsiewicz WJ, Kahrilas PJ, Kwiatek MA, Ghosh SK, Meek A, Pandolfino JE. Esophageal pressure topography criteria indicative of incomplete bolus clearance: a study using high-resolution impedance manometry. Am J Gastroenterol. 2009;104(11):2721–8. https://doi.org/10.1038/ajg.2009.467. Epub 2009 Aug 18. PMID: 19690527; PMCID: PMC2886600
10. Kahrilas PJ, Bredenoord AJ, Fox M, Gyawali CP, Roman S, Smout AJ, Pandolfino JE, International High Resolution Manometry Working Group. The Chicago classification of esophageal motility disorders, v3.0. Neurogastroenterol Motil. 2015;27(2):160–74. https://doi.org/10.1111/nmo.12477. Epub 2014 Dec 3. PMID: 25469569; PMCID: PMC4308501
11. Vitton V, Andrianjafy C, Luciano L, Gonzalez JM, Padovani L. Radio-induced esophageal motility disorders: an unrecognized diagnosis. Cancer Radiother. 2021;25(3):249–53. https://doi.org/10.1016/j.canrad.2020.09.006. Epub 2021 Jan 14. PMID: 33454192
12. Gyawali CP, Sifrim D, Carlson DA, Hawn M, Katzka DA, Pandolfino JE, Penagini R, Roman S, Savarino E, Tatum R, Vaezi M, Clarke JO, Triadafilopoulos G. Ineffective esophageal motility: concepts, future directions, and conclusions from the Stanford 2018 symposium. Neurogastroenterol Motil. 2019;31(9):e13584. https://doi.org/10.1111/nmo.13584. Epub 2019 Apr 11. PMID: 30974032; PMCID: PMC9380027
13. Fernandez AM, Chan WW. Update on extraesophageal manifestations of gastroesophageal reflux. Curr Opin Gastroenterol. 2024;40(4):305–13. https://doi.org/10.1097/MOG.0000000000001037. Epub 2024 Apr 19. PMID: 38662405
14. Samuels TL, Aoun J, Husain I, Figueredo E, Richards D, Johnston N. Advances in laryngopharyngeal reflux: etiology, diagnosis, and management. Ann N Y Acad Sci. 2024;1541(1):53–62.
15. Sawada A, Zhang M, Ustaoglu A, Nikaki K, Lee C, Woodland P, Yazaki E, Takashima S, Ominami M, Tanaka F, Ciafardini C, Nachman F, Ditaranto A, Agotegaray J, Bilder C, Savarino E, Gyawali CP, Penagini R, Fujiwara Y, Sifrim D. Superficial oesophageal mucosal innervation may contribute to severity of symptoms in oesophageal motility disorders. Aliment Pharmacol Ther. 2024;59(1):100–12. https://doi.org/10.1111/apt.17773. Epub 2023 Oct 16. PMID: 37845817
16. Triadafilopoulos G, Mashimo H, Tatum R, O'Clarke J, Hawn M. Mixed Esophageal Disease (MED): a new concept. Dig Dis Sci. 2023;68(9):3542–54. https://doi.org/10.1007/s10620-023-08008-x. Epub 2023 Jul 20. PMID: 37470896
17. Simadibrata DM, Lesmana E, Fass R. Role of endoscopy in gastroesophageal reflux disease. Clin Endosc. 2023;56(6):681–92. https://doi.org/10.5946/ce.2023.182. Epub 2023 Oct 12. PMID: 37822063; PMCID: PMC10665616

18. Triadafilopoulos G. Endoscopic non-ablative radiofrequency treatment (Stretta) for Gastroesophageal Reflux Disease (GERD). Curr Gastroenterol Rep. 2024;26(4):93–8. https://doi.org/10.1007/s11894-024-00917-9. Epub 2024 Feb 23. PMID: 38393432
19. Jaber F, Ayyad M, Ayoub F, Patel KK, Makris KI, Hernaez R, Skef W. Concomitant hiatal hernia repair with transoral incisionless fundoplication for the treatment of refractory gastroesophageal reflux disease: a systematic review. Surg Endosc. 2024;38(10):5528–40. https://doi.org/10.1007/s00464-024-11201-2. Epub 2024 Sep 13. PMID: 39271515
20. Peristeri DV, Room H, Tsironis D, Vasilikostas G, Wan A. Long-term efficacy of total versus posterior partial fundoplication in patients with gastro-oesophageal reflux disease: a systematic review and meta-analysis. Ann R Coll Surg Engl. 2024;106(7):569–75. https://doi.org/10.1308/rcsann.2023.0046. Epub 2023 Oct 16. PMID: 37843095; PMCID: PMC11365733
21. Salvador R, Vittori A, Capovilla G, Riccio F, Nezi G, Forattini F, Provenzano L, Nicoletti L, Moletta L, Costantini A, Valmasoni M, Costantini M. Antireflux surgery's lifespan: 20 years after laparoscopic fundoplication. J Gastrointest Surg. 2023;27(11):2325–35. https://doi.org/10.1007/s11605-023-05797-4. Epub 2023 Aug 14. PMID: 37580489; PMCID: PMC10661768
22. ASGE Standards of Practice Committee, Desai M, Ruan W, Thosani NC, Amaris M, Scott JS, Saeed A, Abu Dayyeh B, Canto MI, Abidi W, Alipour O, Amateau SK, Cosgrove N, Elhanafi SE, Forbes N, Kohli DR, Kwon RS, Fujii-Lau LL, Machicado JD, Marya NB, Ngamruengphong S, Pawa S, Sheth SG, Thiruvengadam NR, Qumseya BJ. ASGE Standards of Practice Committee Chair. American Society for Gastrointestinal Endoscopy guideline on the diagnosis and management of GERD: summary and recommendations. Gastrointest Endosc. 2025;101(2):267–84. https://doi.org/10.1016/j.gie.2024.10.008. Epub 2024 Dec 17. PMID: 39692638
23. Wyman JB, Dent J, Heddle R, et al. Control of belching by the lower esophageal sphincter. Gut. 1990;31:639–46.
24. Straathof JW, Ringers J, Lamers CB, et al. Provocation of transient lower esophageal sphincter relaxations by gastric distention with air. Am J Gastroenterol. 2001;8:2317–23.
25. Lin M, Triadafilopoulos G. Belching: dyspepsia or gastroesophageal reflux disease? Am J Gastroenterol. 2003;98(10):2139–45. https://doi.org/10.1111/j.1572-0241.2003.07627.x. PMID: 14572558
26. Rangan V, Sheth T, Iturrino J, Ballou S, Nee J, Lembo A. Belching: pathogenesis, clinical characteristics, and treatment strategies. J Clin Gastroenterol. 2022;56(1):36–40. https://doi.org/10.1097/MCG.0000000000001631. PMID: 34739403
27. Walker MM, Potter MD, Talley NJ. Tangible pathologies in functional dyspepsia. Best Pract Res Clin Gastroenterol. 2019;40–41:101650. https://doi.org/10.1016/j.bpg.2019.101650. Epub 2019 Aug 16. PMID: 31594648
28. Chang JJ, Gadi SRV, Videnovic A, Kuo B, Pasricha TS. Impact of outpatient gastroenterology consult on pharmacotherapy and management of gastrointestinal symptoms in Parkinson's disease. Clin Park Relat Disord. 2023;29(9):100215. https://doi.org/10.1016/j.prdoa.2023.100215. PMID: 37700817; PMCID: PMC10493246
29. Wysokiński A, Sobów T, Kłoszewska I, Kostka T. Mechanisms of the anorexia of aging – a review. Age (Dordr). 2015;37(4):9821. https://doi.org/10.1007/s11357-015-9821-x. Epub 2015 Aug 1. PMID: 26232135; PMCID: PMC5005824
30. Chowdhury IH, Rahman S, Afroze YJ, Shovah ST. IUPHAR ECR review: cancer-related anorexia-cachexia in cancer patients: pathophysiology and treatment. Pharmacol Res. 2024;203:107129. https://doi.org/10.1016/j.phrs.2024.107129. Epub 2024 Mar 9. PMID: 38461961
31. Kinami S, Takahashi M, Urushihara T, Ikeda M, Yoshida M, Uenosono Y, et al. Background factors influencing postgastrectomy syndromes after various types of gastrectomy. World J Clin Cases. 2018;6(16):1111–20.
32. Shafi MA. Gastrointestinal motility issues in cancer patients. Curr Gastroenterol Rep. 2019;21(12):69. https://doi.org/10.1007/s11894-019-0738-x. PMID: 31823129

33. Camilleri M, Sanders KM. Opiates, the pylorus, and gastroparesis. Gastroenterology. 2020;159(2):414–21. https://doi.org/10.1053/j.gastro.2020.04.072. Epub 2020 May 8. PMID: 32389662
34. Mari A, Abu Backer F, Mahamid M, Amara H, Carter D, Boltin D, Dickman R. Bloating and abdominal distension: clinical approach and management. Adv Ther. 2019;36(5):1075–84. https://doi.org/10.1007/s12325-019-00924-7. Epub 2019 Mar 16. PMID: 30879252; PMCID: PMC6824367
35. Barba E, Burri E, Quiroga S, Accarino A, Azpiroz F. Visible abdominal distension in functional gut disorders: objective evaluation. Neurogastroenterol Motil. 2023;35(2):e14466.
36. Triadafilopoulos G, Lee M, Neshatian L. High prevalence of anorectal dysfunction in ambulatory patients with chronic constipation, regardless of colon transit time. Dig Dis Sci. 2024;69(1):180–8. https://doi.org/10.1007/s10620-023-08072-3. Epub 2023 Aug 9. PMID: 37555883
37. Barba E, Livovsky DM, Accarino A, Azpiroz F. Thoracoabdominal wall motion-guided biofeedback treatment of abdominal distention: a randomized placebo-controlled trial. Gastroenterology. 2024;167(3):538–46.
38. Richmond BK. Biliary dyskinesia-controversies, diagnosis, and management: a review. JAMA Surg. 2024;159(9):1079–84. https://doi.org/10.1001/jamasurg.2024.0818. PMID: 38959007
39. Sharma V, Rana SS, Chaudhary V, Dhaka N, Manrai M, Sivalingam J, Sharma R, Dutta U, Bhasin DK. Opium-related sphincter of Oddi dysfunction causing double duct sign. Endosc. Ultrasound. 2016;5(4):269–71.
40. Cotton PB, Durkalski V, Romagnuolo J, Pauls Q, Fogel E, Tarnasky P, et al. Effect of endoscopic sphincterotomy for suspected sphincter of oddi dysfunction on pain-related disability following cholecystectomy: the EPISOD randomized clinical trial. JAMA. 2014;311:2101–9.
41. Pauls Q, Durkalski-Mauldin V, Brawman-Mintzer O, Lawrence C, Whichard R, Cotton PB. Duloxetine for the treatment of patients with suspected sphincter of oddi dysfunction: a pilot study. Digest Dis Sci. 2016;61:2704–9.
42. Gardner TB, Park WG, Allen PJ. Diagnosis and management of pancreatic cysts. Gastroenterology. 2024;167(3):454–68.
43. Guo A, Poneros JM. The role of Endotherapy in recurrent acute pancreatitis. Gastrointest Endosc Clin N Am. 2018;28(4):455–76.
44. Nwankwo OC, Lara-Salazar FM, Lara-Salazar S, Abdulrahim AO, Chijioke I, Singh J, Koradia I, Gomez NM, Prakash R, Gopagoni R, Joshi M, Rai M. Immune checkpoint inhibitors in cancer treatment and incidence of pancreatitis. Cureus. 2024;16(8):e68043. https://doi.org/10.7759/cureus.68043. PMID: 39347217; PMCID: PMC11433468
45. Pimentel M, Saad RJ, Long MD, Rao SSC. ACG clinical guideline: small intestinal bacterial overgrowth. Am J Gastroenterol. 2020;115(2):165–78. https://doi.org/10.14309/ajg.0000000000000501. PMID: 32023228
46. Mehravar S, Takakura W, Wang J, Pimentel M, Nasser J, Rezaie A. Symptom profile of patients with intestinal methanogen overgrowth: a systematic review and meta-analysis. Clin Gastroenterol Hepatol. 2025;23(7):1111–1122.e9.
47. Damianos JA, Tomar SK, Azpiroz F, Barba E. Abdominophrenic dyssynergia: a narrative review. Am J Gastroenterol. 2023;118(1):41–5. https://doi.org/10.14309/ajg.0000000000002044. Epub 2022 Sep 30. PMID: 36191283; PMCID: PMC9810002
48. Loening-Baucke V, Swidsinski A. Observational study of children with aerophagia. Clin Pediatr (Phila) 2008 Sep;47(7):664–669. doi: https://doi.org/10.1177/0009922808315825. Epub 2008 Apr 29. PMID: 18445758.
49. Sommers T, Petersen T, Singh P, Rangan V, Hirsch W, Katon J, Ballou S, Cheng V, Friedlander D, Nee J, Lembo A, Iturrino J. Significant morbidity and mortality associated with fecal impaction in patients who present to the emergency department. Dig Dis Sci 2019 May;64(5):1320–1327. doi: https://doi.org/10.1007/s10620-018-5394-8. Epub 2018 Dec 8. PMID: 30535766; PMCID: PMC6499648.

50. Abrams P, Andersson KE, Birder L, Brubaker L, Cardozo L, Chapple C, et al. Fourth international consultation on incontinence recommendations of the international scientific committee: evaluation and treatment of urinary incontinence, pelvic organ prolapse, and fecal incontinence. Neurourol Urodyn. 2010;29:213–40. https://doi.org/10.1002/nau.20870.
51. Lewis SJ, Heaton KW. Stool form scale as a useful guide to intestinal transit time. Scand J Gastroenterol. 1997;32:920–4. https://doi.org/10.3109/00365529709011203.
52. Mearin F, Lacy BE, Chang L, Chey WD, Lembo AJ, Simren M, et al. Bowel disorders. Gastroenterology. 2016;150:1393–407. https://doi.org/10.1053/j.gastro.2016.02.031.
53. Jorge JM, Wexner SD. Etiology and management of fecal incontinence. Dis Colon Rectum. 1993;36:77–97. https://doi.org/10.1007/BF02050307.
54. Vaizey CJ, Carapeti E, Cahill JA, Kamm MA. Prospective comparison of faecal incontinence grading systems. Gut. 1999;44:77–80. https://doi.org/10.1136/gut.44.1.77.
55. Rockwood TH, Church JM, Fleshman JW, Kane RL, Mavrantonis C, Thorson AG, Wexner SD, Bliss D, Lowry AC. Fecal incontinence quality of life scale: quality of life instrument for patients with fecal incontinence. Dis Colon Rectum 2000 Jan;43(1):9–16.; discussion 16-7. doi: https://doi.org/10.1007/BF02237236. PMID: 10813117.
56. Hirano I, Pandolfino JE, Boeckxstaens GE. Functional lumen imaging probe for the management of esophageal disorders: expert review from the clinical practice updates committee of the AGA Institute. Clin Gastroenterol Hepatol 2017;15(3):325–334. doi: https://doi.org/10.1016/j.cgh.2016.10.022. PMID: 28212976; PMCID: PMC5757507.
57. Junejo MH, Oyebanji OI, Wang B, Cappello C, Wait B, Farrow E, Nathan M, Bowring J, Cuming T. Early detection of anal squamous cell carcinoma with the use of high-resolution anoscopy. Clin Exp Dermatol. 2025;50(2):395–8. https://doi.org/10.1093/ced/llae362. PMID: 39212481

Tests for Gastrointestinal Sensory-Motor Assessment: Mouth, Tongue, Pharynx, Hypopharynx, Larynx, and Upper Esophageal Sphincter

3

George Triadafilopoulos and David M. Richards

3.1 Mouth, Tongue, Pharynx, Hypopharynx, Larynx, and Upper Esophageal Sphincter

Endoscopy Upper endoscopy is universally the first step in the evaluation of a patient with suspected sensory-motor gastrointestinal disorder to exclude foregut structural pathology that would indirectly compromise function (Fig. 3.1). The use of endoscopy may not be only diagnostic, by providing direct visualization of the mucosa, and histological sampling, but it may also provide therapeutic intervention (i.e., BoTox injection in cricopharyngeal achalasia). Further, endoscopy may be used to facilitate physiologic assessment by placing motility catheters or other probes [1].

Flexible Endoscopic Evaluation of Swallowing (FEES) A fiberoptic, full-color endoscopic evaluation of swallowing (FEES) test assesses how well the patient swallows. During the procedure, a speech-language pathologist (SLP) passes an ultrathin, flexible endoscope through the nose under topical anesthesia and examines exclusively the nasopharynx, pharynx, and larynx while using water, thicker liquids, pureed or soft foods, and even regular foods, noting for any problems chewing, swallowing, or breathing. The findings are given clinical context, differential diagnoses are considered, further diagnostic steps are proposed, treatment options are evaluated, and a timeframe for reassessment to assess evolution is suggested [2]. The success of the DIGEST score for VFSS leads to its adaption to FEES [3].

G. Triadafilopoulos (✉) · D. M. Richards
Department of Gastroenterology, Hepatology and Nutrition, UT MD Anderson Cancer Center, Houston, TX, USA
e-mail: gtriadafilopoulo@mdanderson.org

G. Triadafilopoulos (ed.), *Onco-Neurogastroenterology*,
https://doi.org/10.1007/978-3-031-98848-6_3

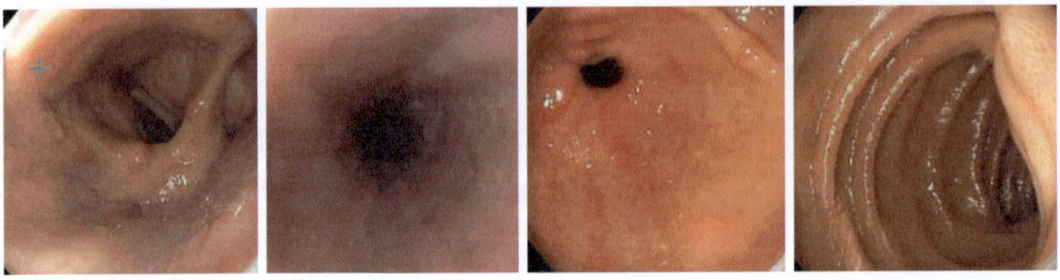

Fig. 3.1 Representative images of a normal endoscopy depicting (left to right) the laryngeal structures, the esophagus, the antrum, and the second portion of the duodenum

Video-Fluorographic Swallowing Study (VFSS) The video-fluorographic swallowing study, also known as a modified barium swallowing examination (MBSS), is the test of choice for the real-time visualization of bolus flow through the upper aerodigestive tract, that is, both the breathing and swallowing systems. Using variable consistencies of barium contrast, VFSS also permits detection of the presence and timing of aspiration, i.e., entry of ingested material through the true vocal folds into the trachea, and it assists in identifying often treatable cause(s) [4]. Penetration can also be observed on the VFSS defined as passage of materials into the larynx, but not through the vocal folds [5]. Further, the VFSS reveals the effects of various bolus volumes, bolus textures, and compensatory strategies on swallowing physiology. This test is particularly important in patients after head and neck radiation therapy or surgery who may suffer from either oropharyngeal, or esophageal dysphagia, or both [6, 7]. Within the head and neck cancer population, the Dynamic Imaging Grade of Swallowing Toxicity (DIGEST) score was developed as a functional-outcome measure. DIGEST provides a clinician-rated measure of the functionality of uncompensated pharyngeal bolus transit on video-fluoroscopy. DIGEST was developed with the intent of mapping existing, widely adopted measures of bolus transport to the CTCAE framework of toxicity grading. DIGEST uses two component scores to quantify pharyngeal bolus transit: (1) a safety profile and (2) an efficiency profile. The summary DIGEST grade is an ideal modified barium study (MBS)-derived endpoint measure for oncology trials (grade 1, mild pharyngeal dysphagia; grade 2, moderate pharyngeal dysphagia; grade 3, severe pharyngeal dysphagia; and grade 4, life-threatening pharyngeal dysphagia) that reflects the combined impairment in swallowing safety and efficiency. Component safety and efficiency scores, however, might be valuable in clinical reporting for describing a profile of the pharyngeal swallow [8].

High-Resolution Pharyngeal Manometry with Impedance (P-HRM-I) During this study, solid-state HRM-impedance catheters incorporating 25–36 1 cm spaced pressure unidirectional sensors and an impedance electrode array are introduced through the nose and the upper esophageal sphincter (UES), and UES relaxation, opening extent, intrabolus pressure, and pharyngeal contractile strength are examined using 10 ml liquid swallows. Typically, three pharyngeal pressurization patterns, which may be indicative of obstructed flow, are characterized:

pan-pressurization (Type 1), distal compartmentalized pressurization (Type 2), and transient pressurization (Type 3). Deglutitive aspiration may also be simultaneously determined using video fluoroscopy. Pharyngeal manometry is an evolving physiologic study with work ongoing to define the optimal metrics to differentiate pathologic swallowing from healthy swallowing and define UES disorders [9]. P-HRM-I adoption is hampered by limited expertise and lack of incorporation of data analysis software into existing manometry platforms. The availability of online data processing software such as Swallow Gateway is helpful but remains a multistep process for data acquisition and review [10].

Impedance Planimetry (EndoFLIP) The EndoFLIP catheter includes a distensible balloon encasing multiple pairs of impedance sensors and a single distal pressure sensor and it is placed through the mouth during a sedated upper endoscopy, such that the balloon traverses the area of interest. The balloon is then distended with a conductive fluid through a mechanical pump while the EndoFLIP system converts the readings into a three-dimensional rendering of the esophageal lumen in real time and measures the relationship between the cross-sectional area (mm^2) over the distensive pressure to generate a luminal distensibility. Hence, impedance planimetry dynamically measures tissue wall distensibility as a function of pressure and cross-sectional area. This novel technique is mostly used in the assessment of esophago-gastric junction (EGJ) distensibility (see below) and more recently in the study of upper esophageal sphincter (UES) distensibility before and after myotomy, using Z-POEM [11]. An emerging role of EndoFLIP in patients with head and neck cancer after chemoradiation and/or surgery is recognized, but it will require further validation. Changes in FLIP distensibility index (DI) may reflect changes in wall mechanics not only within the mucosa but also the submucosal and adjacent structures, perhaps reflecting radiation-related fibrosis with reduced tissue compliance and contributing to dysphagia independent of stricture formation [12]. A key advantage to EndoFLIP in the evaluation of the upper esophageal sphincter is the volume-controlled distention. The UES is closed at baseline and relaxes transiently during swallowing to permit bolus entry to the esophagus. UES opening can be influenced by fibrosis of the cricopharyngeus, pharyngeal propulsive deficiencies, and reduced hyolaryngeal traction, all of which can occur in patients after treatment of head and neck cancer (HNC) [13, 14]. Probe placement across the UES with volume distention during endoscopy is independent of functional disorders that affect UES opening while swallowing.

References

1. Kopelman Y, Triadafilopoulos G. Endoscopy in the diagnosis and management of motility disorders. Dig Dis Sci. 2011;56(3):635–54. https://doi.org/10.1007/s10620-011-1584-3. Epub 2011 Feb 1. PMID: 21286936
2. Dziewas R, Warnecke T, Labeit B, Claus I, Muhle P, Oelenberg S, Ahring S, Wüller C, Jung A, von Itter J, Suntrup-Krueger S. Systematic approach to contextualize findings of flexible endoscopic evaluation of swallowing in neurogenic dysphagia- towards an integrated FEES

report. Neurol Res Pract. 2024;6(1):26. https://doi.org/10.1186/s42466-024-00321-8. PMID: 38720388; PMCID: PMC11080162

3. Starmer HM, Arrese L, Langmore S, Ma Y, Murray J, Patterson J, Pisegna J, Roe J, Tabor-Gray L, Hutcheson K. Adaptation and validation of the dynamic imaging grade of swallowing toxicity for flexible endoscopic evaluation of swallowing: DIGEST-FEES. J Speech Lang Hear Res. 2021;64(6):1802–10. https://doi.org/10.1044/2021_JSLHR-21-00014. Epub 2021 May 25. PMID: 34033498
4. Rosenbek JC, Robbins JA, Roecker EB, Coyle JL, Wood JL. A penetration-aspiration scale. Dysphagia. 1996;11(2):93. https://doi.org/10.1007/BF00417897. PMID: 8721066.
5. Ozaki K, Kagaya H, Yokoyama M, Saitoh E, Okada S, González-Fernández M, Palmer JB, Uematsu AH. The risk of penetration or aspiration during videofluoroscopic examination of swallowing varies depending on food types. Tohoku J Exp Med. 2010;220(1):41–6. https://doi.org/10.1620/tjem.220.41. PMID: 20046051
6. Karnell M, Maccracken E, Moran W, Vokes E, Haraf D, Panje W. Swallowing function following multispecialty organ preservation treatment of advanced head and neck-cancer. Oncol Rep. 1994;1(3):597–601. https://doi.org/10.3892/or.1.3.597. PMID: 21607410
7. Martin-Harris B, Canon CL, Bonilha HS, Murray J, Davidson K, Lefton-Greif MA. Best practices in modified barium swallow studies. Am J Speech Lang Pathol. 2020;29(2S):1078–93. https://doi.org/10.1044/2020_AJSLP-19-00189. Epub 2020 Jul 10. PMID: 32650657; PMCID: PMC7844340.
8. Hutcheson KA, Barrow MP, Barringer DA, Knott JK, Lin HY, Weber RS, Fuller CD, Lai SY, Alvarez CP, Raut J, Lazarus CL, May A, Patterson J, Roe JW, Starmer HM, Lewin JS. Dynamic Imaging Grade of Swallowing Toxicity (DIGEST): Scale development and validation. Cancer. 2017;123(1):62–70. https://doi.org/10.1002/cncr.30283. Epub 2016 Aug 26. PMID: 27564246; PMCID: PMC5161634
9. Omari T, Cock C, Wu P, Szczesniak MM, Schar M, Tack J, Rommel N. Using high resolution manometry impedance to diagnose upper esophageal sphincter and pharyngeal motor disorders. Neurogastroenterol Motil. 2023;35(1):e14461. https://doi.org/10.1111/nmo.14461. Epub 2022 Sep 19. PMID: 36121685
10. Singendonk M, Cock C, Bieckmann L, Szczesniak M, Ferris L, Benninga M, Omari T. Reliability of an online analysis platform for pharyngeal high-resolution impedance manometry recordings. Speech, Lang Hear. 2019;22:195–203. https://doi.org/10.1080/2050571X.2018.1535564.
11. Che SYW, Joseph S, Kuchta K, Amundson JR, Van Druff VN, Ishii S, Zimmermann CJ, Hedberg HM, Ujiki MB. Outcomes after per-oral endoscopic myotomy for Zenker's diverticula (Z-POEM) and correlation with impedance planimetry (FLIP). Surg Endosc. 2024;38(2):957–63. https://doi.org/10.1007/s00464-023-10512-0.
12. Richards DM, Naz S, Triadafilopoulos G, et al. EndoFLIP distensibility index correlates with radiation dose in cancer patients with radiation exposure and dysphagia. Am J Gastronterol (Abstract) ACG. 2024;119:S461.
13. Szczesniak MM, et al. The critical importance of pharyngeal contractile forces on the validity of intrabolus pressure as a predictor of impaired pharyngo-esophageal junction compliance. Neurogastroenterol Motil. 2018;30(10):e13374.
14. Wu PI, et al. Clinical utility of a functional lumen imaging probe in management of dysphagia following head and neck cancer therapies. Endoscopy. 2017;49(9):848–54.

4 Tests for Gastrointestinal Sensory-Motor Assessment: Esophagus

George Triadafilopoulos and David M. Richards

4.1 Esophagus

Endoscopy Several standard classification systems exist and should be used when documenting upper endoscopic findings: The Los Angeles classification for erosive esophagitis, the Prague classification for Barrett's esophagus, the Forrest classification for bleeding peptic ulcers, the Paris classification for superficial neoplastic lesions, the Hill grade classification for gastroesophageal flap valve, and the Eosinophilic Esophagitis Endoscopic Reference System (Figs. 4.1, 4.2, and 4.3) [1]. The American Foregut Society (AFS) uses a broader understanding of the anatomic mechanisms of the antireflux barrier including the crura of the diaphragm, the LES and its sling fibers, and the flap valve and the integral relationship between them. The AFS classification additionally includes assessment of the hiatus aperture, objective extent of hiatal axial length, and the presence or absence of the flap valve [2]. Such standardization is useful at baseline, as well as follow-up, particularly since many patients with motility abnormalities or those with prior surgery may be resistant to therapy.

High-Resolution Esophageal Manometry (HREM) This is a pivotal means to diagnose primary or secondary motility disorders in patients with suspected esophageal dysmotility (i.e., achalasia), since it assesses intraluminal esophageal pressures, peristalsis, and bolus transit. HRM catheters use 20–36 pressure sensors that are highly accurate in assessing pressure changes, better defining esophageal body peristalsis and sphincter relaxation (Fig. 4.4) [3–5].

G. Triadafilopoulos (✉) · D. M. Richards
Department of Gastroenterology, Hepatology and Nutrition, UT MD Anderson Cancer Center, Houston, TX, USA
e-mail: gtriadafilopoulo@mdanderson.org

G. Triadafilopoulos (ed.), *Onco-Neurogastroenterology*,
https://doi.org/10.1007/978-3-031-98848-6_4

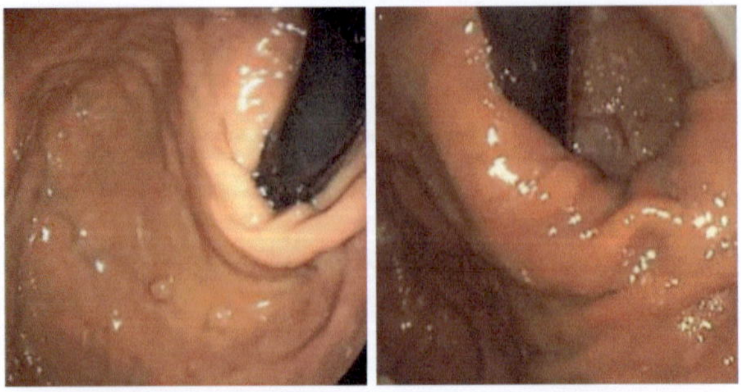

Fig. 4.1 Two retroflexed images of the esophagogastric junction (EGJ) in patients with GERD. Left: Normal. Right: Small (2 cm) sliding hiatal hernia

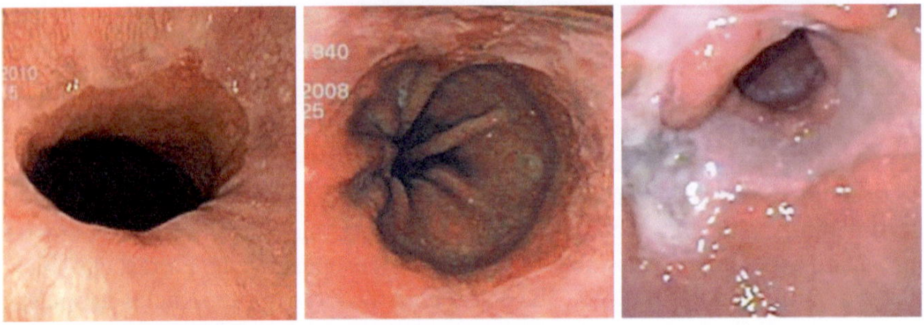

Fig. 4.2 (Left): Patulous EGJ, conducive to GERD without mucosal injury. (Middle) Axial (sliding) hiatal hernia with associated laxity of the EGJ and associated changes of short-segment Barrett's esophagus. (Right): Severe, LA. Grade D esophagitis with circumferential ulceration and stricture in the distal esophagus

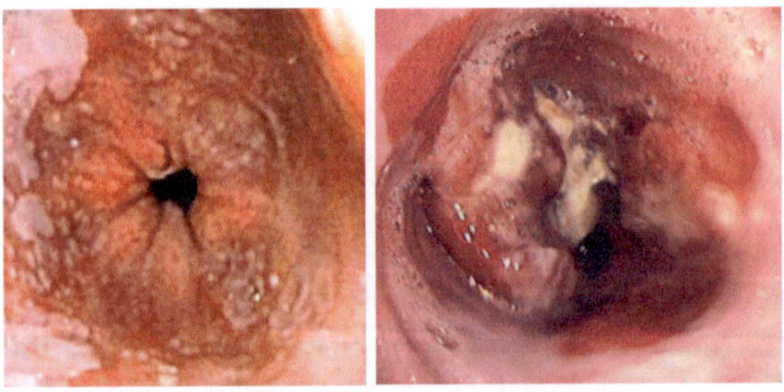

Fig. 4.3 (Left): Long-segment Barrett's esophagus with notable irregularity of the neo-squamocolumnar junction in a patient with long-standing heartburn and regurgitation. (Right): Esophageal adenocarcinoma encroaching upon ¾ of the distal esophageal lumen, causing dysphagia. Areas of visible Barrett's esophagus are seen on the right side of the image

A stepwise approach to a manometric diagnosis is essential (Fig. 4.5). The first step is to reliably define the median integrated relaxation pressure (IRP). If this is high (>15 mmHg), any of the three achalasia types may be present, depending on the contractility pattern of the esophageal body: Type I (classic): 100% failed swallows); type II: Achalasia with esophageal compression (>20% of swallows with panesophageal

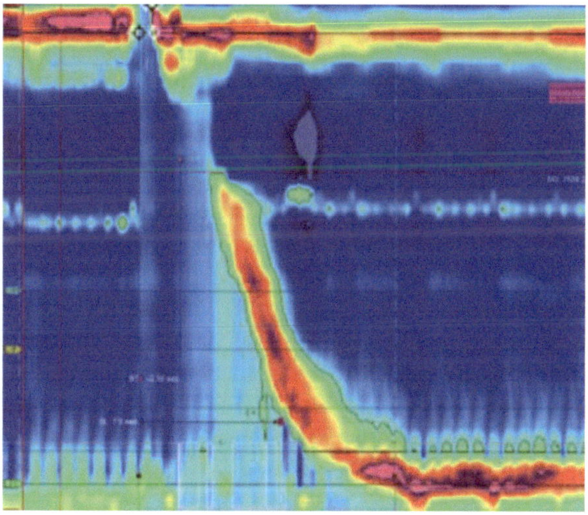

Fig. 4.4 Normal high-resolution esophageal manometry (HREM)

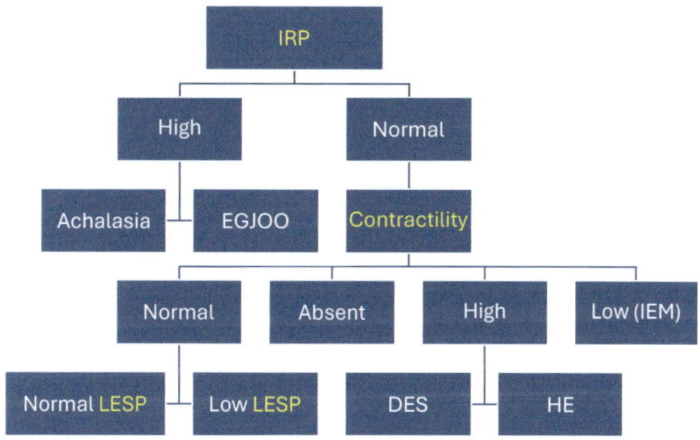

Fig. 4.5 Stepwise approach to manometric diagnosis using high-resolution esophageal manometry

pressurization); and type III (spastic achalasia) (>20% of swallows with premature (spastic) contractions. If there is some peristalsis associated with high IRP, the diagnosis of esophagogastric junction outflow obstruction (EGJOO) is made. In the setting of normal median IRP, the second step is to assess the esophageal body contractility or the distal contractile integral (DCI). This may be normal, absent (100% failed peristalsis), high, or low (<450 mmHg scm; ineffective esophageal motility, IEM, if >50% ineffective swallows). If high and > 20% of swallows are premature, it is distal esophageal spasm (DES); if high and associated with DCI of >8000, it is hypercontractile (jackhammer) esophagus (HE). A final step, the measurement of the lower esophageal sphincter pressure (LESP), is not part of the Chicago classification; may be normal, or low, and associated with sliding hiatal hernia in cases of gastroesophageal reflux disease (GERD); or absent (after esophagectomy or progressive systemic sclerosis (PSS)). Most patients with EGJOO have a coexisting motility disorder and do not have isolated EGJOO. Mixed patterns may occur with a fluidity in the manometric diagnosis that needs to be considered prior to therapy [6].

Impedance Planimetry (EndoFLIP) This tool is mostly used in the assessment of the esophagogastric junction (EGJ) and the evaluation of esophageal achalasia, as an intraoperative tool for the technical optimization of fundoplication for gastroesophageal reflux disease (GERD), as well as during laparoscopic Heller myotomy and peroral endoscopic myotomy (POEM) in esophageal achalasia. FLIP topography converts the readings to color-coded luminal diameter plots over time, enabling evaluation of distensibility across the EGJ, as well as visualizing secondary peristalsis—the esophageal contractile response to distension in the esophageal body. A normal EGJ distensibility index (EGJ-DI) is >2.8 mm^2/mm Hg and normal EGJ diameter is >13 mm. Further, the presence of repetitive antegrade contractions is considered a normal response to distension. Reduced EGJ-DI and/or diameter is often seen in patients with disorders of EGJ outflow, such as achalasia or EGJ outflow obstruction (EGJOO). EGJ-DI of <2 mm^2/mm Hg is definitively abnormal, whereas EGJ diameter of <13 mm is likely abnormal and can serve as a supportive measure when EGJ-DI is indeterminate (2–3 mm^2/mm Hg) [7]. Using the same system, a novel method, termed FLIP topography, may also characterize patterns of contractility in the esophageal body (Figs. 4.6 and 4.7) [8]. Since volume distention by the FLIP probe induces esophageal contractions, rather than a volitional swallow when the patient is awake during manometry, the FLIP motility patterns are likely more representative of secondary peristalsis. Several motility patterns have been observed during FLIP panometry and include repetitive antegrade contractions (RACs), possibly representing the normal response to volume distention, repetitive retrograde contractions, impaired or disordered contractions, spastic contractions, and absent contractile response. Efforts are ongoing to describe patterns seen on FLIP panometry only in controls, patterns seen only in motility disorders, and to correlate findings on FLIP with findings on HRM. FLIP provides the advantage of evaluation in a sedated patient at the time of endoscopy in contrast to HRM typically performed with patient awake and participating in the exam that can be limited by factors such as oropharyngeal dysfunction that can cause aspiration. Since HRM

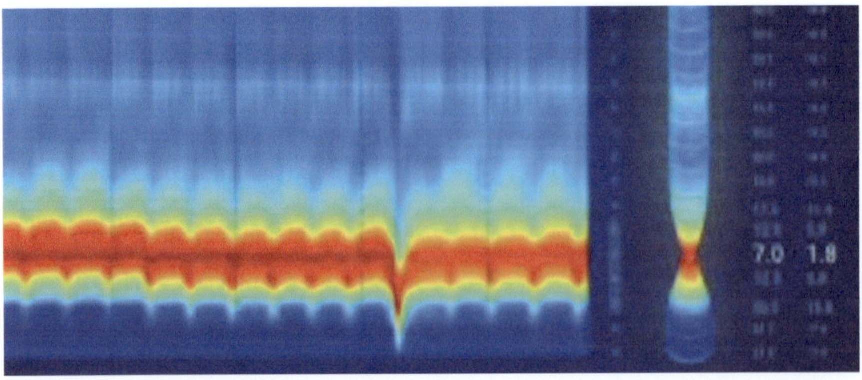

Fig. 4.6 EndoFLIP study showing normal distensibility at 40 ml (up to 60 ml), but absent peristalsis in a patient with scleroderma and GERD symptoms

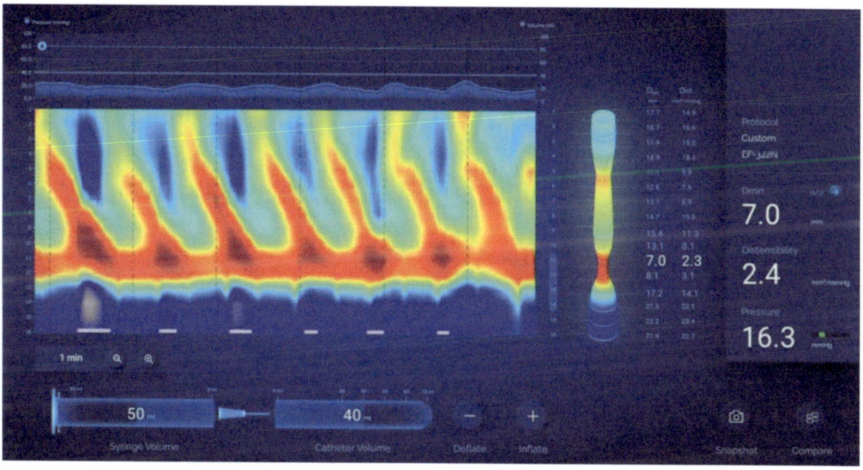

Fig. 4.7 EndoFLIP study showing repetitive antegrade contractions (RACs)

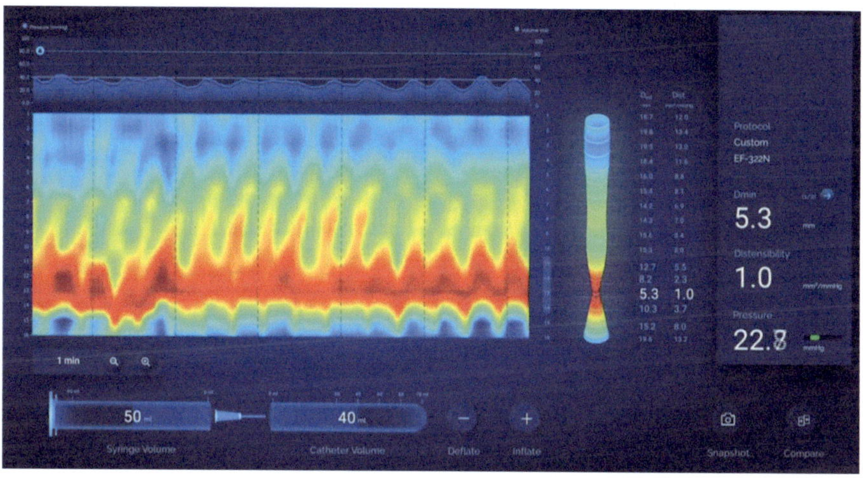

Fig. 4.8 EndoFLIP study showing repetitive retrograde contractions

is evaluating primary peristalsis and FLIP secondary peristalsis, it seems likely that FLIP will not replace HRM, but it will serve as a complimentary study (Figs. 4.6, 4.7, 4.8, and 4.9) [9].

Timed Barium Esophagram (TBE) and Barium Tablet This radiologic test is performed fluoroscopically in the upright position using 8 oz or 236 mL of liquid barium and evaluates the barium column height at 1 and 5 min after ingestion. TBE with oral administration of a 13 mm barium tablet is also performed. The barium column height supports outflow obstruction (such as achalasia), if >5 cm at 1 min or >2 cm at 5 min. The 13-mm barium tablet retention supports

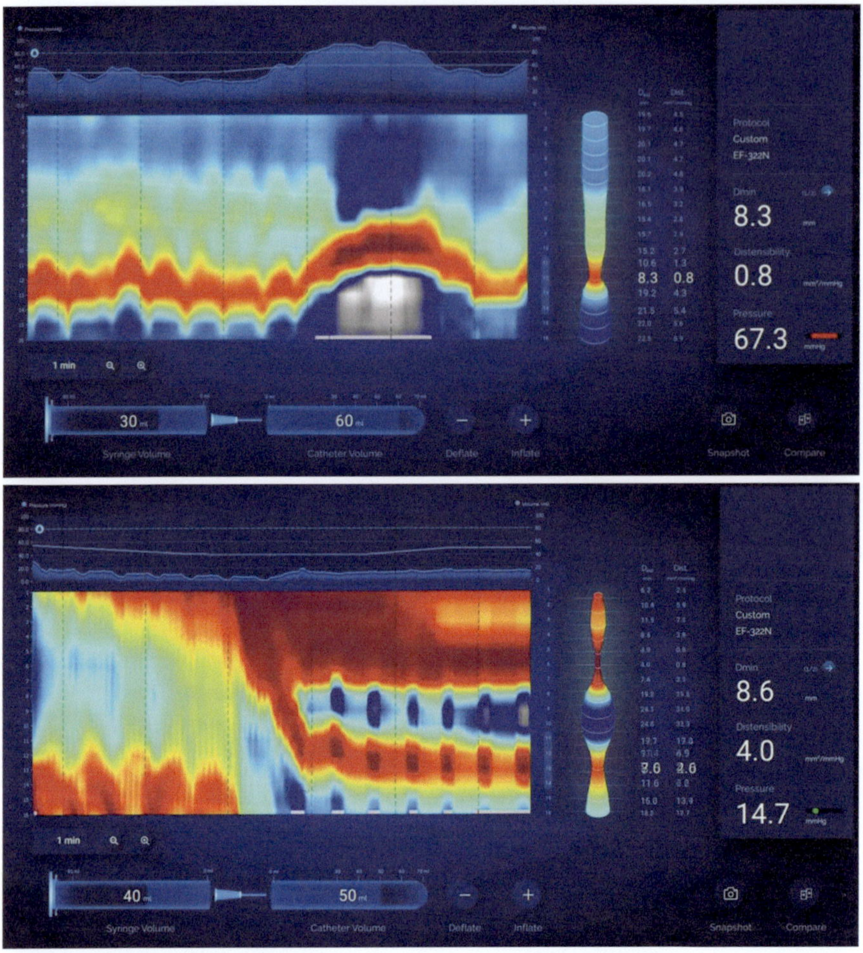

Fig. 4.9 EndoFLIP study showing spastic contractions (top and bottom)

obstructive process. Further, a 3% improvement (decrease) in pre- to posttreatment barium height at 5 min might predict long-term clinical remission in achalasia. Corkscrew appearance may be suggestive of distal esophageal spasm (DES) or hypercontractile esophagus (HE) [10]. Although TBE has been extensively validated in esophageal achalasia and its response to therapeutic intervention, it also provides invaluable information in patients with dysphagia after Ivor-Lewis esophagectomy by identifying subtle anastomotic strictures. Following the barium column beyond the stomach also informs on the possibility of postoperative gastric emptying delay and the possible need of a pyloric intervention. Most commonly, even a single column barium esophagram may identify abnormalities, like a sliding hiatal hernia (Fig. 4.10).

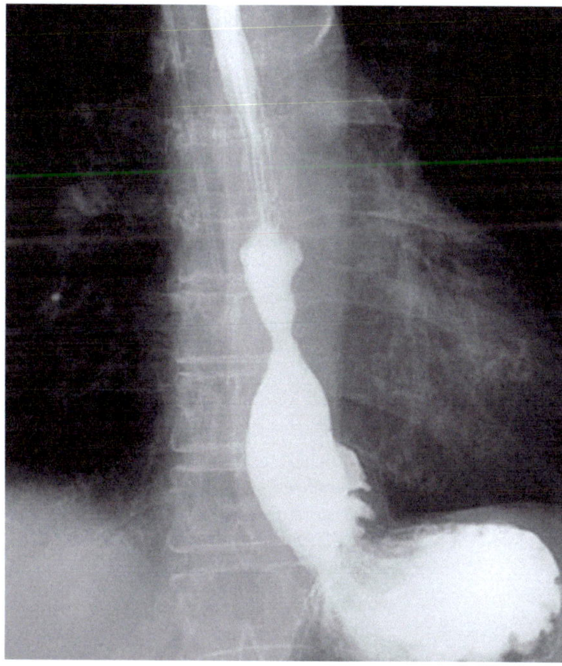

Fig. 4.10 Barium esophagram revealing an esophageal stricture and a large sliding hiatal hernia with significant displacement of the proximal stomach into the chest

24-h Esophageal Impedance-pH Monitoring Since non-erosive reflux disease (NERD) is more prevalent, esophageal pH-impedance monitoring has become a key diagnostic tool to evaluate patients with heartburn, chest pain, and regurgitation. The esophageal impedance-pH sensor is typically positioned 5 cm above the proximal margin of the lower esophageal sphincter (LES) measured by upper endoscopy (location of the squamo-columnar junction), or esophageal manometry (proximal location of the LES pressure zone), and is connected to a portable digital recorder that stores pH data for up to 24 h. Positioning of the catheter is also based on the pH differential between the pH sensors (an intra-gastric one, 10 cm below *the* LES, and a proximal esophageal one, 5 cm above LES). Typically, in patients not receiving acid suppressive therapy, the gastric sensor reveals low pH (~1–2), while the esophageal sensor exhibits higher pH (~4–5). Patients are instructed to keep a diary of symptoms, meal intake times, and body position, such as supine position at night, regardless of sleep (nocturnal supine period). Acid suppressive drugs, typically PPI (taken qd or bid before meals), may or may not be used during the study, depending on the reason for the pH monitoring (diagnosis, response to therapy, or symptom persistence). The parallel impedance monitoring helps identify non-acid reflux in many cases of normal pH monitoring (Fig. 4.11) [11]. Positive symptom association probability (>95%) and/or symptom index (SI) >50% increase confidence that symptoms may be linked to reflux episodes [12]. Sometimes, a dual sensor (proximal and distal esophageal) pH monitoring is performed to explore for proximal esophageal acid exposure, contributing to laryngo-esophageal or extraesophageal

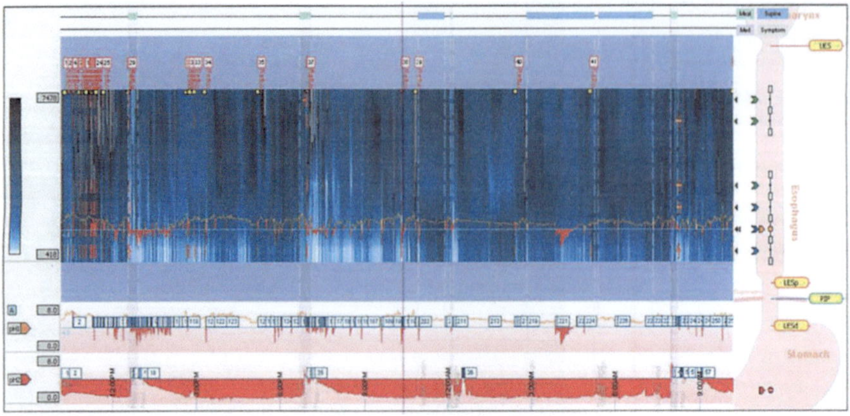

Fig. 4.11 Dual sensor (esophageal and gastric) 24-h esophageal impedance-pH monitoring. Top part of the image shows the impedance tracing. The pH tracing of the distal esophagus sensor (top red line, middle) shows moderately abnormal acid reflux (% pH <4.0 of 12.8; normal <6), mostly in the upright position, while the stomach sensor (bottom red line) shows normal stomach acidity (% pH <4.0 of 96%), throughout the 24-h period, evidence against lack of gastric acidity

symptoms. Alternatively, continuous proximal gastric pH monitoring may be performed to validate and quantify gastric hypochlohydria (usually a result of acid suppressive therapy), or achlorhydria, a result of autoimmune or *H. pylori*-related atrophic gastritis and pernicious anemia, both precursors to gastric cancer [13, 14].

96-h Wireless Ambulatory Esophageal pH Monitoring By convention, the 96-h wireless esophageal pH recording capsule is attached to the mucosa, 6 cm above the endoscopically identifiable squamo-columnar junction. The subsequent wireless esophageal ambulatory pH monitoring is better tolerated, allowing patients to eat freely and thereby achieving more real-life data and for longer recording period (96 h), which allows for measurement of the effect of diet or drugs on esophageal acid exposure. The study should be considered when trying to establish the presence of abnormal acid exposure. It may also be useful when a catheter-based pH monitoring cannot be tolerated. Patients are studied while on- or off-acid suppressant therapy, keeping record of their symptoms, meals, and position (Figs. 4.12, 4.13, and 4.14) [15]. As with standard pH monitoring, a positive symptom association probability (>95%) and/or symptom index >50% increase confidence that symptoms may be linked to reflux episodes.

Esophageal ambulatory pH monitoring is also useful in guiding the need for postural measures aimed at preventing heartburn and acid reflux. These general recommendations aim at preventing acid reflux through an incompetent lower esophageal sphincter (LES) and improving esophageal clearance by gravity. However, low LES pressure is found only in a minority of patients with GERD, while frequent transient LES relaxations (tLESRs), primarily in the upright position, are the main pathophysiological abnormality in GERD. Raising the head of

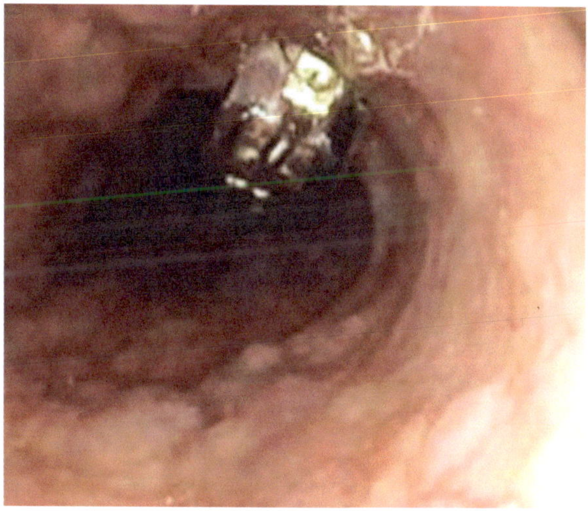

Fig. 4.12 Endoscopic appearance of the Bravo pH capsule shortly after its placement 6 cm above the endoscopically identified squamo-columnar junction. The capsule communicates wirelessly with a recording device to generate a tracing of the distal esophageal pH over 4 days (96 h)

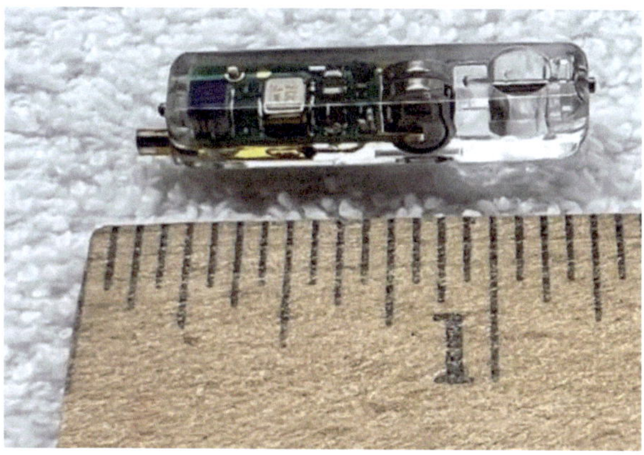

Fig. 4.13 Bravo pH capsule adjacent to a ruler for scale. Note the small ~1/8-in circular opening in the top right of the capsule that permits mucosal entry and placement of the pin to adhere the capsule to the esophageal mucosa

the entire bed frame on 8-inch bed blocks, or using a commercially available foam wedge, providing a 22° angle, are not favored by patients or their spouses who often slide to the end of the bed in an uncomfortable position during sleep. Transient lower esophageal relaxations (tLESRs) appear without an antecedent pharyngeal contraction, persist for longer periods (5–30 s) than swallow-induced LES relaxations, and usually are unaccompanied by esophageal peristalsis. The frequency of tLESRs is greatly increased by the distension of the stomach by gas, as occurs in the upright versus the supine position. In contrast, LES incompetence may be associated with GERD by two mechanisms: stress and free reflux. Stress reflux may occur when a relatively hypotensive LES is overcome by a sudden increase in intra-abdominal pressure, and it is more likely to occur in the upright than in the supine position. Stress reflux is unlikely when the LESP is greater than 10 mmHg. Free reflux is noted when the resting LESP is less than 4 mmHg above the intragastric pressure. In general, LESP is lowest in the postprandial period and

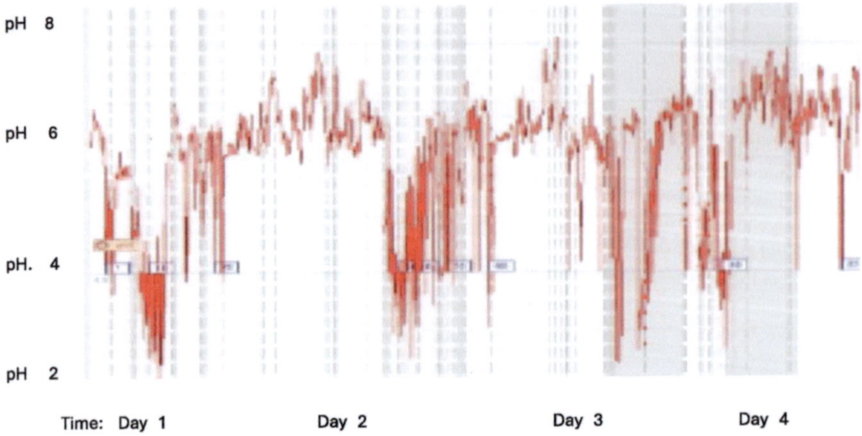

Fig. 4.14 A 96-h wireless ambulatory esophageal pH-monitoring study consistent with severe, bipositional GERD that occurs throughout the 4-day study. Distal esophageal pH (range 0–8) is depicted on the Y axis; time (4 days) on the X axis. Acid events are depicted everytime the red line crosses pH 4. A symptom diary allows for symptom reporting and correlation with acid reflux events

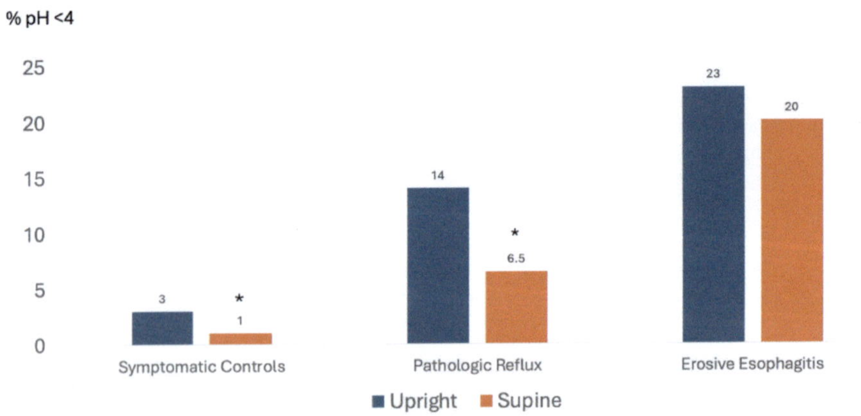

Fig. 4.15 Percent time with esophageal pH < 4 in symptomatic controls without abnormal esophageal acid exposure, in patients with pathologic acid reflux without esophagitis, and those with erosive disease. Supine reflux is dominant mostly in the erosive esophagitis group

highest at night, making supine reflux a less common occurrence. However, as shown in Fig. 4.15, patients with reflux symptoms but normal 24-h pH studies and endoscopy as well as in patients with symptomatic GERD without esophagitis, supine reflux is rare and limited. Supine or bipositional acid reflux by pH monitoring is mainly seen in patients with ulcerative and/or complicated esophagitis, who also have reduced LES tone, and it is in this group that postural measures might be useful [16].

References

1. Nagula S, Parasa S, Laine L, Shah SC. AGA clinical practice update on high-quality upper endoscopy: expert review. Clin Gastroenterol Hepatol 2024;22(5):933–943. https://doi.org/10.1016/j.cgh.2023.10.034. Epub 2024 Feb 22. PMID: 38385942.
2. Nguyen NT, Thosani NC, Canto MI, et al. The American Foregut Society white paper on the endoscopic classification of esophagogastric junction integrity. Foregut. 2022;2(4):339–48. https://doi.org/10.1177/26345161221126961.
3. Tack J, Pauwels A, Roman S, Savarino E, Smout A; ESNM HRM consensus group. European Society for Neurogastroenterology and Motility (ESNM) recommendations for the use of high-resolution manometry of the esophagus. Neurogastroenterol Motil 2021;33(5):e14043. https://doi.org/10.1111/nmo.14043. Epub 2020 Dec 4. PMID: 33274525.
4. Sharma P, Yadlapati R. Evaluation of esophageal motility and lessons from Chicago classification version 4.0. Curr Gastroenterol Rep. 2022;24(1):10–17. https://doi.org/10.1007/s11894-022-00836-7. PMID: 35084643; PMCID: PMC9380285.
5. Carlson DA, Pandolfino JE. High-Resolution Manometry in Clinical Practice. Gastroenterol Hepatol (NY). 2015;11(6):374–84.
6. Triadafilopoulos G, Clarke JO. Clinical and manometric characteristics of patients with oesophagogastric outflow obstruction: towards a new classification. BMJ Open Gastroenterol. 2018;5(1):e000210. https://doi.org/10.1136/bmjgast-2018-000210.
7. Savarino E, di Pietro M, Bredenoord AJ, et al. Use of the functional lumen imaging probe in clinical esophagology. Am J Gastroenterol. 2020;115:1786–96.
8. Ahuja NK, Clarke JO. The role of impedance Planimetry in the evaluation of esophageal disorders. Curr Gastroenterol Rep 2017;19(2):7. https://doi.org/10.1007/s11894-017-0544-2. PMID: 28220362.
9. Carlson DA, Baumann AJ, Prescott JE, Donnan EN, Yadlapati R, Khan A, Gyawali CP, Kou W, Kahrilas PJ, Pandolfino JE. Validation of secondary peristalsis classification using FLIP panometry in 741 subjects undergoing manometry. Neurogastroenterol Motil 2022;34(1):e14192. https://doi.org/10.1111/nmo.14192. Epub 2021 Jun 13. PMID: 34120383; PMCID: PMC8666463.
10. Patel DA, Yadlapati R, Vaezi MF. Esophageal motility disorders: current approach to diagnostics and therapeutics. Gastroenterology 2022;162(6):1617–1634. https://doi.org/10.1053/j.gastro.2021.12.289. Epub 2022 Feb 25. PMID: 35227779; PMCID: PMC9405585.
11. Pohl D, Tutuian R. Reflux monitoring: pH-metry, bilitec and oesophageal impedance measurements. Best Pract Res Clin Gastroenterol. 2009;23:299–311.
12. Gyawali CP, Kahrilas PJ, Savarino E, et al. Modern diagnosis of GERD: the Lyon consensus. Gut. 2018;67:1351–62. https://doi.org/10.1136/gutjnl-2017-314722.
13. Gomez Cifuentes JD, Sparkman J, Graham DY. Management of upper gastrointestinal symptoms in patients with autoimmune gastritis. Curr Opin Gastroenterol. 2022;38(6):600–606. https://doi.org/10.1097/MOG.0000000000000878. Epub 2022 Sep 9. PMID: 36165039; PMCID: PMC9561041.
14. Khan MY, Aslam A, Mihali AB, Shabbir Rawala M, Dirweesh A, Khan S, Adler DG, Siddiqui A. Effectiveness of *Helicobacter pylori* eradication in preventing metachronous gastric cancer and preneoplastic lesions. A systematic review and meta-analysis. Eur J Gastroenterol Hepatol 2020;32(6):686–694. https://doi.org/10.1097/MEG.0000000000001740. PMID: 32355093.
15. Triadafilopoulos G, Kamal A, Clarke JO. Value of 96-hour ambulatory esophageal pH monitoring in the assessment of patients with refractory acid reflux symptoms and their response to anti-reflux diet. Dis Esophagus. 2022;36(7):doac102. https://doi.org/10.1093/dote/doac102. Epub ahead of print. PMID: 36567531.
16. Ouatu-Lascar R, Lin OS, Fitzgerald RC, Triadafilopoulos G. Upright versus supine reflux in gastroesophageal reflux disease. J Gastroenterol Hepatol 2001;16(11):1184–1190. https://doi.org/10.1046/j.1440-1746.2001.02581.x. PMID: 11903733.

Tests for Gastrointestinal Sensory-Motor Assessment: Stomach

5

George Triadafilopoulos and Mehnaz A. Shafi

5.1 Stomach

Endoscopy Upper endoscopy is universally the first step in the evaluation of a patient with suspected foregut sensory-motor gastrointestinal disorder (i.e., dyspepsia) to exclude structural pathology that would indirectly compromise function (Fig. 5.1). The use of endoscopy may not be only diagnostic, providing direct visualization of the mucosa and histological sampling (Fig. 5.2); it may also provide therapeutic intervention (i.e., pyloric BoTox injection in gastroparesis) (Fig. 5.3) [1]. In conjunction with laparoscopy, endoscopy also serves as a guide in the proper placement of the Enterra electrical stimulator [2].

Upper GI Series An upper gastrointestinal (GI) series is a set of X-rays that examines the throat, esophagus, stomach, and the first part of the small intestine. The examination helps identify the cause of swallowing problems, unexplained nausea and vomiting, abdominal discomfort, and severe indigestion, by detecting ulcers, gastroesophageal reflux, hiatal hernia, obstructions, or benign or malignant narrowing of the upper GI tract. The patient drinks a barium suspension, which coats the GI tract and makes it radiologically visible. X-rays are taken in various positions to capture specific images. The radiologist may also use fluoroscopy, a real-time imaging technique, to observe the movement of the barium and assess the function of the upper GI tract. Upper GI series does not provide the mucosal detail of an endoscopy and does not provide a reliable quantitative means of transit, compared to gastric emptying scan.

G. Triadafilopoulos (✉) · M. A. Shafi
Department of Gastroenterology, Hepatology and Nutrition, UT MD Anderson Cancer Center, Houston, TX, USA
e-mail: gtriadafilopoulo@mdanderson.org

G. Triadafilopoulos (ed.), *Onco-Neurogastroenterology*,
https://doi.org/10.1007/978-3-031-98848-6_5

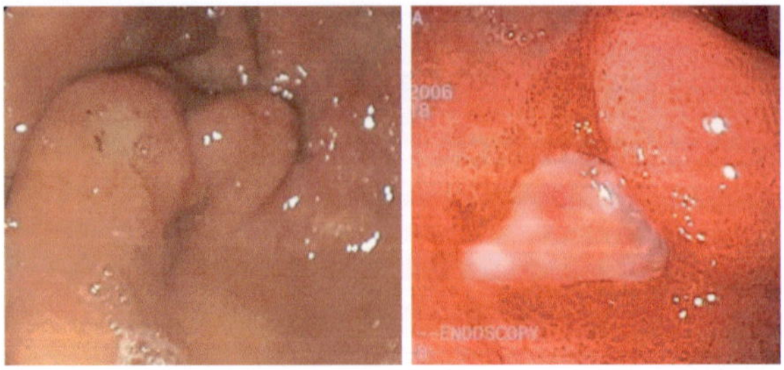

Fig. 5.1 Endoscopic images of *Helicobacter pylori* infection causing dyspepsia. (Left) Prepyloric region exhibiting erosive gastritis secondary to the infection. (Right) *H. pylori*-related duodenal ulcer (white crater, surrounded by inflammation of the duodenal bulb). This ulcer will require therapy against *H. pylori* infection and is expected to heal within 2–3 months

Fig. 5.2 Close-up view of antral gastritis (patchy erythema) from *H. pylori* infection

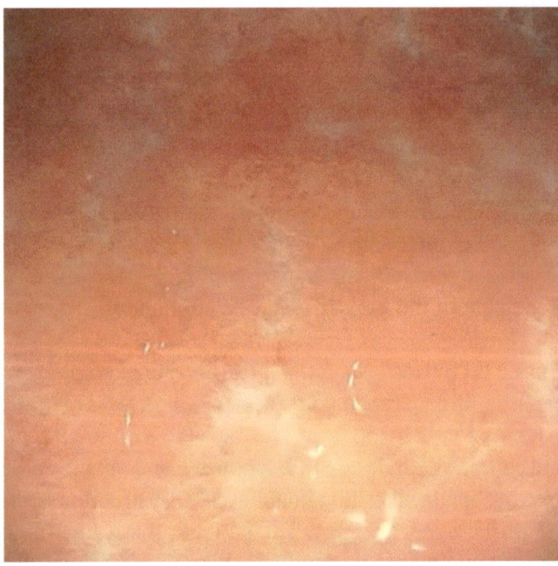

Endoscopic Ultrasound (EUS) and Biopsy EUS can help diagnose conditions in the upper and lower GI tract, as well as nearby organs, such as the lungs, pancreas, liver, and gallbladder. Endoscopic ultrasound can be used to better examine areas of concern identified by other imaging tests, such as an X-ray, MRI, or CT. As a procedure that examines the GI tract by combining two imaging techniques, endoscopy and ultrasound, it is particularly useful in patients with functional symptoms of neuroendocrine tumors (NETs), a group of rare neoplasms originating from dispersed neuroendocrine cells, mainly of the digestive and respiratory tract. EUS can also be helpful in diagnosing submucosal lesions that are symptomatic due to their size and location. Depending on the type of lesion and location within the stomach, submucosal lesions can present with dysphagia, early satiety, or organ outflow obstructions (Fig. 5.4).

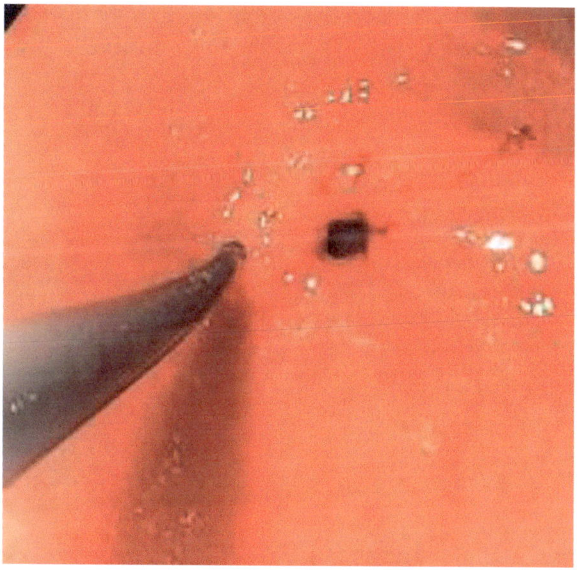

Fig. 5.3 Endoscopic image of a normal pylorus being injected with botulinum toxin (100 IU in 4 quadrants) using a standard sclerotherapy needle for the management of gastroparesis

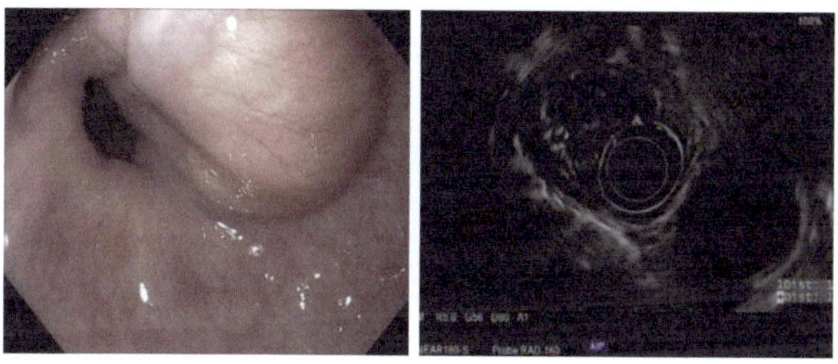

Fig. 5.4 Endoscopic (left) and EUS (right) images from a patient with dysphagia from a large distal esophageal leiomyoma. EUS-FNA revealed a spindle cell proliferation without cytologic atypia and the patient was managed conservatively for several years. Progressive dysphagia led to surgical resection confirming the diagnosis of leiomyoma and resolving dysphagia

Gastric Emptying Scintigraphy In patients with suspected delayed or accelerated gastric emptying resulting from prior surgery of the gastroesophageal junction (i.e., Ivor-Lewis esophagectomy), partial gastrectomy, or primary invasion of the gastric muscularis propria by primary cancer or neoplastic peritoneal involvement, gastric scintigraphy may noninvasively assess gastric emptying and guide therapy. The test involves ingestion of a standard test meal (typically >200 kcal) labeled with a radioactive isotope (99mTc for solids and 111 Indium for liquids) and measurement of the % gastric emptying hourly over 4 h. The patient ingests the standard egg sandwich meal over 10 min. Images of the abdomen are then taken in the front and back positions immediately after completion of the meal and at 30 min (normally, <96% retention), 1 h (normally <90% retention), 2 h (normally <60%), 3 h (normally <30%), and 4 h (normally <10% retention) (Figs. 5.5 and 5.6). Symptom severity does not always correlate with the rate gastric emptying. Delayed emptying serves

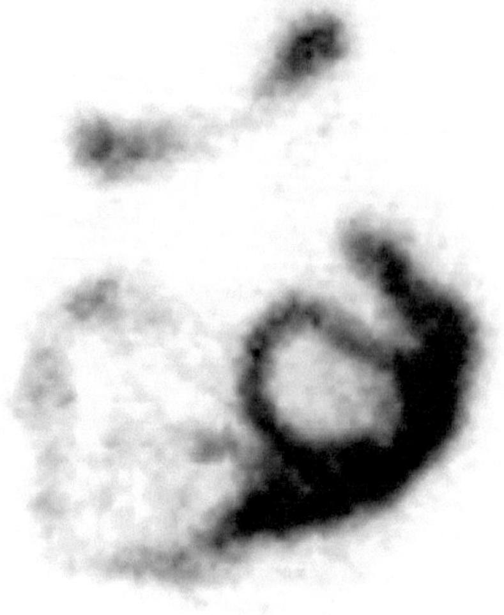

Fig. 5.5 Normal gastric scintigraphy with expected activity at 2 h (14%) that was seen within the stomach on the immediate imaging with activity extending into the small bowel loops on the 30-min imaging that continued over time. There is no suggestion of esophageal reflux. For the study, 1 mCi of Technetium 99 m unfiltered sulfur colloid was mixed/cooked with one egg. The patient ingested the standard egg sandwich meal over 8 min. Static images of the abdomen were obtained immediately after completion of the meal and at 30 min, 1 h, 2 h (this image), 3 h, and 4 h delay. Gastric % retention at 30 min was 77% and at 1 h 54% (ULN 90%), at 2 h 14% (this image) (ULN 60%), at 3 h 3% (ULN 30%), and at 4 h 0% (ULN 10%)

Fig. 5.6 Abnormal gastric emptying scan, suggestive of gastroparesis. Most of the radioactivity (in black) is retained and outlining the stomach in both the front (left) and back (right) projections, with very little escaping in the esophagus and small bowel. Specifically, stomach % retention was 96%, at 1 h 93%, at 2 h 88%, at 3 h 74%, and at 4 h 64%, suggesting significant delay in stomach emptying

as a guide to the magnitude of dysfunction, while rapid gastric emptying may be associated with dyspeptic symptoms in some patients, particularly postoperatively. Notably, in the postoperative setting, calibration of the regions of interest (ROI) to accurately measure gastric emptying may be technically challenging [3].

Gastric Emptying Breath Test (GEBT) The carbon-13 spirulina gastric emptying breath test (GEBT) is approved to identify normal, delayed, or accelerated gastric emptying. This is a safe, non-radioactive, FDA-approved, and commercially available alternative to nuclear scintigraphy-based gastric emptying evaluation that can be administered locally or through a telehealth program. For the test, patients consume a 230-kcal test meal labeled with technetium 99 m and ^{13}C-spirulina, after which ten scintigraphic images and breath samples (baseline, 15, 30, 45, 60, 90, 120, 150, 180, 210, and 240 min) are collected [4].

Cutaneous Electrogastrography (EGG) This noninvasive technique involves placement of surface electrodes to record the electrical control activity of the stomach. Altered frequency (bradygastria, tachygastria, or mixed) and reduction in the amplitude of the postprandial electrical gastric signal are seen in patients with gastroparesis and nausea. Such dysrhythmias may be seen in patients with dyspepsia, with or without evidence of gastric emptying delay. EGG has not been adequately explored in the clinical evaluation and management of patients with cancer, but it could provide an easy, noninvasive management tool [5].

Gastric Alimetry (GA) Gastric alimetry (GA; Alimetry, Auckland, New Zealand) is a new test of gastric function that combines noninvasive body surface gastric mapping (BSGM) with concurrent validated symptom profiling. GA enables high-resolution characterization of gastric myoelectrical activity, being optimized to maximally separate the weak gastric signals from noise, and in achieving a critical advance over conventional electrogastrography. The technique has been validated against antroduodenal manometry and invasive gastric electrical recordings and can identify specific patient subgroups with gastric neuromuscular dysfunction, including with symptom correlations. The merits of this new technology have not been fully shown [6]. It is plausible that GA and GET will play a complementary role in clinical practice.

The GutTracker Wireless Patch System (WPS) The wireless patch system (GTech Medical, Mountain View, CA USA) is a novel diagnostic tool that uses three small cutaneous patches applied to the abdominal wall to measure electrical activity from the stomach, intestines, and colon. Information is relayed through a low-energy Bluetooth system from the patches to a paired iPhone (Fig. 5.7). Ambulatory monitoring is performed for up to 6 days, during which time the patient records mealtimes, symptoms, and bowel habits. Small studies and case reports have shown

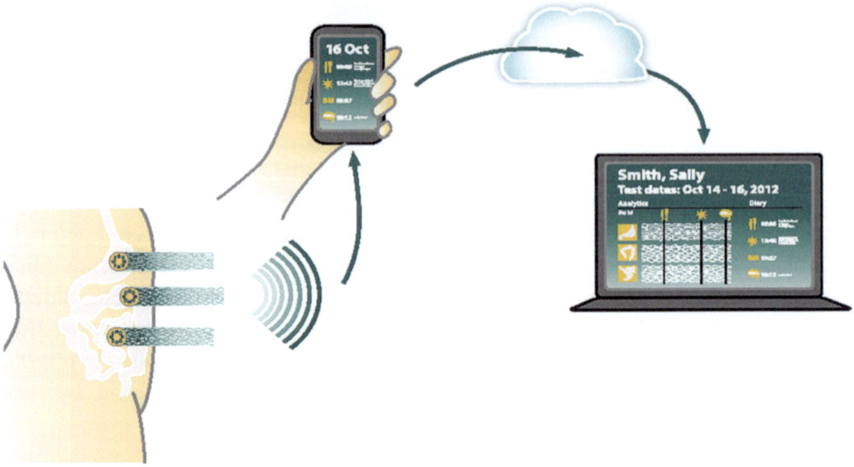

Fig. 5.7 Schematic diagram of the wireless patch system. Patches on patient's abdomen collect myoelectrical signals that are transferred via Bluetooth to an iOS-based mobile device. The app transfers the data to a secure cloud server for processing and reporting. The app also allows patients to enter events, such as meals, pain, bowel movements, and activities, which are time-stamped and transferred to the cloud along with the measurement data

that this system is safe and provides reliable data. The system is promising in our understanding of gastric sensory-motor function in patients with nausea and vomiting (Figs. 5.8 and 5.9) [7] and as measuring tool for gut transit under physiologic conditions [8], as well as in postoperative patients with suspected ileus [9]. Because of its noninvasive, ambulatory nature, this technology has many applications in patients with cancer, but currently validation studies are lacking.

Whole Gut Transit Scintigraphy (WGTS) Whole gut transit scintigraphy assesses gastric emptying, small bowel transit, and colonic transit, but it is not generally available [10]. Patients with predominant constipation frequently experience colonic transit delay, whereas those with upper GI symptoms often exhibit delayed gastric emptying. Patients undergo WGTS utilizing a standard egg sandwich meal radiolabeled with Tc-99 m SC (short half-life for radioactive decay and short imaging time) and water radiolabeled with 111In-DTPA (longer half-life for radioactive decay and more prolonged imaging up to 72 h) as part of a standard solid-liquid gastric emptying meal. Gastric emptying is assessed for the first 4 h of the study. Small bowel transit analysis utilizes the liquid water phase for the next 2 h. Small bowel transit is considered delayed if less than 40% of the meal accumulates in the terminal ileum/ascending colon area at 6 h. Colon transit images are acquired at 24, 48, and 72 h after meal ingestion using the In-111, which was administered in water. To calculate the colonic geometric center, the colon is divided into seven anatomic regions, each of which has a numeric value: cecum–ascending colon (1), hepatic flexure

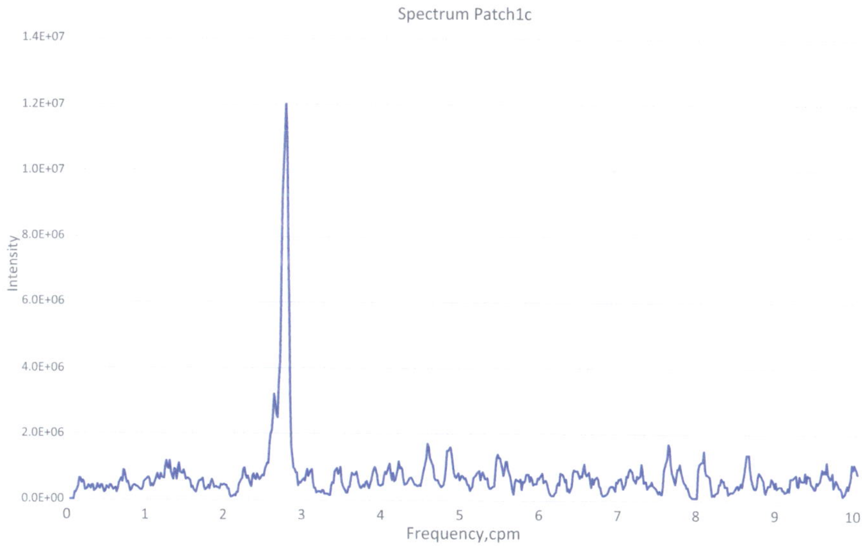

Fig. 5.8 Spectra from a data channel following a meal showing a strong 3 cpm (normal) stomach peak

(2), transverse colon (3), splenic flexure (4), descending colon (5), rectosigmoid colon (6), and, by calculation, excreted stool. The geometric center is the weighted average of the counts in each region. The normal mean values (± SD) for geometric center are 4.6 ± 1.5 at 24 h, 6.1 ± 1.0 at 48 h, and 6.6 ± 0.19 at 72 h [11].

Wireless Motility Capsule (WMC; Smartpill) This is an ambulatory, noninvasive diagnostic sensor (Smartpill; Medtronic, Sunnyvale, California, USA) that samples intraluminal pH, temperature, and pressure as it moves through the GI tract. Patients first ingest a meal to initiate the postprandial motility pattern, they then swallow the capsule that wirelessly connects to a data receiver, and they keep a diary for recording bowel movements, food intake, sleep, and GI symptoms while continuing their regular diet and life routines. After 5 days, patients return the data receiver and the diary, and the downloaded data are analyzed using the display software. This technology quantifies transit through the stomach (primarily using the pH transition from acidic (gastric) to alkaline (duodenal) but also assesses transit through all gut regions in a single test, and it has been used for the diagnosis of functional GI symptoms, such as bloating, early postprandial fullness, nausea, and constipation, by measuring gastric emptying time, as well as small bowel and colonic transit times (Fig. 5.10) [12]. The technology is currently not commercially available and its use in cancer patients, albeit very promising, has not been formally studied.

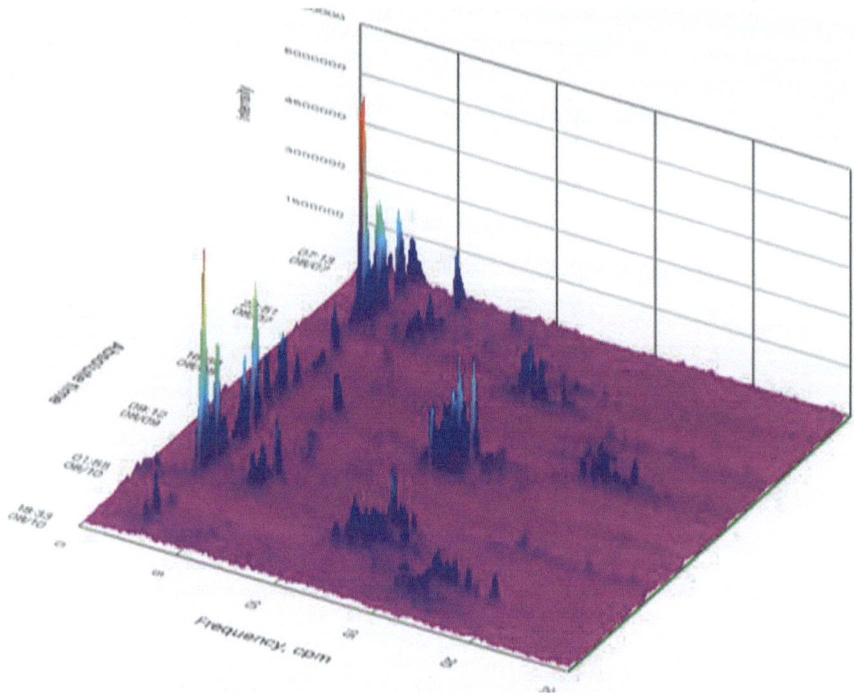

Fig. 5.9 Normal, waterfall spectral plot of 3 days of data in one channel. Frequency runs from left to right, time from back to front. Narrow line of peaks on the left is from the stomach, while the clusters of peaks on the right are from the colon. Repetitive nature of the colon peaks is readily apparent and occurs during the nighttime hours. Figure exemplifies the potential of a noninvasive recording beyond the stomach, to the small intestine and ultimately the colon, over time and under physiologic conditions

Point-of-Care Gastric Ultrasound In patients suspected of gastric emptying delay, such as those with diabetic, postoperative, neoplasia-associated gastroparesis, or in patients on GLP1 agonists, gastric ultrasound can be used preoperatively to assess high gastric residual imposing an aspiration risk [13]. This is particularly important when the onset of fasting prior to anesthesia for an endoscopic procedure or surgery is uncertain, such as for patients with an altered mental status or conflicting histories from patients and caretakers. Caution should also be utilized in cancer patients with altered gastric anatomy, in those using glucagon-like-peptide-1 receptor agonists, users of cannabis, and those participating in Enhanced Recovery programs using carbohydrate beverages aimed at mitigating exaggerated stress response, reducing postoperative complications, and achieving earlier recovery [14].

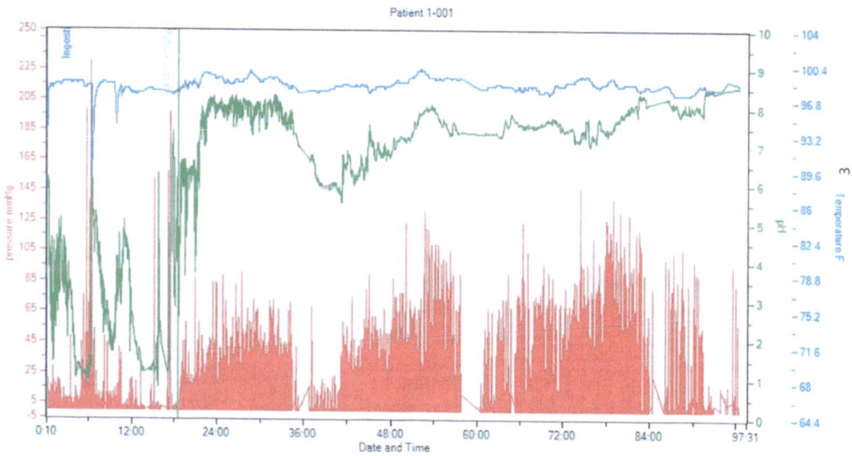

Fig. 5.10 WMC tracing revealing delayed gastric emptying time, prolonged small intestinal, and colonic transit times, suggestive of a diffuse gastrointestinal dysmotility and delayed transit that is not confined to one organ. The blue line traces the temperature sensed by the capsule (it drops when the capsule leaves the body). The green line traces the pH sensed by the capsule as it passes through the stomach (low pH), the duodenum and small bowel (alkaline pH), and the colon (pH increases toward the ileum and then drops again upon the transition to the colon). The red line represents the pressure sensed by the capsule, reflecting gut contractility throughout the study

References

1. Ahuja NK, Clarke JO. Pyloric therapies for gastroparesis. Curr Treat Options Gastroenterol. 2017;15(1):230–40. https://doi.org/10.1007/s11938-017-0124-4. PMID: 28124202
2. Soliman H, Gourcerol G. Gastric electrical stimulation: role and clinical impact on chronic nausea and vomiting. Front Neurosci. 2022;16:909149. https://doi.org/10.3389/fnins.2022.909149. PMID: 35620661; PMCID: PMC9127333
3. Maurer AH. Enhancing scintigraphy for evaluation of gastric, small bowel, and colonic motility. Gastroenterol Clin N Am. 2020;49(3):499–517. https://doi.org/10.1016/j.gtc.2020.04.006. Epub 2020 Jun 14. PMID: 32718567
4. Varma R, Williams CE, McClain ES, Bailey KR, Ordog T, Bharucha AE. Utility of a ^{13}C-spirulina stable isotope gastric emptying breath test in diabetes mellitus. Neurogastroenterol Motil. 2025;28:e15008. https://doi.org/10.1111/nmo.15008. Epub ahead of print. PMID: 39873950
5. Camilleri M, Hasler WL, Parkman HP, Quigley EM, Soffer E. Measurement of gastrointestinal motility in the GI laboratory. Gastroenterology. 1998;115(3):747–62. https://doi.org/10.1016/s0016-5085(98)70155-6. PMID: 9721173
6. Wang WJ, Foong D, Calder S, Schamberg G, Varghese C, Tack J, Xu W, Daker C, Carson D, Waite S, Hayes T, Du P, Abell TL, Parkman HP, Huang IH, Fernandes V, Andrews CN, Gharibans AA, Ho V, O'Grady G. Gastric Alimetry expands patient phenotyping in gastroduodenal disorders compared with gastric emptying scintigraphy. Am J Gastroenterol. 2024;119(2):331–41.
7. Lacy BE, Cangemi DJ, Accurso JM, Axelrod S, Axelrod L, Navalgund A. A novel pilot study to evaluate the efficacy and safety of a wireless patch system in patients with chronic nausea and vomiting. Neurogastroenterol Motil. 2024;36(9):e14862.

8. Axelrod L, Axelrod S, Navalgund A, Triadafilopoulos G. Pilot validation of a new wireless patch system as an ambulatory, noninvasive tool that measures gut Myoelectrical signals: physiologic and disease correlations. Dig Dis Sci. 2021;66(10):3505–15.
9. Navalgund A, Axelrod S, Axelrod L, et al. Colon myoelectric activity measured after open abdominal surgery with a noninvasive wireless patch system predicts time to first flatus. J Gastrointest Surg. 2019;23(5):982–9.
10. Maurer AH, Camilleri M, Donohoe K, et al. The SNMMI and EANM practice guideline for small-bowel and colon transit 1.0. J Nucl Med. 2013;54:2004–13.
11. Bonapace ES, Maurer AH, Davidoff S, Krevsky B, Fisher RS, Parkman HP. Whole gut transit scintigraphy in the clinical evaluation of patients with upper and lower gastrointestinal symptoms. Am J Gastroenterol. 2000;95:2838–47.
12. Saad RJ. The wireless motility capsule: a one-stop shop for the evaluation of GI motility disorders. Curr Gastroenterol Rep. 2016;18(3):14. https://doi.org/10.1007/s11894-016-0489-x. PMID: 26908282
13. Razak A, Baburyan S, Lee E, Costa A, Bergese SD. Role of point-of-care gastric ultrasound in advancing perioperative fasting guidelines. Diagnostics (Basel). 2024;14(21):2366. https://doi.org/10.3390/diagnostics14212366. PMID: 39518332; PMCID: PMC11545054
14. Ljungqvist O, Scott M, Fearon KC. Enhanced recovery after surgery: a review. JAMA Surg. 2017;152(3):292–8. https://doi.org/10.1001/jamasurg.2016.4952. PMID: 28097305

6 Tests for Gastrointestinal Sensory-Motor Assessment: Biliary-Pancreas

George Triadafilopoulos

6.1 Biliary-Pancreas

Biliary Scintigraphy (HIDA Scan) Also called hepatobiliary scan, this is a non-invasive nuclear medicine scan that tracks the flow of bile from the liver into the small intestine and is used to identify the reason for biliary emesis. The test can help diagnose certain conditions, such as cholecystitis, biliary leak, or other abnormalities that may occur after complex reconstructive hepatobiliary surgery [1]. Biliary obstruction can occur in the cancer patient from malignancy and benign causes. Conditions causing hemolysis or surgical resection of the ileum can favor formation of pigment stones. Biliary scintigraphy can also help to understand complications from biliary surgery such as bile leaks. There can be difficulty in interpreting HIDA scans in this context. It is critical to interpret the findings in the context of the type of prior surgery, presence and location of drains, and the time between surgery and the HIDA scan [2]. Interpretation of HIDA scans requires knowledge of the patient's surgical history and clinical condition in general since false positive results can occur in several scenarios, including critical illness (cholestasis) and hepatocyte dysfunction [3].

ERCP with Sphincter of Oddi Manometry (SOM) This invasive test involves passing a catheter into the bile and/or pancreatic duct(s) during endoscopic cholangiopancreatography (ERCP) to measure the pressures of the biliary and/or pancreatic sphincters. The results of SOM can guide the decision as to whether to perform sphincter ablation. Sphincter of Oddi dysfunction (SOD) refers to a smooth muscle dysfunction that may result in an abnormal contractility of the sphincter, impeding biliary and pancreatic duct flow, causing pain, elevated liver test results, dilated bile

G. Triadafilopoulos (✉)
Department of Gastroenterology, Hepatology and Nutrition, UT MD Anderson Cancer Center, Houston, TX, USA
e-mail: gtriadafilopoulo@mdanderson.org

G. Triadafilopoulos (ed.), *Onco-Neurogastroenterology*,
https://doi.org/10.1007/978-3-031-98848-6_6

and pancreatic ducts, or pancreatitis. SOD may be encountered in patients who chronically use narcotics, particularly morphine for pain, since these drugs may induce SO spasm. Proof of SOD may then guide the clinician to alter their pain management strategy by using other agents or consider using endoscopic ampullary BoTox injection or sphincterotomy [4]. The popularity of this test has diminished due to its risks and the lack of robust evidence of the various methods used to treat SOD.

EUS with Biopsies Endoscopic ultrasound is particularly valuable in the diagnosis of submucosal lesions. Neuroendocrine tumors (NETs) are gastro-entero-pancreatic (GEP), in 70% of all cases. These tumors can remain asymptomatic or present with nonspecific symptoms through the release of chromogranin A (CgA), serotonin, insulin, glucagon, and others. Symptoms vary depending on the location of the tumor and the specific hormones produced, which can include flushing, diarrhea, pain, and weight loss [5]. The occurrence of the classic carcinoid syndrome in GEP NETs is rare without liver metastasis or some other form of bypass, since serotonin and other substances undergo hepatic metabolism.

MRCP with Secretin Stimulation Secretin-enhanced MRCP (S-MRCP) provides several advantages compared with standard MRCP for imaging the pancreaticobiliary tree. By using secretin to induce fluid production from the pancreas, and leveraging fluid-sensitive MRCP sequences, S-MRCP increases the visualization of pancreatic ductal anatomy and provides insight into pancreatic function. Such imaging provides qualitative demonstration of dynamic changes to main pancreatic duct dilation after secretin administration and readily demonstrates any increase in dilation of side branches. It may also show indicators of ductal communication of cystic lesions or side branches. In response to secretin stimulation and pancreatic fluid release, one may identify variable amounts of duodenal fluid accumulation and the presence or absence of any communication with the main duct or side branches [6].

References

1. Lambie H, Cook AM, Scarsbrook AF, Lodge JP, Robinson PJ, Chowdhury FU. Tc99m-hepatobiliary iminodiacetic acid (HIDA) scintigraphy in clinical practice. Clin Radiol. 2011;66(11):1094–105. https://doi.org/10.1016/j.crad.2011.07.045. Epub 2011 Aug 20. PMID: 21861996
2. Matesan M, Bermo M, Cruite I, Shih CH, Elojeimy S, Behnia F, Lewis D, Vesselle H. Biliary leak in the postsurgical abdomen: a primer to HIDA scan interpretation. Semin Nucl Med. 2017;47(6):618–29. https://doi.org/10.1053/j.semnuclmed.2017.06.002. Epub 2017 Jul 25.PMID: 28969760
3. David Q-H, Wang, Afdhal NH. Gallstone disease. Sleisenger and Fordtran's Gastrointestinal and Liver Disease. 65:1016–1046.e7.
4. Villavicencio Kim J, Wu GY. Update on Sphincter of Oddi dysfunction: a review. J Clin Transl Hepatol. 2022;10(3):515–21. https://doi.org/10.14218/JCTH.2021.00167. Epub 2022 Jan 11. PMID: 35836767; PMCID: PMC9240241

5. Sansone A, Lauretta R, Vottari S, Chiefari A, Barnabei A, Romanelli F, Appetecchia M. Specific and non-specific biomarkers in neuroendocrine gastroenteropancreatic tumors. Cancers (Basel). 2019;11:1113.
6. Swensson J, Zaheer A, Conwell D, Sandrasegaran K, Manfredi R. Tirkes T. Secretin-enhanced MRCP: how and why-*AJR* expert panel narrative review. AJR Am J Roentgenol. 2021;216(5):1139–49. https://doi.org/10.2214/AJR.20.24857. Epub 2021 Mar 11. PMID: 33263419; PMCID: PMC8068672

Tests for Gastrointestinal Sensory-Motor Assessment: Small Intestine

7

George Triadafilopoulos, Mehnaz A. Shafi, and Lavanya Viswanathan

7.1 Small Intestine

Enteroscopy Deep enteroscopy, typically reaching the small intestine beyond the ligament of Treitz, can be accomplished using a pediatric colonoscope or a dedicated small bowel endoscope. Deep enteroscopy allows for more than visual diagnosis (Fig. 7.1). Tissue can be obtained for histology, lesions like angioectasias ablated, and endoscopic resection can be performed. While small bowel tumors are rare, several conditions like Crohn's disease and hereditary non-polyposis colorectal cancer syndrome (HNPCC) can increase the risk of small bowel cancers (Fig. 7.2) [1, 2].

MR Enterography (MRE) The main indication for MR enterography is the assessment of the small intestine for inflammation and its complications, such as stricture and fistula, postoperative adhesions radiation enteritis, and small bowel tumors causing isolated or scattered partial small obstruction. Its advantages include the lack of ionizing radiation and excellent soft tissue contrast resolution [3].

CT Enterography (CTE) Like MRE, CTE assesses mainly the structure of the small intestine using oral contrast, ruling out inflammatory and neoplastic processes, but also providing clues to the presence of an underlying motility disorder by demonstrating slow transit and dilation of intestinal loops in the absence of strictures [4]. PET/CT enterography is increasingly being integrated into the field of nuclear medicine to resolve controversial findings arising from bowel folds, flexures, variant redundancy, decompressed bowel segments, and physiological uptake.

G. Triadafilopoulos (✉) · M. A. Shafi · L. Viswanathan
Department of Gastroenterology, Hepatology and Nutrition, UT MD Anderson Cancer Center, Houston, TX, USA
e-mail: gtriadafilopoulo@mdanderson.org

G. Triadafilopoulos (ed.), *Onco-Neurogastroenterology*,
https://doi.org/10.1007/978-3-031-98848-6_7

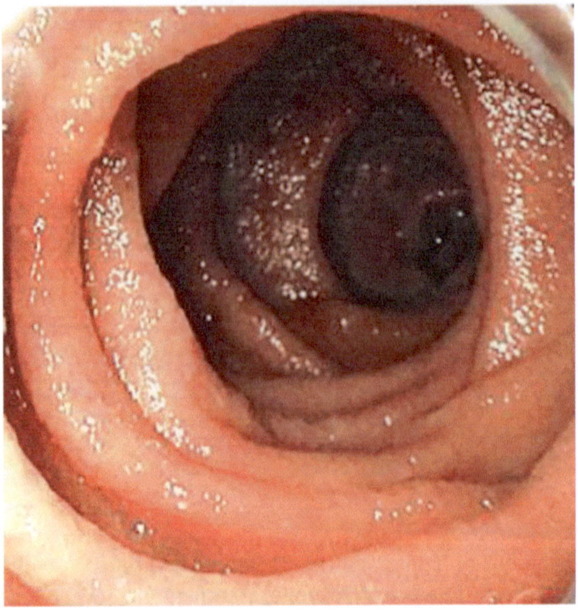

Fig. 7.1 Normal endoscopic appearance of small bowel where the valvulae conniventes and the fine villous mucosal architecture can be assessed, particularly with high-definition and magnification endoscopes

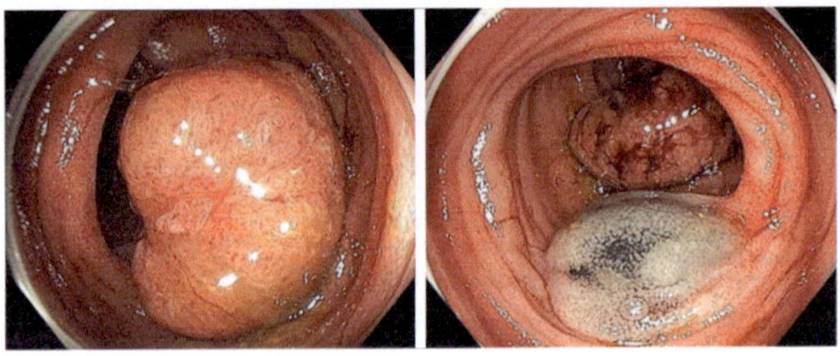

Fig. 7.2 Large ileal tubulovillous adenoma with high-grade dysplasia in a patient with HNPCC (left). The same lesion after biopsies were taken and tattoo placed (right)

This technique combines negative/neutral contrast to distend the lumen of the gut and iodinated contrast to enhance the gastrointestinal wall and pathological findings [5].

Video Capsule Endoscopy (VCE) Also known as wireless capsule endoscopy, this is a noninvasive study that uses a pill camera to visualize the entire length of the small intestinal lumen (Fig. 7.3). The capsule is ingested and transmits images over 8 to 12 h until its battery expires. It generates high-resolution images that allow detailed inspection of the gastrointestinal mucosa. VCE is purely a diagnostic procedure. Most commonly, VCE is used in the evaluation of obscure gastrointestinal bleeding thought to originate in the small bowel, after endoscopy and colonoscopy have failed to find the source. VCE is also useful in exploring small bowel etiologies for chronic diarrhea, such as Crohn's disease, carcinoid tumor, or refractory sprue. It also provides information about small bowel transit [6, 7].

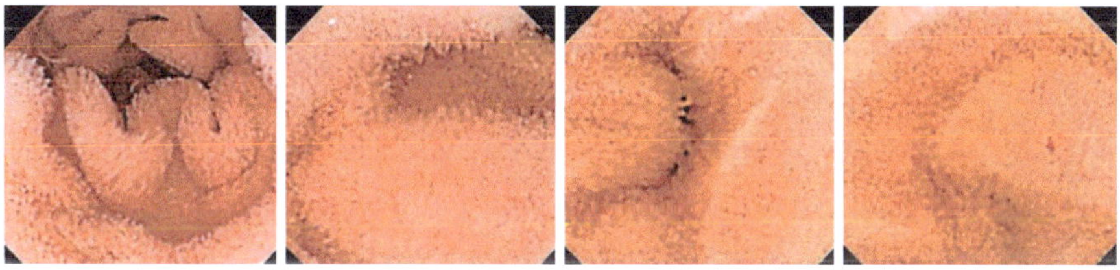

Fig. 7.3 Normal video capsule endoscopy, excluding inflammatory or neoplastic causes accounting for the patient's symptoms

Wireless Motility Capsule (WMC) This is an ambulatory, noninvasive diagnostic sensor (Smartpill; Medtronic, Minneapolis, MN, USA) that samples intraluminal pH, temperature, and pressure as it moves through the GI tract. Patients first ingest a meal to initiate the postprandial motility pattern, they then swallow the capsule that wirelessly connects to a data receiver, and they keep a diary for recording bowel movements, food intake, sleep, and GI symptoms while continuing their regular diet and life routines. After 5 days, patients return the data receiver and the diary, and the downloaded data are analyzed using the display software. This technology quantifies transit in all gut regions in a single test and it has been increasingly used for the diagnosis of functional GI symptoms, such as bloating, early postprandial fullness, nausea, and constipation, by measuring gastric emptying time, as well as small bowel and colonic transit times [8]. The technology is not currently commercially available, and it has not been validated in patients with cancer.

Small Intestinal Manometry Also called antro-duodenal manometry (ADM), this specialized manometry is not widely used or standardized, but it may help differentiate a myopathic from a neuropathic foregut process (i.e., visceral or autonomic neuropathy). Myopathic disorders are typically associated with low-amplitude contractions (mean < 20 mmHg), whereas in neuropathic disorders, the amplitude of contractions is typically normal, but there is disorganization of the contractile response to a simulated meal with associated persistence of fasting motor patterns after meal ingestion [9, 10]. Normally, small intestinal manometry plots are analyzed for normal fasting and postprandial motility. Antral motility (when captured) is characterized by high-amplitude contractions with a maximal contraction rate of ~3 per min. Amplitudes of contraction in the small intestine are lower, but frequency is higher frequency (up to ~12 per min). During the fasting state, there is a constant transition between phases I and III of the inter-digestive migrating motor complex (MMC), with motor quiescence during phase I, irregular contractions that are propagated over only smaller segments during phase II, and regular, aborally propagated contractions that usually start in the stomach and traverse long segments of the small bowel during phase III. Postprandially, the MMC activity is interrupted and replaced by irregular contractions that serve to mix the luminal contents and to slowly propel them distally. Figure 7.4 highlights the findings on small intestinal

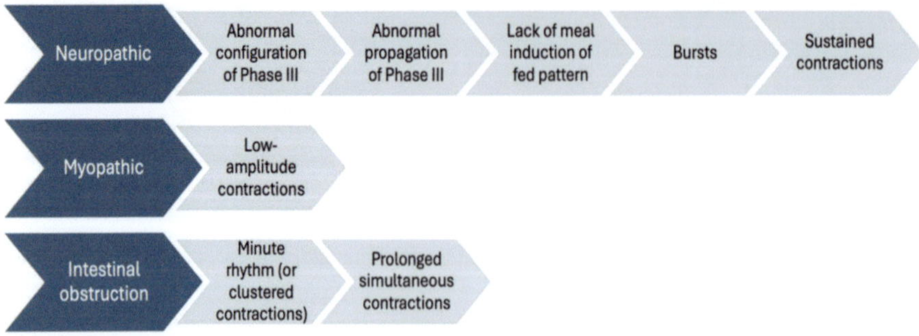

Fig. 7.4 Small intestinal manometry findings typically characterizing a neuropathic from a myopathic abnormality or suggestive of partial small bowel obstruction

Fig. 7.5 Positive lactulose breath test, diagnostic of SIBO

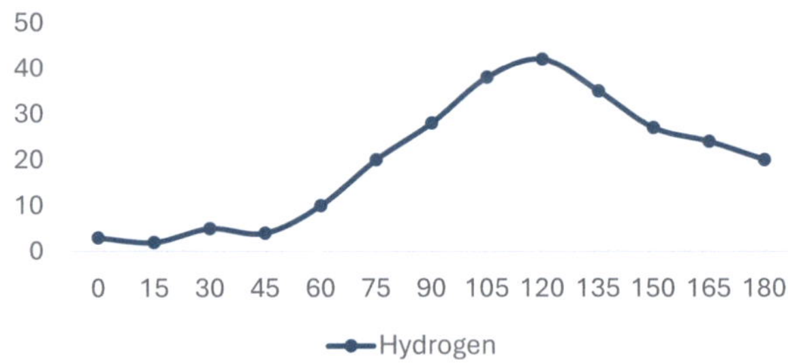

manometry, supporting the underlying abnormal small intestinal motility as the putative source of the patients' symptoms.

The presence of non-propagating clustered contractions (>30 min duration) and simultaneous prolonged (>8 s) or summated contractions suggest partial mechanical obstruction. However, modern, high-resolution CT or MR enterography make small bowel manometry rarely necessary for this indication in clinical practice [11].

Glucose or Lactulose Breath Tests In these tests, glucose or lactulose are swallowed and hydrogen and methane gases are measured in the exhaled breath. Gas levels rise as the sugar solution passes through the intestine resulting from fermentation of the sugar by bacteria. If the gas levels rise quickly and to an abnormal level, a diagnosis of small intestinal bacterial overgrowth (SIBO) can be made and treated [11]. By convention, an increase of greater or equal to 20 parts per million (ppm) from baseline in hydrogen by 90 min is considered a positive test to diagnose SIBO. A level of greater than or equal to 10 ppm in methane is considered positive for methanogenic overgrowth (Fig. 7.5). Although hydrogen is only produced by anaerobic bacteria normally found in the colon, methanogens are not actually bacteria but Archaea, a species that do not cause disease. Thus, instead of SIBO, the term intestinal methanogen overgrowth (IMO) is used for a positive methane breath test, which has been associated with constipation because methane blocks intestinal transit. Ideally, in patients who frequently suffer from constipation and bloating, both hydrogen (for SIBO) and methane (for IMO) should be measured during breath testing (Fig. 7.6). Before the breath test is performed, antibiotics should be avoided for 4 weeks and laxatives should be avoided for 1 week. Diet, smoking, and physical activity may also need to be altered [12].

Small Bowel Aspiration with Quantitative Cultures Aspiration of small bowel fluid for analysis of total bacterial count (TBC) and bacterial species identification is considered the benchmark diagnostic test for diagnosing SIBO. SIBO is defined as $\geq 10^5$ colony-forming unit (CFU) mL^{-1} of TBC grown from the jejunum aspiration based on traditional microbiological standards for bacterial culture [13]. The North American consensus and ACG guidelines both recommend a threshold of $\geq 10^3$ CFU mL^{-1} via small bowel aspirates as positive for SIBO, since a TBC $\geq 10^3$ CFU mL^{-1} is rarely seen in asymptomatic subjects [14]. However, limitations of endoscopic aspiration include its invasiveness, cost (endoscopy, sedation), lack of availability and standardization, and sample contamination. Further, few laboratories are equipped to perform sensitive TBC assays locally.

Smart Capsule Bacterial Detection System (SCBDS) This is a novel ingestible device in development (Biora Therapeutics Inc. San Diego, CA) and is similar in size to a fish-oil pill. It consists of a targeted sampling technology and a miniature fluorescent SCBDS assay onboard to detect metabolically active bacteria and it has been validated [15]. Upon detecting entry into the jejunum, the device acquires a sample of jejunal fluid absorbed into the sampling pad. Bacterial concentrations in the sample can be determined directly by the onboard miniature fluorometer within the SCBDS. Real-time data is then transmitted to a wearable device to facilitate SIBO diagnosis. The novel localization, site-specific sampling, and onboard assay technology of the SCBDS device may avoid the complexities of the endoscopic aspiration technique and provides a noninvasive and rapid screening tool for the diagnosis of SIBO [16]. The technology is still in its early phases and has not been validated in patients with cancer.

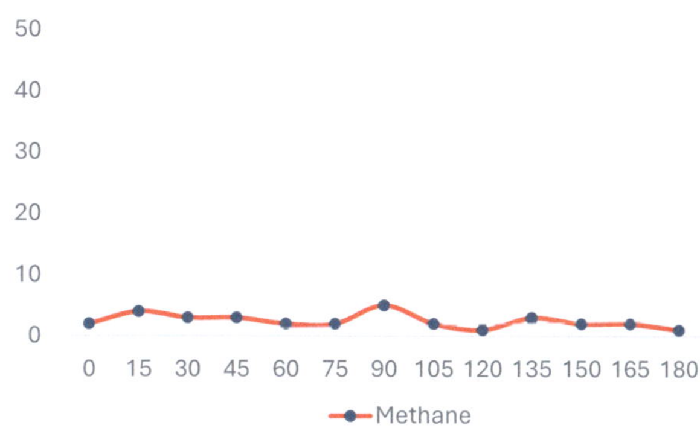

Fig. 7.6 Negative breath test for methane, thereby excluding IMO

CapScan This sampling capsule is a single-use, passive device that collects fluid from the human intestines at multiple locations (duodenum, jejunum, ileum, and cecum) for ex vivo analysis. Currently the device is used for research purposes only and has not been validated in patients with cancer. The device contains a collapsed collection bladder capped by a one-way valve inside a dissolvable capsule with an enteric coating that prevents contact between the collection bladder and the surrounding environment before entry into the intestines. The pH of the intestines typically rises from 4–6 in the duodenum to 7–8 in the ileum· Once the device reaches a pre-set pH sufficient to dissolve the enteric coating, the collection bladder expands and draws in luminal contents through the one-way valve. The first-generation device was pH-driven, and the second was time-driven (Fig. 7.7).

Early use of the second-generation device in patients with SIBO has shown significant differences in bacterial abundance when comparing intestinal (CapScan) and corresponding stool samples and significant differences between baseline and post-rifaximin sampling at multiple time points (Fig. 7.8) [17].

Disaccharidase Assays Disaccharidase deficiency, once thought to be unique to the pediatric population, has more recently been recognized as prevalent in the adult population [18]. Approximately 10% of the adult population presenting with

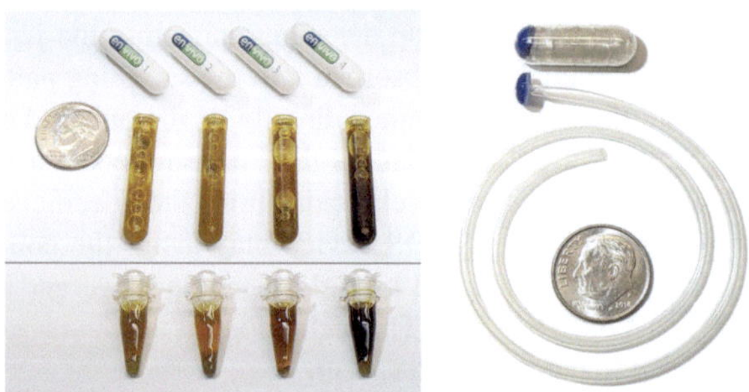

Fig. 7.7 First- and second-generation CapScan devices to assess multi-omics along the intestine

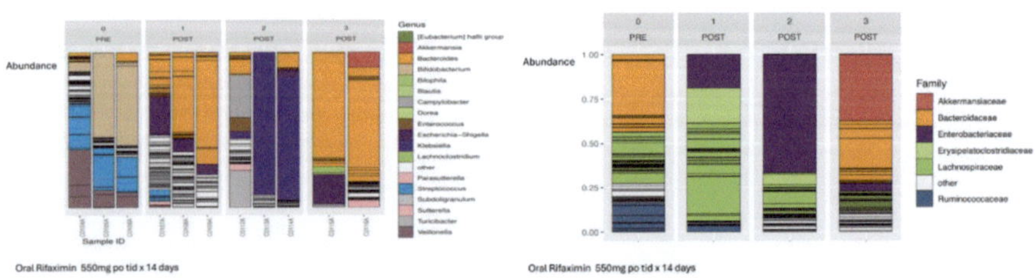

Fig. 7.8 Composite graphs of microbial abundance in intestinal samples extracted from CapScan samples of jejunum, ileum, cecum) at baseline (Day 0) and on days 14, 28, 42 after rifaximin day 14, 28, 42 (left). Reciprocal stool samples are also shown (right) and highlight significant differences in relative bacterial abundance before and after therapy. Prior to CapScan, the patient was given the diagnosis of SIBO, due to symptoms and positive hydrogen breath test

unexplained GI symptoms, to include pain, bloating, and variable bowel habits have a deficiency in all four disaccharidase enzymes (i.e., lactase, maltase, sucrase, and palatinase) and these patients may often be mislabeled as having IBS. The gold standard for testing disaccharidase deficiencies is endoscopically obtaining two biopsies from the third portion of the duodenum. One biopsy is used to histologically study the mucosal integrity, and the other is used for analysis of sucrase, maltase, lactase, and isomaltase levels, using the Dahlqvist method with the caveat that enzyme distribution may be patchy. Current reports of these assays from specialty labs also include alpha-glucosidase and alpha-amylase levels. Although not reviewed by the FDA for safety and effectiveness, taking lactase enzyme (Lactaid) with milk products can help prevent upset stomach, abdominal bloating/cramping, gas, and diarrhea that is caused by lactose-containing products. The only FDA-approved treatment at present is sacrosidase (trade name: Sucraid), which is a liquid enzyme replacement derived from baker's yeast. This only contains sucrase, so additional dietary modification limiting starches and carbohydrates is needed for these patients [19].

Laparoscopy In cases where diffuse peritoneal carcinomatosis is suspected to affect the small bowel motility and causing prolonged paralytic ileus, a diagnostic laparoscopy, with direct visualization and biopsies of the peritoneal surface, is useful in clarifying the diagnosis, prognosis, and management. This is often the case with tumors of gynecologic origin that might benefit from debulking or cytoreductive therapies. An abdominopelvic CT imaging is used first, since it may reveal areas of multiregional infiltration or focal points of partial obstruction, most commonly in the small intestine, but also involving the colon.

References

1. Korekawa K, Naito T, Fujishima F, Nagai H, Shimoyama Y, Moroi R, Shiga H, Kakuta Y, Masamune A. Small bowel cancer in a patient with Crohn's disease diagnosed preoperatively by double-balloon enteroscopy. Clin J Gastroenterol. 2023;16(6):836–41. https://doi.org/10.1007/s12328-023-01846-2. Epub 2023 Aug 19. PMID: 37597132
2. Yamamoto H. Top tips for balloon enteroscopy. Gastrointest Endosc. 2023;98(3):432–6. https://doi.org/10.1016/j.gie.2023.01.056. Epub 2023 Feb 4. PMID: 36739995
3. Khatri G, Coleman J, Leyendecker JR. Magnetic resonance enterography for inflammatory and noninflammatory conditions of the small bowel. Radiol Clin North Am. 2018;56(5):671–89.
4. Delgado-Barriga K, Medina C, Gomez-Quiles L, Marco-Domenech SF, Escrig J, Llueca A. CT enterography for preoperative evaluation of peritoneal carcinomatosis index in advanced ovarian cancer. J Clin Med. 2022;11(3):476. https://doi.org/10.3390/jcm11030476. PMID: 35159927; PMCID: PMC8836697
5. Sharma A, Phulia A, Sethi RS. PET/computed tomography enterography. Nucl Med Commun. 2021;42(6):694–8. https://doi.org/10.1097/MNM.0000000000001373. PMID: 33560721
6. Kim SH, Yang DH, Kim JS. Current status of interpretation of small bowel capsule endoscopy. Clin Endosc. 2018;51(4):329–33.

7. Sonu I, Oh SJ, Rao SSC. Capsules for the diagnosis and treatment of gastrointestinal motility disorders—a game changer. Curr Gastroenterol Rep. 2024;26(6):157–65. https://doi.org/10.1007/s11894-024-00926-8. Epub 2024 Apr 17. PMID: 38630422
8. Saad RJ. The wireless motility capsule: a one-stop shop for the evaluation of GI motility disorders. Curr Gastroenterol Rep. 2016;18(3):14. https://doi.org/10.1007/s11894-016-0489-x. PMID: 26908282
9. O'Grady G, Carbone F, Tack J. Gastric sensorimotor function and its clinical measurement. Neurogastroenterol Motil. 2022;34:e14489. https://doi.org/10.1111/nmo.14489. Epub ahead of print. PMID: 36371709.
10. Frank JW, Sarr MG, Camilleri M. Use of gastroduodenal manometry to differentiate mechanical and functional intestinal obstruction: an analysis of clinical outcome. Am J Gastroenterol. 1994;89(3):339–44. PMID: 8122641
11. Triadafilopoulos G. Utility of wireless motility capsule and lactulose breath testing in the evaluation of patients with chronic functional bloating. BMJ Open Gastroenterol. 2016;3(1):e000110. https://doi.org/10.1136/bmjgast-2016-000110. PMID: 27648298; PMCID: PMC5013333
12. Mehravar S, Takakura W, Wang J, Pimentel M, Nasser J, Rezaie A. Symptom profile of patients with intestinal methanogen overgrowth
13. Saad RJ, Chey WD. Breath testing for small intestinal bacterial overgrowth: maximizing test accuracy. Clin Gastroenterol Hepatol. 2014;12(12):1964–72.
14. Pimentel M, Saad RJ, Long MD, et al. Clinical guideline: small intestinal bacterial overgrowth. Am J Gastroenterol. 2020;115(2):165–78.
15. Huntsman M, Lee SN, Stylli J, et al. Development of a novel drug delivery system to deliver drugs directly to the colonic mucosa, resulting in improved efficacy and reduced systemic exposure for the treatment of ulcerative colitis. Crohn's & Colitis. 2021;360(3, 4):1–5.
16. Lee SN, Rahimian P, Stork C, Moshiree B, Jones M, Chuang E, Wahl C, Singh S, Rao SSC. Evaluation of a novel smart capsule bacterial detection system device for diagnosis of small intestinal bacterial overgrowth. Neurogastroenterol Motil. 2024;25:e14965. https://doi.org/10.1111/nmo.14965. Epub ahead of print. PMID: 39587802
17. Shalon D, Culver RN, Grembi JA, Folz J, Treit PV, Shi H, Rosenberger FA, Dethlefsen L, Meng X, Yaffe E, Aranda-Díaz A, Geyer PE, Mueller-Reif JB, Spencer S, Patterson AD, Triadafilopoulos G, Holmes SP, Mann M, Fiehn O, Relman DA, Huang KC. Profiling the human intestinal environment under physiological conditions. Nature. 2023;617(7961):581–91. https://doi.org/10.1038/s41586-023-05989-7. Epub 2023 May 10. PMID: 37165188; PMCID: PMC10191855
18. Viswanathan L, Rao SSC, Kennedy K, Sharma A, Yan Y, Jimenez E. Prevalence of disaccharidase deficiency in adults with unexplained gastrointestinal symptoms. J Neurogastroenterol Motil. 2020;26(3):384–90. https://doi.org/10.5056/jnm19167. PMID: 32380581; PMCID: PMC7329151
19. Viswanathan L, Rao SS. Intestinal disaccharidase deficiency in adults: evaluation and treatment. Curr Gastroenterol Rep. 2023;25(6):134–9. https://doi.org/10.1007/s11894-023-00870-z. Epub 2023 May 18. PMID: 37199899; PMCID: PMC10226910

Tests for Gastrointestinal Sensory-Motor Assessment: Colon

8

George Triadafilopoulos and Lavanya Viswanathan

8.1 Colon

Colonoscopy Colonoscopy is a diagnostic and therapeutic procedure to evaluate the colon and distal terminal ileum. It employs a handheld, flexible fiberoptic tube with a high-definition camera and light mounted at its tip to visualize the GI tract as well as accessory channels to perform diagnostic and therapeutic interventions (Fig. 8.1). In onco-neuro-gastroenterology, colonoscopy with biopsies is essential for the structural evaluation of the large intestine, cancer recognition, and the diagnosis of disorders related to diarrhea and constipation, such as immune-mediated colitis, graft-versus-host disease, and stercoral ulcers. As a therapeutic tool, colonoscopy can be used for oncological (i.e., benign or malignant stricture management) and non-oncological indications, such as the treatment of sigmoid volvulus, acute colonic pseudo-obstruction, gastrointestinal bleeding, and colonic impactions (Fig. 8.2) [1].

Barium or Gastrografin Enema A barium enema is an X-ray procedure that uses barium, a contrast agent, to visualize the large intestine (colon) and rectum. The procedure does not require sedation, but requires a cooperative patient who is able to change positions or hold their breath for the X-ray imaging process to get different views of the colon. X-rays are taken as the barium flows through the colon, allowing the radiologist to visualize the structure and any abnormalities. Sometimes, air is introduced into the colon after the barium, creating a double contrast study. Barium enema does not have the sensitivity or specificity of a colonoscopy; it is mostly used in cases in which colonoscopy is unsuccessful, mostly to delineate strictures. Gastrografin is frequently used as an alternative to barium when there is an obstruction. It is a water-soluble,

G. Triadafilopoulos (✉) · L. Viswanathan
Department of Gastroenterology, Hepatology and Nutrition, UT MD Anderson Cancer Center, Houston, TX, USA
e-mail: gtriadafilopoulo@mdanderson.org

G. Triadafilopoulos (ed.), *Onco-Neurogastroenterology*,
https://doi.org/10.1007/978-3-031-98848-6_8

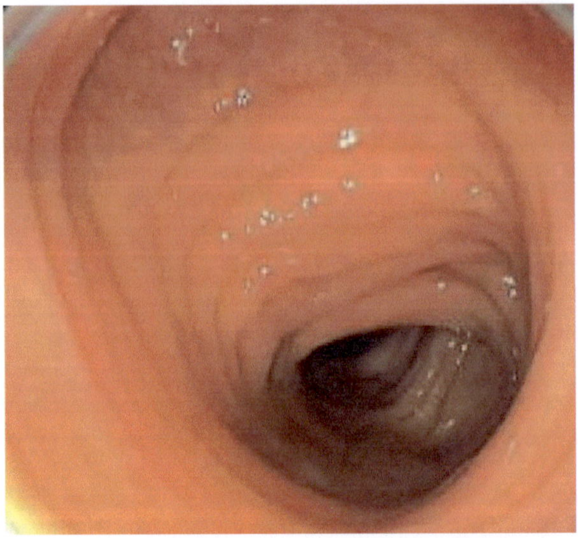

Fig. 8.1 Normal, glistening appearance of the colonic mucosa at colonoscopy. In patients with chronic diarrhea, multiple biopsies should be taken from the right and left colon to rule out microscopic (lymphocytic) or collagenous colitis

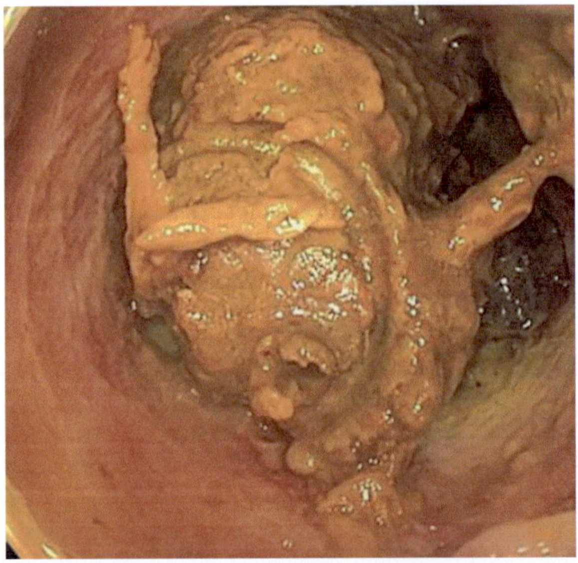

Fig. 8.2 Colonoscopic appearance of fecal impaction, with hard stool completely obliterating the rectal lumen and causing severe constipation

hyperosmolar contrast agent which draws water into the colon, potentially relieving a colonic obstruction. Further, gastrografin is highly beneficial as a pretreatment for colonoscopy due to its ability to enhance intestinal motility, provide excellent cleansing effects, and maintain visualization during endoscopy [2].

Abdominal and Pelvic CT Imaging CT imaging is most frequently used for the diagnosis of acute or chronic abdominal and pelvic pain with or without other symptoms, such as diarrhea, constipation, or bleeding. The study guides the clinician to diagnose inflammatory or infectious diseases of small bowel and colon, such as appendicitis, diverticulitis, or infected fluid collections. The study may be performed with or without oral or intravenous contrast depending on the indication and underlying risk of contrast-induced nephrotoxicity. At a minimum, a non-contrast study may focus attention to a particular area of disease involvement (Fig. 8.3).

CT Colonography (CTC) CT colonography is a screening modality that uses a CT scan to visualize colon polyps and masses while the colon is insufflated. Current protocols generally require bowel preparation, oral contrast, and colon insufflation, without sedation. It is used mostly for colon cancer screening, but it may also provide valuable information about the structural integrity of the colon when colonoscopy is not technically possible or unsafe (i.e., in cancer patients with severe pelvic adhesive disease or sigmoid diverticulosis). Sensitivity for adenomas ≥1 cm and CRC are estimated to be 95% [3].

Radio-Opaque Marker (Sitzmarks) Study Sitzmarks study is a useful diagnostic tool in patients who suffer from chronic constipation (typically less than three bowel movements per week). Radio-opaque "markers" are used as a surrogate marker for colon transit. The patient swallows one gelatin capsule that contains 24 small plastic ring markers easily identifiable on abdominal radiographs. After capsule ingestion, the patient is asked to return for an abdominal X-ray 5 days later, to see if any of the markers are left in the colon. The test is normal (less than five markers are seen at day 5) or abnormal (five or more markers are present). If the constipation is a result of a generally sluggish colon (slow transit), the markers are found dispersed throughout the abdomen. If colon transit is normal but there is outlet obstruction from poor coordination and tone of the pelvic floor and the anal canal (pelvic floor

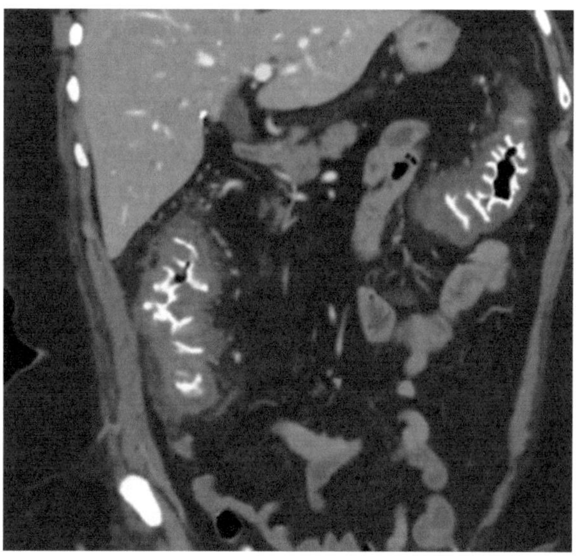

Fig. 8.3 Abdominal CT imaging depicting thickening of the ascending and transverse colon in a patient who presented with abdominal pain and diarrhea caused by *C. difficile*. Note the thickness of the colonic wall compressing the lumen, as highlighted by the oral contrast (white)

dyssynergia or an evacuation disorder), a predominance of markers may be seen within the rectum. In cases of overlapping colon transit and dyssynergic defecatory disorders affecting the colon and anorectum, the markers can appear both diffusely throughout the colon and within the pelvis. Anorectal manometry can help distinguish between the two. The physician can then initiate and adjust therapy accordingly. For an accurate test, patients should abstain from using any substances that can alter colon transit, such as laxatives or opiates during the study. There is good diagnostic agreement between the radio-opaque marker study and wireless motility capsule (WMC) in patients with chronic constipation [4].

Wireless Motility Capsule (WMC) This is an ambulatory, noninvasive diagnostic sensor (Smartpill; Medtronic, Minneapolis, MN, USA) that samples intraluminal pH, temperature, and pressure as it moves through the GI tract. Currently this modality is not commercially available. For this test, patients first ingest a meal to initiate the postprandial motility pattern, they then swallow the capsule that wirelessly connects to a data receiver, and they keep a diary for recording bowel movements, food intake, sleep, and GI symptoms while continuing their regular diet and life routines. After 5 days, patients return the data receiver and the diary, and the downloaded data are analyzed using the display software (Fig. 8.4).

It is important to note that values may fluctuate either as a result of the natural history of the underlying condition or in response to therapy (pharmacologic, endoscopic BoTox injection, G-POEM, or surgery (Fig. 8.5). This technology measures whole gut transit in a single test and it has been increasingly used for the diagnosis of functional GI symptoms, such as bloating, abdominal fullness, and constipation,

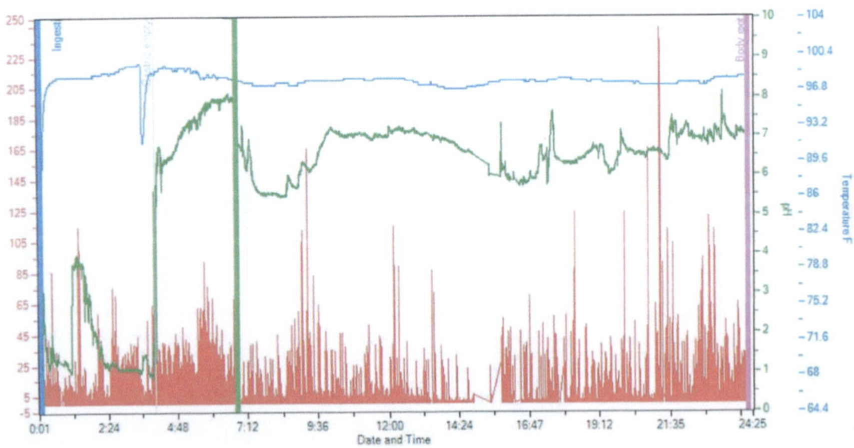

Fig. 8.4 Wireless motility capsule study, revealing normal gastric emptying time (GET), and small bowel transit (SBT) as well as colonic transit time (CTT). This patient presented with recurrent bloating and abdominal pain. She was diagnosed with a disorder of brain-gut interaction (DBGI) and treated with the neuromodulator desipramine 25 mg at bedtime to address her pain symptoms

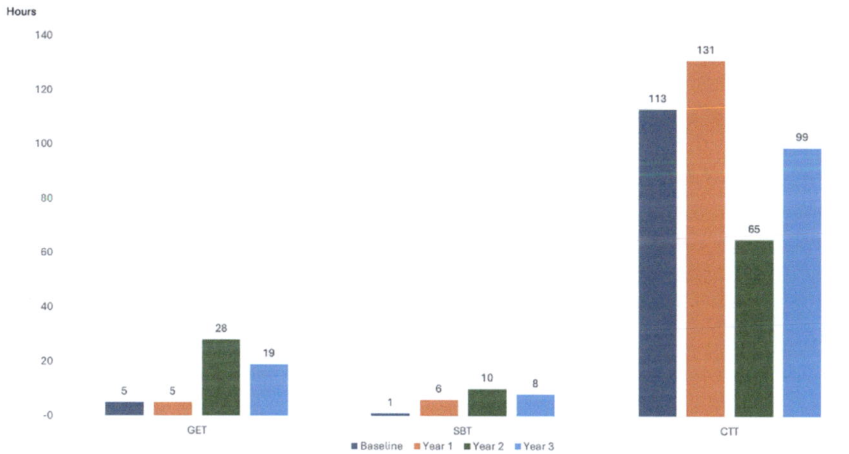

Fig. 8.5 Serial emptying times in a patient with diffuse gastrointestinal dysmotility who underwent WMC testing on a yearly basis over 4 years in response to various pharmacological treatments. Although the values for gastric emptying time (GET), small bowel transit (SBT), and colonic transit time (CTT) remained mostly in the abnormal range, there were fluctuations. Normal values: GET <4 h; SBT: 2.5–6 h; CTT < 59 h. Of note, treatment was interrupted for 3 days before and 5 days during the test. If one wishes to assess response to therapy, WMC should be performed without interruption of such therapy

by measuring colonic transit time. If the colon transit time of the WMC exceeds 59 h after its ingestion, the diagnosis of slow-transit constipation is made [5].

Gas-Sensing Capsule Until recently, the wireless motility capsule (WMC) (SmartPill, Medtronic, Minneapolis, MN, USA) was our main outpatient assessment tool for GI transit assessment. WMC (SmartPill) is no longer available on the market, but a promising replacement is a gas-sensing capsule (Atmo Capsule; Atmo Biosciences, Melbourne, VIC, Australia). A recent study showed excellent interobserver agreement in landmarks between WMC and Atmo (mean ICC ICC ≥0.97) in 50 healthy subjects [6].

Another comparative study of 48 patients with functional dyspepsia and/or functional constipation showed significant correlation between WMC and the Atmo gas-sensing capsule (gastric emptying time $r = 0.79$, $P < 0.001$ and colonic transit time $r = 0.66$, $P < 0.001$) [7]. In a larger, multicenter US trial, in which 177 patients underwent testing with both WMC and Atmo, Atmo assessment showed significant agreement with WMC times [overall agreement in GET of 83.62% (SE: 2.78%) and CTT of 84.35% (SE 3.00)]. Moreover, 11% of participants displayed isolated GET delay, 20% displayed delayed CTT only, and 18% displayed multiregional delay. Notable differences between the two technologies include battery life (WMC is 120 min, while Atmo is 100 min) and ingestion of carbonated beverages will interfere with the gas-sensing capsule function [8]. This attractive, noninvasive modality will require further validation in patients with cancer.

Whole Gut Transit Scintigraphy (WGTS) This scintigraphic study may be useful in patients with symptomatic constipation by documenting delayed colonic transit (CT), assessing the pattern of such transit delay, and determining if there are potential upper GI transit abnormalities contributing to symptoms. Depending on the focus of clinical interest, several gastrointestinal transit (GIT) scintigraphic examinations may be clinically used to assess transit through the esophagus, stomach, small bowel, and colon, all of which can be performed separately (more commonly), or collectively, using a whole-gut transit scintigraphy. It is important to keep in mind that overlap states are common, particularly when a multifactorial etiology is involved (i.e., opioid use and possibly peritoneal malignancy) [9]. In a recent retrospective study of patients with symptomatic constipation, WGTS assessment showed delayed colonic transit in 68% of patients, with 31% having colonic inertia, 28% functional rectosigmoid obstruction pattern, and 9% generalized delay in colonic transit. Abnormalities in gastric emptying and small intestinal transit were present in 36% and 19%, respectively [10].

High-Resolution Anorectal Manometry (HRAM), Rectal Sensation (RST), and Balloon Expulsion Test (BET) High-resolution anorectal manometry (HRAM) is a catheter-based outpatient test that objectively assesses anorectal dysfunction leading to dyssynergic defecation. Intrarectal solid-state catheters can measure anal sphincter pressure, rectal compliance and sensation, and the recto-anal inhibitory reflex (RAIR). During normal defecation, the rectal pressure should increase, and anal sphincter pressure should decrease (Fig. 8.6). However, if there is an incoordination between the two pressure bands, this suggests a defecatory disorder that is often clinically significant (Fig. 8.7). There are four main patterns of dyssynergia that are summarized in Fig. 8.8. The patient is positioned in the left lateral decubitus position, similar to the positioning during a colonoscopy, and this unsedated procedure last 30 min. A rectal exam is done first, to detect anything that may prevent safe catheter insertion i.e. anal fissure, anal stricture. Next, the catheter (4-6 cm in length) is inserted through the rectum and the external catheter with a deflated balloon at the tip is taped in place along the patient's thigh. Resting pressure and anal sphincter length are recorded first, followed by the patient performing several maneuvers such as squeeze, cough, and push or bear-down. Each maneuver is done at least twice. The recto-anal inhibitory reflex (RAIR) is an involuntary relaxation of the IAS in response to a transient increase in anal pressure. The balloon is inflated to evoke this response. The RAIR is absent in Hirschsprung's disease (congenital colonic aganglionosis), and it may also be absent in cases of muscle or nerve injury due to surgery (i.e., lower anterior resection) or pelvic radiation. Rectal sensation is evaluated by measuring the lowest perceived volume of balloon distention, desire to defecate, and the maximum tolerable volume. IAS hypotonicity and shortened sphincter length may contribute to patients' urgency, frequency, and occasional fecal incontinence after pelvic radiotherapy; 75% of such patients exhibit one or more abnormal manometric parameters for sensory or motor functions, either in isolation or

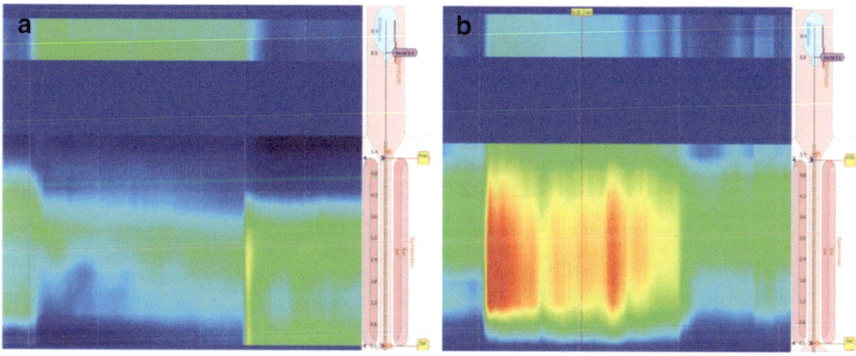

Fig. 8.6 Two high-resolution anorectal manometry pressure tracings. A schematic view of the position of the anorectal manometry catheter sensors is shown on the right of each image. Shown are the rectal (top) and anal (bottom) pressures recorded by the sensors (deep blue = low pressure; green = intermediate pressure; red = high pressure) as recorded by the sensors. An inflatable balloon is stationed in the rectum. (**a**) Normal anal relaxation during simulated defecation in a healthy subject. Note adequate rectal push effort (top pressure band) with decrease in the anal sphincter pressure (bottom pressure band). (**b**) This reading shows paradoxical anal sphincter contraction during simulated defecation, consistent with dyssynergic (poorly coordinated) defecation

Fig. 8.7 Diagnostic considerations in patients with constipation, specifically effective v. ineffective (dyssynergic) defecation

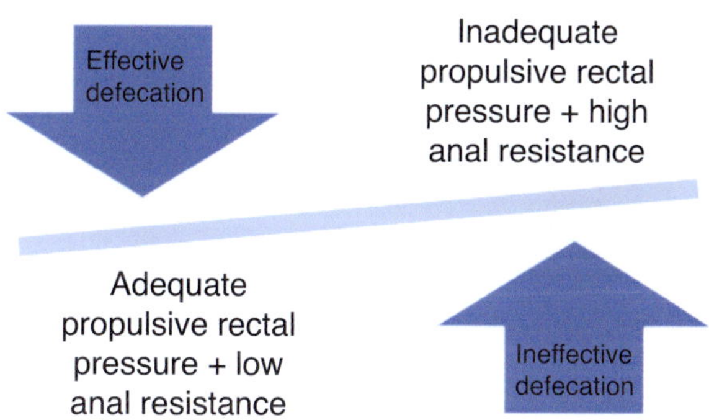

combination, while the RAIR may be absent or abnormal in up to 40% of patients. HRAM, RST, and BET are all performed in one visit [11]. However, when the durability and reproducibility of HRAM was examined in a recent study, only a minority of patients who underwent repeat anorectal manometry—as analyzed by the London Classification—had stable manometric findings, raising questions regarding the validity of a single manometric measurement for clinical decision-making at the point of care [12].

High-resolution anorectal manometry (HRAM) identifies coordination or incoordination of the defecatory muscles and classifies dyssynergic defecation into one of four types (Fig. 8.8). The rectal sensation test (RST) assesses sensitivity to progressive intrarectal balloon distention, which may be normal, hyper-, or

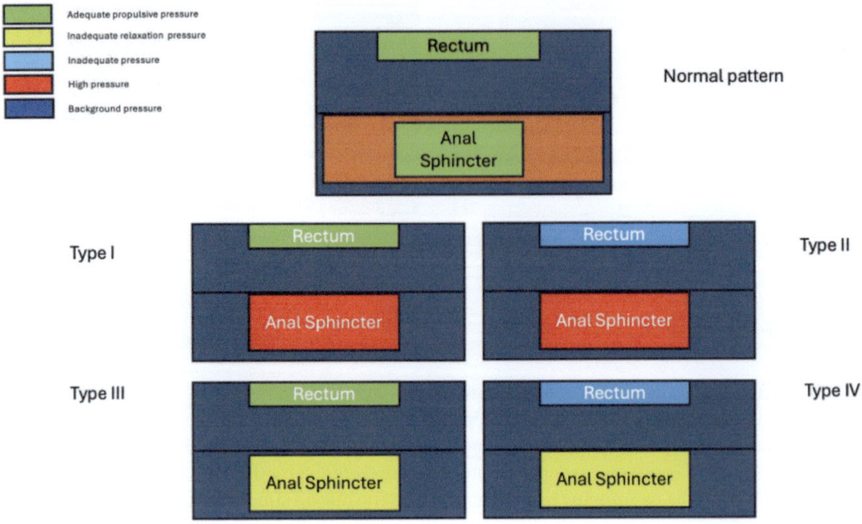

Fig. 8.8 Practical classification of defecatory disturbances and the four dyssynergia subtypes (I–IV). Their recognition assists in patient management

Table 8.1 Typical HRAM finding in patients with chronic constipation

Variable	Value
HPZ length (n = 4.1–4.5 cm)	Normal
Resting pressure (n = 83–96 mmHg)	Normal or high
Squeeze pressure (n = 245–287 mmHg)	Normal or high
Squeeze duration (n = 28–30 s)	Normal or high
Residual anal pressure (n = 28–52)	Normal or high
RAIR (n = present)	Present or absent
First rectal sensation (n = 20–25 ml)	Normal or high
Urge to defecate (n = 140–167 ml)	Normal or high
Discomfort (n = 192–222 ml)	Normal or high
Balloon expulsion (50 cc expulsion in <60 s)	Normal or absent

hyposensitive. The balloon expulsion test (BET) defines the ability of the patient to expel a 50 ml rectal balloon in 60 s, and it is considered a measure of the global ability of the rectum to expel stool (Table 8.1). If a patient displays dyssynergia on HRAM along with a failed BET, he/she can be diagnosed with dyssynergic defecation.

In type I dyssynergia, the subject can generate an adequate propulsive force (rise in intrarectal pressure ≥ 40 mmHg) along with paradoxical increase in anal sphincter pressure. In type II dyssynergia, the subject is unable to generate an adequate propulsive force; additionally there is paradoxical anal contraction. In type III dyssynergia, the subject can generate an adequate propulsive force, but there is either absent relaxation (a flat line) or inadequate (≤20%) relaxation of anal sphincter. In type IV dyssynergia, the subject is unable to generate an adequate propulsive force together with an absent or inadequate relaxation of anal sphincter (Fig. 8.9) [13].

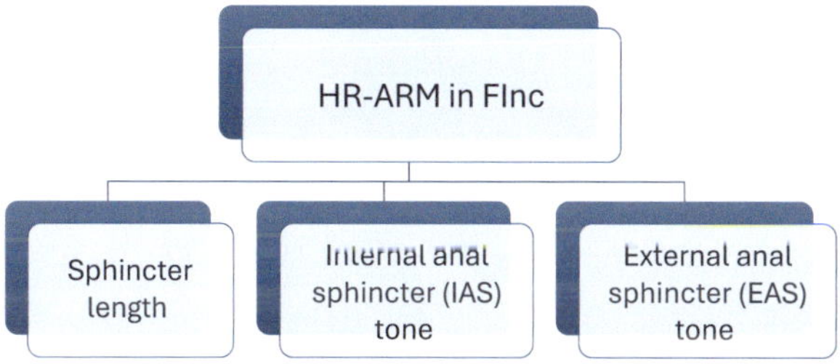

Fig. 8.9 Important findings upon anorectal manometric evaluation of patients suffering from bowel urgency and fecal incontinence (FInc). Based on the assessment of these parameters, pertinent therapeutic decisions are made

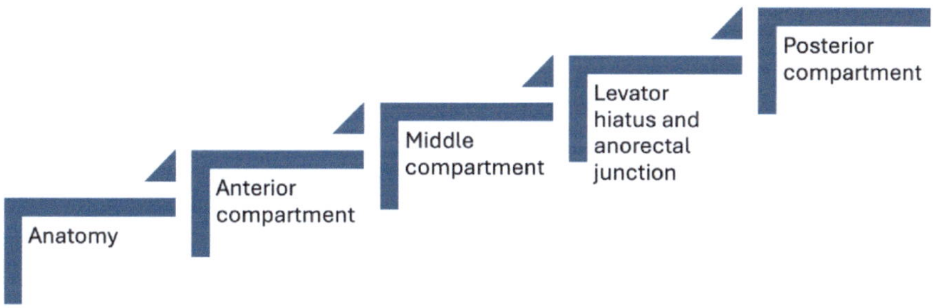

Fig. 8.10 Outline of a full assessment of pelvic floor structure and function by dynamic MR defecography

Dynamic MR Defecography In general, MR imaging of the female pelvis can characterize and differentiate benign from malignant adnexal masses, and it is useful in the staging of malignancy and the evaluation of benign gynecologic and pelvic floor processes [14]. Dynamic pelvic floor MR imaging, or MR defecography with rectal contrast, can evaluate all pelvic compartments (anterior, middle, and posterior), muscles, ligaments, and fascia and is particularly useful in patients with suspected defecatory dysfunction or pelvic organ prolapse, with or without urinary dysfunction (Fig. 8.10) [15].

The study should be performed in at least a 1.5 T closed MR imaging unit, with the patient supine and knees elevated, using 120 to 250 mL of ultrasound gel for rectal contrast and vaginal gel as appropriate. The urinary bladder should be partially distended. The study involves the acquisition of high-resolution T2WI through the pelvis in the coronal, axial, and sagittal planes in addition to dynamic sagittal sequences during squeezing (Kegel), straining (Valsalva), and evacuation (defecation) maneuvers [16].

A full assessment of anorectal function involves the use of four complimentary tests: high-resolution anorectal manometry, rectal sensation test, balloon expulsion test, and MR defecography. All four tests may be performed in tandem, as part of one visit to a specialized anorectal motility unit. MR defecography is performed in

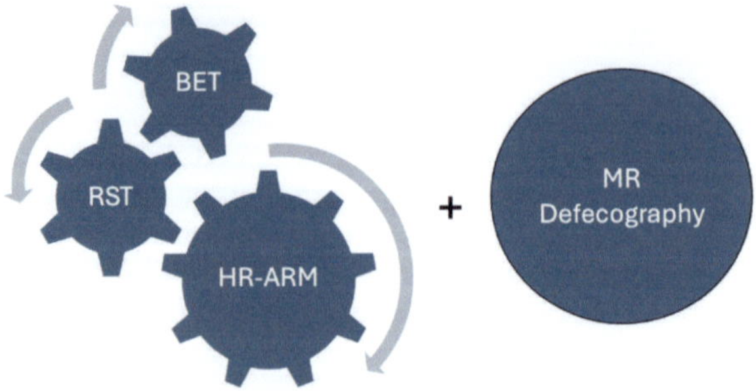

Fig. 8.11 Four well-validated tools in the evaluation and management of chronic rectal evacuation disorders

the Radiology department. They are important and well-validated tools to evaluate evacuation disorder (ED), chronic constipation, stool impaction, and fecal incontinence (Fig. 8.11).

Colonic Manometry Colonic high-resolution manometry is a novel diagnostic method used in the final workup of chronic refractory constipation before surgery. After placing a catheter in the colon, motor patterns consisting of short, cyclic, long, or slow antegrade or retrograde motor patterns, or high-amplitude propagating contractions, and pancolonic pressurizations are assessed [17].

Endoscopic Ultrasound (EUS) Forward-viewing echoendoscopes and through the scope EUS miniprobes allow for EUS imaging of lesions through the entire colon to assess perianal disease and provide detailed information about the anatomy and physiology of the anorectal region and sphincter integrity [18].

Point-of-Care Intestinal Ultrasound (POCUS) This modality is mainly used to quantify inflammation in patients with inflammatory bowel disease (IBD), and it is increasingly validated in patients with diarrhea and suspected ICI colitis in patients with cancer. Standard parameters assessed during this procedure include the bowel wall thickness (BWT), bowel wall layers stratification, blood flow (by Doppler signal), luminal diameters and motility, and the assessment of fistulas and abscesses, if present [19].

POCUS can recognize bowel obstruction early and identify thickened bowel wall, luminal narrowing, and proximal bowel dilation. Fixed luminal narrowing with upstream bowel dilation >3 cm is considered an unequivocal stricture sometimes revealing to-and-fro motion of bowel contents at the stricture site, whereas diminished peristalsis supports adynamic ileus. A meta-analysis of 11 studies reported ultrasound has a sensitivity and specificity of 92% and 97%, respectively, for a diagnosis of small bowel obstruction, compared with abdominal CT. Abdominal radiographs have a reported sensitivity and specificity of 75% and 66%, respectively [20].

While constipation is a clinical diagnosis, there can be uncertainty as to whether it is the final diagnosis, a symptom of another process, or unrelated to acute symptoms in the emergency care setting. While, abdominal radiography may be less specific, POCUS may be used to evaluate artifacts caused by high tissue impedance of hard stool in the rectum behind the bladder to qualitatively evaluate for stool burden and the transrectal diameter. Trans-rectal diameter can be measured before and after enema administration, in order to reevaluate patients for symptom resolution or improvement [21].

References

1. Naveed M, Jamil LH, Fujii-Lau LL, Al-Haddad M, Buxbaum JL, Fishman DS, Jue TL, Law JK, Lee JK, Qumseya BJ, Sawhney MS, Thosani N, Storm AC, Calderwood AH, Khashab MA, Wani SB. American Society for Gastrointestinal Endoscopy guideline on the role of endoscopy in the management of acute colonic pseudo-obstruction and colonic volvulus. Gastrointest Endosc. 2020;91(2):228–35.
2. Kato H, Kobayashi M, Tagawa R, Tominaga S, Maruyama A, Takeshima H, Nakayabu H. The usefulness of barium enema using a water-soluble contrast medium as an emergency examination. Rev Esp Enferm Dig. 2025:9. https://doi.org/10.17235/reed.2024.10968/2024. Epub ahead of print. PMID: 39784733
3. Gupta S. Screening for colorectal cancer. Hematol Oncol Clin North Am. 2022;36(3):393–414. https://doi.org/10.1016/j.hoc.2022.02.001. Epub 2022 Apr 30. PMID: 35501176; PMCID: PMC9167799
4. Rao SS, Coss-Adame E, Valestin J, Mysore K. Evaluation of constipation in older adults: radioopaque markers (ROMs) versus wireless motility capsule (WMC). Arch Gerontol Geriatr. 2012;55(2):289–94. https://doi.org/10.1016/j.archger.2012.04.003. Epub 2012 May 7. PMID: 22572600
5. Saad RJ. The wireless motility capsule: a one-stop shop for the evaluation of GI motility disorders. Curr Gastroenterol Rep. 2016;18(3):14. https://doi.org/10.1007/s11894-016-0489-x. PMID: 26908282
6. Thwaites PA, Yao CK, Maggo J, et al. Comparison of gastrointestinal landmarks using the gas-sensing capsule and wireless motility capsule. Aliment Pharmacol Ther. 2022;56:1337–48.
7. Zhou J, Thwaites PA, Gibson PR, et al. Comparison of gas-sensing capsule with wireless motility capsule in motility disorder patients. J Neurogastroenterol Motil. 2024;30(3):303–12.
8. Kuo B, Lee A, Abell T, Attaluri A, Cline M, Hasler WL, Ho V, Lembo AJ, Masoud A, McCallum R, Moshiree B, Quigley E, Rao SSC, Sanchez MM, Sarosiek I, Stocker A, Surjanhata B, Zhou J, Chey W. S729 Comparative evaluation of gas-sensing capsule and wireless motility capsule for transit time assessment in motility disorders. Am J Gastroenterol. 2024;119(10S):S500–1.
9. Banks KP, Revels JW, Tafti D, Moshiri M, Shah N, Moran SK, Wang SS, Solnes LB, Sheikhbahaei S, Elojeimy S. Scintigraphy of gastrointestinal motility: best practices in assessment of gastric and bowel transit in adults. Radiographics. 2024;44(6):e230127. https://doi.org/10.1148/rg.230127. Erratum in: Radiographics 2024;44(7):e249005. https://doi.org/10.1148/rg.249005. PMID: 38814800
10. Ifrah A, Kanaparthi J, Fromer R, Gayner AH, Maurer AH, Dadparvar S, Parkman HP. Whole gut transit scintigraphy for the assessment of patients with symptoms of chronic constipation. Dig Dis Sci. 2024;69(10):3875–81.
11. Carrington EV, Heinrich H, Knowles CH, Fox M, Rao S, Altomare DF, Bharucha AE, Burgell R, Chey WD, Chiarioni G, Dinning P, Emmanuel A, Farouk R, Felt-Bersma RJF, Jung KW, Lembo A, Malcolm A, Mittal RK, Mion F, Myung SJ, O'Connell PR, Pehl C, Remes-Troche JM, Reveille RM, Vaizey CJ, Vitton V, Whitehead WE, Wong RK, Scott SM. All members of the international anorectal physiology working group. The international anorectal physiology working group (IAPWG) recommendations: standardized testing protocol and the London classification for disorders of anorectal function. Neurogastroenterol

Motil. 2020;32(1):e13679. https://doi.org/10.1111/nmo.13679. Epub 2019 Aug 12. PMID: 31407463; PMCID: PMC6923590

12. Triadafilopoulos G, Clarke JO, Kamal A, Neshatian L. Intra-subject variability in high resolution anorectal manometry using the London classification: diagnostic and therapeutic implications. Dig Dis Sci. 2022;67(11):5014–8. https://doi.org/10.1007/s10620-021-07373-9. Epub 2022 Feb 22. PMID: 35194706
13. Rao SS, Patcharatrakul T. Diagnosis and treatment of dyssynergic defecation. J Neurogastroenterol Motil. 2016;22(3):423–35. https://doi.org/10.5056/jnm16060. PMID: 27270989; PMCID: PMC4930297
14. Sakala MD, Shampain KL, Wasnik AP. Advances in MR imaging of the female pelvis. Magn Reson Imaging Clin N Am. 2020;28(3):415–31. https://doi.org/10.1016/j.mric.2020.03.007. Epub 2020 Jun 6. PMID: 32624159
15. Gurland BH, Khatri G, Ram R, Hull TL, Kocjancic E, Quiroz LH, El Sayed RF, Jambhekar KR, Chernyak V, Paspulati RM, Sheth VR, Steiner AM, Kamath A, Shobeiri SA, Weinstein MM, Bordeianou L, Members of the Expert Workgroup on Magnetic Resonance Imaging of Pelvic Floor Disorders. Consensus Definitions and Interpretation Templates for Magnetic Resonance Imaging of Defecatory Pelvic Floor Disorders. Proceedings of the Consensus Meeting of the Pelvic Floor Disorders Consortium of the American Society of Colon and Rectal Surgeons, the Society of Abdominal Radiology, the International Continence Society, the American Urogynecologic Society, the International Urogynecological Association, and the Society of Gynecologic Surgeons. Female Pelvic Med Reconstr Surg. 2021;27(10):e645–56. https://doi.org/10.1097/SPV.0000000000001111. PMID: 34506350
16. El Sayed RF, Alt CD, Maccioni F, et al. Magnetic resonance imaging of pelvic floor dysfunction—joint recommendations of the ESUR and ESGAR Pelvic Floor Working Group. Eur Radiol. 2017;27:2067–85.
17. Pannemans J, Vanuytsel T, Pauwels A, Rommel N, De Schepper H, Lam TJ, Thys A, Tack J. High-resolution colonic manometry interobserver analysis trial. Neurogastroenterol Motil. 2022;34(1):e14285.
18. Kumar S, Chaudhary RK, Shah SS, Kumar D, Nepal P, Ojili V. Current update on the role of endoanal ultrasound: a primer for radiologists. Abdom Radiol (NY). 2024;49(8):2873–90.
19. Shankar N, Kuo L, Krugliak Cleveland N, Galen B, Samel NS, Perez-Sanchez A, Nathanson R, Coss E, Echavarria J, Rubin DT, Soni NJ. Point-of-care ultrasound in gastroenterology and hepatology. Clin Gastroenterol Hepatol. 2025;23(8):S1542-3565(25)00019-9. https://doi.org/10.1016/j.cgh.2024.09.040. Epub ahead of print. PMID: 39793722.
20. Gottlieb M, Peksa GD, Pandurangadu AV, et al. Utilization of ultrasound for the evaluation of small bowel obstruction: a systematic review and meta-analysis. Am J Emerg Med. 2018;36:234–42.
21. Riera A, Phatak UP. Qualitative point-of-care ultrasound enema management for constipation. Pediatr Emerg Care. 2024;40(3):239–42. https://doi.org/10.1097/PEC.0000000000003081. Epub 2023 Oct 30. PMID: 37890187

9 Tests for Gastrointestinal Sensory-Motor Assessment: Ancillary Tests

George Triadafilopoulos

9.1 Ancillary Tests

Fecal Elastase A fecal elastase test measures the amount of elastase in a stool sample and is a noninvasive test that helps diagnose and monitor pancreatic function. The test is useful in diagnosing exocrine pancreatic insufficiency (EPI); monitoring pancreatic function in people with cystic fibrosis, diabetes, or chronic pancreatitis; and identifying pancreatic causes of chronic diarrhea. A normal fecal elastase level is 200 micrograms per gram (mcg/g) or higher. Levels between 100 and 200 mcg/g indicate mild to moderate exocrine pancreatic insufficiency, while levels below 100 mcg/g indicate severe exocrine pancreatic insufficiency [1].

72-H Stool Collection for Fat This test measures the amount of fat in the stool over a 3-day period. It is used to diagnose fat maldigestion or malabsorption. The test is laborious and infrequently used. It involves a high-fat diet intake (at least 100 g of fat per day) for 3 days, followed by collection of all the stool that is stored in the refrigerator or freezer until ready to be sent to the laboratory. A normal result is less than 7 g of fat per day. Higher values indicate fat malabsorption of any cause; values higher than 15 suggest fat maldigestion, usually a result of chronic pancreatic exocrine insufficiency [2].

Fecal Calprotectin Calprotectin is a protein released by neutrophils that accumulate in areas of inflammation. When there is inflammation in the gastrointestinal tract, more neutrophils, shedding from the mucosa, are present, leading to elevated levels of calprotectin in the stool (>50 μg/g). Unless associated with inflammation, patients with motor or sensory dysfunction should have normal calprotectin levels [3].

G. Triadafilopoulos (✉)
Department of Gastroenterology, Hepatology and Nutrition, UT MD Anderson Cancer Center, Houston, TX, USA
e-mail: gtriadafilopoulo@mdanderson.org

G. Triadafilopoulos (ed.), *Onco-Neurogastroenterology*,
https://doi.org/10.1007/978-3-031-98848-6_9

Fecal Bile Acid Test The fecal bile acid excretion test quantifies individual and total bile acids in a 48-h stool collection sample, using high-performance liquid chromatography and mass spectrometry. Increased total fecal bile acids are seen in patients with chronic functional diarrhea, and higher levels of the primary bile acids, cholic acid (CA), and chenodeoxycholic acid (CDCA) are associated with IBS-D. Either total bile acids above the reference range or CA + CDCA above 3.7% are consistent with bile acid malabsorption (BAM). The test requires a diet containing 100 g of fat for 2 days before and during the 48-h collection period. Fecal bile acid measurement is useful in the evaluation of patients who have diarrhea after ileal resection or radiation that impedes bile acid absorption in the distal ileum and in those patients with post-cholecystectomy diarrhea [4].

C-Reactive Protein This test measures the level of C-reactive protein in the blood. CRP is a protein produced by the liver in response to inflammation, typically caused by an infection or autoimmune disorders, like rheumatoid arthritis or inflammatory bowel disease. Elevated CRP levels may also be found in several cancers, such as breast, lung, stomach, colon, liver, or kidney. Low CRP levels (less than 1 mg/dL) indicate no significant inflammation. Moderate levels (1–3 mg/dL) may indicate mild inflammation, such as an infection or injury. High levels (greater than 3 mg/dL) may indicate severe inflammation, such as an autoimmune disease, heart attack, or stroke. Patients with isolated motor or sensory dysfunction should have normal calprotectin levels [5].

Autonomic Function Tests Autonomic testing includes measurements of heart rate variability with deep breathing, Valsalva maneuver, and head-up tilt table testing. Most patients who are suspected of autonomic dysfunction also undergo evaluation of sweat production with quantitative sudomotor axon reflex (QSART) testing [6].

Paraneoplastic Markers Paraneoplastic cases of gastrointestinal dysmotility, where autoimmune antibodies against neuronal antigens expressed by tumor cells cross-react with native neurons leading to dysfunction, have been described. Antineuronal antibodies (AAbs) have also been found in autoimmune gastrointestinal dysmotility (AGID), a clinically heterogeneous group of disorders in which symptoms are presumed to result from ENS dysfunction, and, as such, potentially affecting every level of the gut, include (neuronal) gAChR, (muscle) nicotinic AChR, VGKC complex, P/Q type VGCC, N type VGCC, and GAD65. AAbs specific for neuronal antigens, which are known to be pathogenic in some peripheral neuromuscular diseases, are present in some individuals with gut dysmotility [7]. Serological evaluation of patients who present with a subacute neurological disorder of undetermined etiology, especially those with known risk factors for cancer, is available through the Mayo Clinic laboratories under the acronym PAVAL (Paraneoplastic, Autoantibody Evaluation, Serum). The test investigates neurological symptoms that appear during, or after, cancer therapy; they are not explainable by metastasis and may help differentiating autoimmune neuropathies from neurotoxic effects of chemotherapy. It may also facilitate monitoring the immune response of seropositive patients during cancer therapy and in the detection of cancer recurrence in previously seropositive patients.

Blood and Urine Tests The serum chromogranin A (CgA) test detects this protein released by neuroendocrine tumors (NETs). 5-HIAA urine test is a 24-h urine sample that measures this substance produced from serotonin [8].

Transvaginal Pelvic Ultrasound Ultrasound is a useful tool in the evaluation of women with lower abdominal pain often mixed with pelvic complaints. The onco-neurogastroenterologist is frequently called upon to clarify the origin of overlapping symptoms of defecatory dysfunction, urinary frequency, or dyspareunia. Point-of-care, transabdominal, and transvaginal approaches may be employed to assess a variety of obstetric or gynecologic pathologies. Transvaginal ultrasound (TVUS) with the high-frequency endocavitary probe has superior near-field resolution and is useful in the evaluation of the adnexa and ovaries in women with pelvic pain. Fibroids, or leiomyomas, are common benign gynecologic tumors that can be vascular or calcified, isoechoic, hyperechoic, or hypoechoic to the surrounding myometrium. They can distort the contour of the uterus, project into the endometrial lumen, or locate within the myometrium or the cervix. If a patient has an ovarian cyst greater than 10 cm, or is postmenopausal, follow-up is appropriate to assess for malignancy. Features of malignant ovarian masses include larger size, multilocular appearance with septa, solid components, papillary projections, irregular thick walls, and increased blood flow in solid areas and ascites [9].

Pelvic MRI Dynamic pelvic MRI (MR defecography) can significantly impact management, particularly for patients with cancer and concurrent urogynecological and colorectal complaints, previous pelvic reconstructive surgery, or when symptoms do not correlate with physical examination. To characterize pelvic organ prolapse using this imaging technique, several lines have been proposed. The pubococcygeal line (PCL) is helpful, particularly for cul-de-sac hernias, such as peritoneoceles, sigmoidoceles, and enteroceles. The "hiatus" or "H line" demonstrates the anteroposterior width of the levator hiatus and is a line drawn from the inferior border of the pubic symphysis to the posterior wall of the rectum at the level of the anorectal junction. The "muscle" or "M line" represents the vertical descent of the levator hiatus, and it is drawn perpendicularly from the PCL to the most-posterior aspect of the H line. In case of a defect in the rectovaginal fascia, herniation of small bowel, peritoneum, and sigmoid colon can occur, in turn causing symptoms. Posterior compartment abnormalities include rectocele and rectal prolapse. With the rectum prolapsing distal to the external anal sphincter and left untreated for a period as short as 2 years, permanent damage to the pudendal nerve can result, causing permanent fecal incontinence. Descending perineal syndrome involves the descent of the anorectal junction greater than 2.5 cm from the PCL. Pelvic MRI can also evaluate functional disorders, such as the paradoxical contraction of the puborectalis muscle or anismus. The anorectal angle is the angle between the posterior border of the rectum and the central axis of the anal canal, is approximately 110–125° at rest, and normally increases by 15–20° with evacuation. In cases of paradoxical contraction, the angle would not change or becomes more acute and is also associated with a lack of pelvic floor descent, leading to prolonged and incomplete evacuation [10].

References

1. Nelson HA. Preanalytical and analytical factors affecting elastase quantitation in stool. Clin Biochem. 2024;131-132:110811. https://doi.org/10.1016/j.clinbiochem.2024.110811. Epub 2024 Aug 15. PMID: 39153524
2. Khan A, Vege SS, Dudeja V, Chari ST. Staging exocrine pancreatic dysfunction. Pancreatology. 2022;22(1):168–72. https://doi.org/10.1016/j.pan.2021.11.005. Epub 2021 Nov 19. PMID: 34916141
3. Murray J, Kok KB, Ayling RM. Fecal calprotectin in gastrointestinal disease. Clin Chem. 2023;69(7):699–710. https://doi.org/10.1093/clinchem/hvad051. PMID: 37228058
4. Hughes LE, Ford C, Brookes MJ, Gama R. Bile acid diarrhoea: current and potential methods of diagnosis. Ann Clin Biochem. 2021;58(1):22–8. https://doi.org/10.1177/0004563220966139. Epub 2020 Oct 28. PMID: 32998535
5. Plebani M. Why C-reactive protein is one of the most requested tests in clinical laboratories? Clin Chem Lab Med. 2023;61(9):1540–5. https://doi.org/10.1515/cclm-2023-0086. PMID: 36745137
6. Zhou W, Zikos TA, Clarke JO, Nguyen LA, Triadafilopoulos G, Neshatian L. Regional gastrointestinal transit and contractility patterns vary in postural orthostatic tachycardia syndrome (POTS). Dig Dis Sci. 2021;66(12):4406–13. https://doi.org/10.1007/s10620-020-06808-z. Epub 2021 Jan 11. PMID: 33428036
7. Nakane S, Mukaino A, Ihara E, Ogawa Y. Autoimmune gastrointestinal dysmotility: the interface between clinical immunology and neurogastroenterology. Immunol Med. 2021;44(2):74–85. https://doi.org/10.1080/25785826.2020.1797319. Epub 2020 Jul 27. PMID: 32715927
8. Ma ZY, Gong YF, Zhuang HK, Zhou ZX, Huang SZ, Zou YP, Huang BW, Sun ZH, Zhang CZ, Tang YQ, Hou BH. Pancreatic neuroendocrine tumors: a review of serum biomarkers, staging, and management. World J Gastroenterol. 2020;26(19):2305–22. https://doi.org/10.3748/wjg.v26.i19.2305. PMID: 32476795; PMCID: PMC7243647
9. Shibata J, Liu YT. Clinical ultrasound in obstetrics and gynecology. Emerg Med Clin North Am. 2024;42(4):839–62. https://doi.org/10.1016/j.emc.2024.05.008. Epub 2024 Aug 17. PMID: 39326991
10. Welch EK, Ross W, Dengler KL, Gruber DD, Lamb S. The "Ins and Outs" of dynamic magnetic resonance imaging for female pelvic organ prolapse. Int Urogynecol J. 2024;35(11):2223–5. https://doi.org/10.1007/s00192-024-05935-9. Epub 2024 Sep 28. PMID: 39340644; PMCID: PMC11638283

Regional Disorders of Sensory-Motor Dysfunction: Oropharynx, Hypopharynx, and Upper Esophageal Sphincter

10

George Triadafilopoulos and David M. Richards

10.1 Oropharynx, Hypopharynx, and Upper Esophageal Sphincter

Myasthenia Gravis Thymic epithelial tumors are rare neoplasms that include thymomas, thymic carcinomas, and thymic neuroendocrine neoplasms. These tumors differ in aggressiveness, their recurrence rates after resection, and outcomes [1]. Myasthenia gravis is characterized by fatigable weakness due to failure of neuromuscular junction transmission that is caused by antibodies against the acetylcholine receptor, and it is associated with thymomas in 15% of cases. By definition, this predominantly affects skeletal muscles, such as those in the oropharynx, tongue, hypopharynx, and proximal esophagus. This may manifest with bulbar effects, such as dysarthria, dysphagia, and dysphonia, ptosis and diplopia, frequent eyelid closure, or proximal muscle weakness. Weakness in the proximal structure swallowing muscles can result in poor clearance of pharyngeal residue, as well as disturb laryngeal elevation and can thus lead to aspiration. This itself can precipitate a myasthenic crisis. Aspiration in these patients can be silent [2]. High-resolution manometry may show fatigue as reduced-amplitude contractions with repetitive swallows and increased amplitude with administration of the anticholinesterase edrophonium [3]. Pharyngeal manometry, while not widely available, has been used to demonstrate the contributions of the oropharyngeal through proximal esophageal structures, as well as to assess the improvement in parameters, like the duration of relaxation pressure at the UES using maneuvers, like a chin-down position [2]. There is also autonomic dysfunction, such as pupillary fatigability, gastroparesis [4], or paraneoplastic intestinal pseudo-obstruction [5].

G. Triadafilopoulos (✉) · D. M. Richards
Department of Gastroenterology, Hepatology and Nutrition, UT MD Anderson Cancer Center, Houston, TX, USA
e-mail: gtriadafilopoulo@mdanderson.org

G. Triadafilopoulos (ed.), *Onco-Neurogastroenterology*,
https://doi.org/10.1007/978-3-031-98848-6_10

Lambert-Eaton Syndrome The Lambert-Eaton myasthenic syndrome (LEMS) is a rare autoimmune disorder that affects the neuromuscular junction, characterized by proximal muscle weakness, reduction of tendon reflexes, and autonomic dysfunction [6]. The muscle weakness in these patients is due to pathogenic autoantibodies directed against voltage-gated calcium channels (VGCC) present on the presynaptic nerve terminal. More than 50% of patients with LEMS have small-cell lung carcinoma (SCLC), which also expresses functional voltage-gated calcium channels. VGCC antibody positivity strongly supports the diagnosis. Oncological therapy against the primary tumor, immunotherapy, and symptomatic treatments can improve LEMS in patients with small-cell lung carcinoma. Most patients benefit from 3,4-diaminopyridine administration for symptomatic treatment [7].

Dermatomyositis Dermatomyositis (DM) is a rare systemic autoimmune disease that is characterized by skin rash (typically on face and hands, such as the shawl sign, V sign, "mechanics hands," Gottron papules, and Gottron sign), proximal muscle weakness, and oropharyngeal dysphagia. It is an idiopathic inflammatory myopathy—closely linked to malignancy—that is often found within the first 3 years of the dermatomyositis diagnosis. Typically, the disease improves after treatment of cancer; otherwise, the muscle and skin changes might occur upon relapse of malignant disease, further supporting that it is a paraneoplastic phenomenon [8]. The dysphagia in these patients reflects weak, ineffective peristalsis of the proximal (striated) portion of the esophageal body, detected on HREM.

Acute and Late Oropharyngeal Radiation Injury Radiation therapy (XRT) can be a critical part of the treatment of head and neck cancers, thyroid cancers, proximal esophageal malignancies, and the treatment of cancers in adjacent or adjoining organs, like the lungs and breast. Dysphagia related to radiation therapy can be thought of occurring in phases: There is an initial phase of acute injury during and for several weeks after radiation is received, a period of relative quiescence or a "honeymoon period," and a late radiation injury phase. Injury during the acute and late phases can lead to dysphagia.

Acute radiation toxicity induces mucositis that can cause dysphagia and odynophagia, in turn resulting in weight loss, dehydration, and malnutrition. To support patients nutritionally, prophylactic gastrostomy tube placement has been used. However, such intervention carries surgical/procedural risks related to tube insertion, tumor seeding if placement is performed endoscopically. Further, when prolonged tube feedings are given, there is a risk of prolongation of dysphagia related to oropharyngeal muscle disuse and atrophy. There may be a correlation between acute, severe radiation-induced dysphagia and the dose absorbed by the cricopharyngeus and cervical esophagus muscles. Radiation may cause a volume enlargement of the pharyngeal muscles, in turn leading to a reduction of the lumen at the cricopharyngeus, producing a mechanical dysphagia. Radiation to the mucosa may also lead to mucositis, resulting in odynophagia. The radiation dose absorbed by the pharyngeal mucosa and the dose absorbed by the pharyngeal muscles in the lower part of the pharyngeal axis may be key variables [9]. Although chemotherapy and XRT increase the incidence and severity of acute radiation toxicity, such combination therapy is widely used to improve survival and organ preservation. Radiation techniques, such as intensity-modulated radiation therapy (IMRT), aim to spare the off-target organs and reduce acute and late radiation toxicity [10].

While newer XRT techniques aim to limit toxicity, there is still controversy over the idea of prophylactic versus reactive G-tube placement, given that only a fraction of patients will require a G-tube to get through the acute toxicity. The reactive approach may be favorable, since these patients receive G-tube feedings for shorter time periods while managing to maintain their weight similarly to patients with prophylactic tubes. One study showed prophylactic tubes were used for less than 2 weeks in almost half of patients. Prophylactic G-tube placement may be placing patients through unnecessary procedures [11]. A systematic review suggested that prophylactic PEG placement may reduce the number of patients malnourished during treatment, despite average weight loss not differing from a reactive PEG strategy. Reactive PEGs appear to be feasible with minimal interruption to treatment although there may be an increased risk of aspiration and stricture formation. There does not seem to be inferior tumor control or effects on overall survival with reactive PEG placement. The impact of the two strategies on long-term swallow function is unclear. It may be best to look at risk factors for the need for PEG placement and consider honing a prophylactic strategy in those patients at highest risk for feeding tube placement, given tumor site, age, pretreatment weight, treatment volume, and perhaps utilizing information on modified barium swallow studies to look at pretreatment oropharyngeal function [12].

Radiation techniques continue to evolve in balancing treatment effect and toxicity. Proton therapy, as compared to intensity-modulated radiation therapy, holds the promise of more optimal dose distribution. There is a suggestion that proton therapy may have largely favorable outcomes in terms of disease control and toxicities, such as reduced need for feeding tube placement, less weight loss, and reduced symptom severity in the subacute recovery period with proton therapy compared to intensity-modulated radiation therapy. The novelty of this technique may have not allowed enough time lapse to yet provide insight into the late toxicity effects of proton therapy [13].

The acute side effects of XRT usually resolve within weeks or months after its completion. The definition of late radiation toxicity are side effects emerging more than 3 months after completion XRT. The window between the acute toxicity and its resolution and the emergence of late radiation sequelae can be variable and related to the dose of radiation received, as well as the location of the tumor. Late radiation toxicity may lead to xerostomia, dysphagia, osteoradionecrosis, trismus, and hearing loss [14].

Xerostomia is related to damage to salivary glands from XRT. The damaged glands produce thicker or small volumes of saliva. The composition of the saliva can also be altered affecting swallowing, speech, and oral health. Xerostomia and dysphagia are both associated with worse health-related quality of life (HRQoL). Management of xerostomia can be difficult. Pilocarpine is a nonselective cholinergic parasympathomimetic agonist that has been used prophylactically to enhance proliferation of undamaged acinar cells and progenitor cells as well as increase saliva production and stimulate salivary flow rates. Its use is typically limited by side effects related to cholinergic stimulation, including bronchospasm, bradycardia, vasodilation, and diarrhea. Cevimeline is also a cholinergic agonist, used post XRT, that can improve salivary flow rate and oral dryness, but its use is also limited by side effects. Acupuncture can also provide some relief if there is still a portion of functional salivary gland. Many patients use saliva substitutes for symptomatic relief. Several agents are available over the counter as gels, mouthwashes, and sprays [15].

Chronic dysphagia can occur months to many years after XRT for head and neck malignancies, but its severity is not predicted by tumor site or stage, nor by the time since therapy, age, gender, or adjuvant chemotherapy. Fibrosis of soft tissues can restrict compliance, cause luminal strictures, and restrict muscle contractility, at times all compounded by lymphedema. Muscle atrophy can result from disuse during the acute phase or occur in patients who are suffering from aspiration and are placed on modified or restricted diets. Sensory and motor nerve damage can occur leading to dysfunction and aspiration [16]. Aspiration pneumonia may account for about 20% of non-cancer-related deaths, underscoring the need for timely diagnosis and implementation of preventive measures, mostly using speech therapy rehabilitation, combined with dietary and postural measures [17].

Beyond just XRT, the treatment of head and neck and proximal esophageal cancers using combinations of chemotherapy, surgery, and XRT can result in neural damage, anastomotic strictures, and damage to brain structures that control aspects of the swallowing mechanism. One series of head and neck cancer survivors with up to 8 years of follow-up after radiotherapy with curative intent reported a high prevalence of dysphagia, with 59% with patients newly presenting to clinic with dysphagia 5 years or more after radiotherapy [17]. It is helpful to think of dysphagia after XRT as occurring from the "pump," the "pipe," or both. The pump refers to the oropharyngeal, tongue, and hypopharyngeal structures involved in swallowing that are responsible for controlling and manipulating the bolus, propelling it to and through the UES and into esophagus. This initiates the swallow and primary peristalsis in the esophagus. Management of this portion of the swallow falls largely on speech pathologists who work to optimize and stabilize, if unable to improve, the function of these structures using motor exercises, patterning, and postural or sensory techniques. Goals are to minimize aspiration, improve swallow safety, and improve swallow efficiency. Some of these measures have been shown to have more of an impact on the patient perceptions of swallowing and quality of life than on objective parameters. More intensive swallow therapy programs like the McNeil Dysphagia Therapy Program and biofeedback show promise in improving compensation for deficits and may have some functional gains [15].

Esophageal strictures (luminal narrowings) occur in 7% of patients treated with head and neck radiation therapy, with some subgroups having an even higher incidence. For example, intensity-modulated radiotherapy (IMRT) has a 16% risk of stricture and the risk is 19% among patients treated with total laryngectomy [18].

Strictures are an attractive target for improving dysphagia, since there are effective interventions (i.e., esophageal dilation) available to address them. A recent systematic review found studies reported between 42 and 100% success for the treatment of postradiation strictures using endoscopic dilation [19]. This is consistent with prior guidelines that reported adequate dysphagia relief in patients with postradiation strictures of up to 84%. While dilation is effective, much remains unknown. There is limited consensus on the adequate esophageal luminal diameter that is needed for relief of dysphagia. Some studies have used an endpoint of 42 French (14 mm) while guidelines on dysphagia have defined refractory strictures as those that have failed to achieve 14 mm after 5 dilation sessions at 2-week intervals [20]. The number and cadence of dilations needed to achieve these diameters is variable. In a study of 19 head and neck cancer survivors, 6 required 5–7 dilation sessions and 5 required more than 10 dilations. One patient required 24 dilations over the course of 3 years [21]. Current evidence is lacking as to why some patients have repeated formation of fibrosis after initial therapy, while others manage with one or two dilations. Risk factors for refractory strictures include complex strictures (>2 cm, angulated, irregular, severe luminal narrowing), postsurgical anastomotic strictures, and radiation-induced strictures [22]. Cancer survivors commonly have strictures that fall into these difficult to treat categories. The combination of a mechanical barrier to swallowing can cause dysphagia in a patient who may otherwise have compensated for reduced pharyngeal function.

The precise luminal diameter needed to avoid dysphagia in the setting of reduced oropharyngeal function is unclear. Even the working definition of refractory stricture in 2005 excluded inflammatory strictures and dysphagia based on neuromuscular dysfunction (e.g., those with postoperative and postradiation therapy dysphagia) [23]. It may be that patients with reduced oropharyngeal function need even large diameter lumens to avoid dysphagia. While many techniques have been tried for refractory and recurrent strictures, including needle knife incision, or stenting of benign strictures, serial dilation may be the best approach. In a recent study at a referral center, weekly serial dilation was performed on two cohorts of complex benign esophageal strictures—a group who had failed therapy with endoscopic dilation done greater than or equal to 2-week intervals and a group of newly diagnosed strictures. Over 55% of patients who had failed dilations at greater than or equal to 2-week intervals achieved long-term relief without needing stents or electrocautery incisions. The success of this strategy in newly diagnosed strictures was higher, ~83%. The authors hypothesized that after breaking the mucosal barrier with dilation, fibrosis sets in by the second week, even if reepithelization takes over 5 weeks. Hence, dilating before the fibrosis sets in may lead to better success [24]. Both balloons and Savary dilators can be used, occasionally in the same session. Dilation has been associated with weight gain in 47%, feeding tube removal in 38.3%, and perforation in 3.3% of patients. Few patients may require stenting for refractory strictures [25].

Many of these strictures occur at the junction of the hypopharynx and esophagus, the pharyngoesophageal segment (PES). This area is vulnerable to radiation exposure during treatment of head and neck (H&N) malignancies, thyroid cancers, and proximal esophageal cancers. While it seems intuitive that modified barium swallow study may visualize this area, it has overall poor diagnostic accuracy in detecting strictures [26]. This is likely because opening the UES is a complex process and relaxation of the muscles included in the UES, like the cricopharyngeus, is only part of the process. In addition to the relaxation of the cricopharyngeus, opening the PES requires elevation of the laryngeal cartilages off the cervical spine (traction) and an intra-bolus pressure generated by contraction of the tongue and pharynx [27]. Endoscopically this is a difficult area to evaluate since the UES is closed at baseline, and unless the stricture is narrower than the endoscope, the collapsed/closed UES region may not reveal any resistance to scope passage or allow for the stricture to be visualized. The functional lumen imaging probe (FLIP) is an intriguing technology to evaluate this area by utilizing an infinitely compliant bag that is filled with a conductive fluid. During volume-controlled distension, the FLIP uses impedance planimetry to measure luminal cross-sectional area (thus diameter). Synchronizing this with a singular pressure measured within the probe bag allows visualization of luminal geometry and pressure, akin to compliance. This is expressed as the distensibility index (DI)—calculated by dividing the median narrowest cross-sectional area by the median intra-bag pressure over a set timeframe or distention volume. The DI is therefore an assessment of the mechanical properties of the measured structure [28, 29]. Since the FLIP measurements are taken during endoscopy, not related to a swallow, and involve filling the probe across the area of interest, the assessment at the UES reflects properties related to the structure, independent of the actions of the tongue, pharynx, hyolaryngeal complex, and intra-bolus pressures. FLIP is highly accurate for the detection of PES strictures with a sensitivity and specificity of 100%, given a FLIP diameter of 12 mm. Defining strictures by visualizing a mucosal tear after passing dilators up to 16 mm in diameter, there was moderate correlation between the largest dilator passed and the FLIP-derived diameter, measured immediately after dilation, which were systematically ~2 mm lower than the size of the largest dilator passed [26]. A recent small study showed a correlation between the distensibility index measured by FLIP and the dose of radiation received in Gy, but there was no correlation between diameter and radiation dose, presumably a reflection of radiation-induced esophageal wall mechanics [30].

Esophageal self-dilation therapy (ESDT) is a complement to endoscopic dilation, in which patients learn to independently pass a flexible tapered dilator (Maloney bougie) transorally to maintain luminal patency. Based on small studies, ESDT is effective for resistant benign esophageal strictures, reducing the number of endoscopic dilations and increasing the intervention-free interval. In general, ESDT is an underutilized treatment option, due to several factors, such as physician and provider awareness, lack of physician training, lack of structural guidelines, and paucity of high-quality research data on safety and efficacy [31].

The ideal selection of patients for ESDT requires a personalized approach. The approach intends to maintain, not achieve, luminal patency. Hence, the amenability of a stricture to achieving at least temporary luminal patency by endoscopic dilation predicts the success of ESDT. Further, the ability of a patient to pass a dilator is essential, and significant esophageal angulation, the presence of esophageal diverticula, or altered postsurgical pharyngeal anatomy may be limiting. In general, proximal strictures are more amenable to ESDT. Anticoagulation does not absolutely contraindicate ESDT because the dilator acts to maintain patency, with little tissue disruption. ESDT must be performed frequently, often daily, to achieve success. The notion of passing a dilator is daunting, and patient motivation is critical. Yet, the repeated failure of endoscopic therapy, the cost and risks, often strongly motivates patients.

Laryngectomy Total laryngectomy, usually followed by chemoradiotherapy, is performed to treat advanced laryngeal cancer. Dysphagia following total laryngectomy is common, ranging from 17% to 72%, is often multifactorial, and it reflects stenosis at the pharyngoesophageal anastomosis or chemoradiation-related pharyngeal dysfunction [32]. Patients undergoing laryngectomy are often treated with multiple modalities, that is, not just surgical resection and reconstruction, but combinations of neoadjuvant and adjuvant radiation and/or chemotherapy. As a result, stricture formation is not uncommon and may occur in up to one half of these cases [32]. Studies have examined endoscopic dilation as a treatment modality, and it can be effective. These strictures can be refractory and may require serial dilations [33]. Beyond radiation and chemotherapy exposure, the type of reconstruction required can influence stricture formation in the laryngectomized patient. Patients with tube-free flap reconstruction may require more dilations than patients with partial tubulation or primary reconstruction. Further, the need for multiple dilations may be higher in patients with pharyngo-cutaneous fistulas and primary chemoradiotherapy [34]. Small retrospective studies report no major complications (i.e., perforation or pneumothorax), but minor, self-limited bleeding may be seen. Dilation techniques in laryngectomized patients involve endoscopic and radiologic guidance using wire-guided Savary bougies, or Maloney or Jackson bougies, and balloon dilators. There is no consensus on the need for trachea-esophageal prosthesis removal prior to dilation [35]. Clinical and technical success can vary [33].

When patients were assessed for possible esophageal dysmotility following total laryngectomy, minor disorders of peristalsis were noted in 50%. Absent peristalsis was the next most common finding (21.7%), followed by jackhammer esophagus in twp patients and esophageal spasm, EGJOO, and type I achalasia [32]. Therefore, patients after laryngectomy without response to endoscopic dilation or without apparent strictures should undergo HRAM, especially those with poor trachea-esophageal speech, leakage from trachea-esophageal puncture sites, or aspiration, since they have poor esophageal clearance, acid reflux, and/or LES incompetence.

FLIP probe placement is feasible in the total laryngectomy population. Interestingly, the probe may be placed transnasally after topical anesthesia in awake patients. Most (70%) tolerate probe placement, while failure is attributed to strictures within the neo-pharynx. The bolus volume has an impact on the opening diameter, with larger diameters seen with larger bolus volumes [36].

Radiation-induced complete pharyngoesophageal stricture (CPS) or occlusion is a challenging clinical problem that requires a rendezvous procedure to re-establish the esophageal lumen. In this approach, two endoscopes are passed simultaneously antegrade and retrograde (one via the mouth and the other via a gastrostomy tract) to gain access to the proximal and distal sides of the stricture aiming to pass a guidewire across the occlusion. Re-establishing the lumen is done using endoscopic devices like forceps to cross the occluded segment or burrow a new tract through the scar tissue with fluoroscopic guidance. Once a wire is placed, the stricture is dilated using bougies. Rendezvous has a high technical success rate (88.9%)—defined as ability to traverse the occlusion—but a lower clinical success rate (58.4%) in terms of improvement of dysphagia. A smaller portion of patients will become feeding tube free (43.5%) [37]. Regular antegrade dilation in the post-rendezvous period may produce greater improvements in swallowing function [38]. The utilization of a standardized clinical pathway, with multidisciplinary input from speech pathologists to help achieve early diet advancement and swallow therapy, may help improve outcomes. Figure 10.1 shows endoscopic appearance of a CPS during the sequence of a rendezvous intervention.

Laryngopharyngeal Reflux Disease (LPRD) Laryngopharyngeal reflux disease results from the direct and/or indirect effects of gastroduodenal content reflux, inducing morphological and/or neurological changes in the upper aerodigestive tract. LPR is etiologically linked to many laryngeal disorders and plays a role in chronic cough, laryngeal leukoplakia, dysphonia, and laryngeal tumors. Although there is clear evidence for GERD-related dysphagia, a direct connection between dysphagia and LPRD is not as clear. Up to 60–80% of patients with globus have LPRD, but the response of globu to PPI therapy is low. LPRD-related laryngopharygeal inflammation and globus may require longer courses of high-dose PPI and resolution of inflammation before symptoms abate [39]. Screening is often performed using the Reflux Symptom Index (RSI), a self-administered 9-item outcomes instrument, where LPRD is defined as RSI >13 [40]. The hypopharyngeal-esophageal multichannel intraluminal impedance-pH testing can suggest the diagnosis of LPRD when there is >1 acid, weakly acid, or nonacid hypopharyngeal reflux event in 24 h [41]. It is likely that LPRD results from a combination of alterations of reflexes in the UES and poor esophageal clearance of refluxate. Reflux of contents into the esophagus can trigger reflexes designed to prevent aspiration. The UES pressure increases and is further augmented by the acidity of the refluxate. There are also

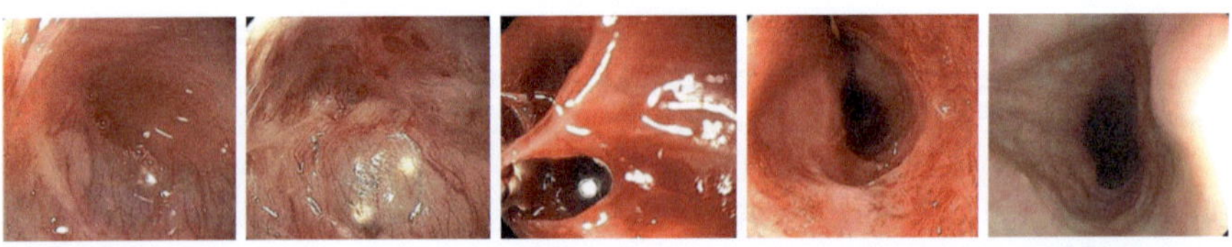

Fig. 10.1 Serial endoscopic images of a CPS. From left to right: (1) Antegrade view of membrane with complete luminal occlusion (esophageal side); (2) retrograde view of membrane with complete luminal occlusion (gastric side); (3) use of forceps to re-establish the lumen followed by stricture dilation over guidewire; (4) lumen after dilation; (5) stricture 4.5 years after the rendezvous procedure

esophagus-stimulated pharyngeal swallow responses and esophageal peristaltic contractions that function to sweep and clear refluxed material out of the hypopharynx and esophagus. Patients with LPRD are less likely to exhibit an esophago-UES contractile reflex in response to reflux, regardless of acidity. An esophago-UES relaxation reflex has been observed in LPRD that is not seen in patients with GERD without LPRD or in healthy controls. LPRD can also affect the UES itself making it shorter and hypotonic. Together these changes impair the sphincter's barrier function and reduce the clearance of refluxate leading to LPRD [39].

References

1. Romi F. Thymoma in myasthenia gravis: from diagnosis to treatment. Autoimmune Dis. 2011;2011:474512. https://doi.org/10.4061/2011/474512. Epub 2011 Aug 10. PMID: 21860784; PMCID: PMC3155972
2. Kumai Y, Miyamoto T, Matsubara K, Satoh C, Yamashita S, Orita Y. Swallowing dysfunction in myasthenia gravis patients examined with high-resolution manometry. Auris Nasus Larynx. 2021;48(6):1135–9. https://doi.org/10.1016/j.anl.2021.05.002. Epub 2021 Jun 5. PMID: 34103207
3. Torres-Barrera G, Herrera-Quiñones G, Scharrer SI, Benavides-Salgado DE, Maldonado-Garza HJ, Achem SR. High-resolution esophageal manometry in myasthenia gravis. ACG Case Rep J. 2020;7(3):e00340. https://doi.org/10.14309/crj.0000000000000340. PMID: 32337306; PMCID: PMC7162132
4. Vernino S, Cheshire WP, Lennon VA. Myasthenia gravis with autoimmune autonomic neuropathy. Auton Neurosci. 2001;88(3):187–92. https://doi.org/10.1016/S1566-0702(01)00239-9. PMID: 11474561
5. Anderson NE, Hutchinson DO, Nicholson GJ, Aitcheson F, Nixon JM. Intestinal pseudo-obstruction, myasthenia gravis, and thymoma. Neurology. 1996;47(4):985–7. https://doi.org/10.1212/wnl.47.4.985. PMID: 8857731
6. Lipka AF, Verschuuren JJGM. Lambert-Eaton myasthenic syndrome. Handb Clin Neurol. 2024;200:307–25. https://doi.org/10.1016/B978-0-12-823912-4.00012-8. PMID: 38494285
7. Matsuo H. Lambert-Eaton myasthenic syndrome. Brain Nerve. 2024;76(5):630–4. https://doi.org/10.11477/mf.1416202653. Japanese. PMID: 38741506
8. Chang L, Zhang L, Jia H, Nie Z, Zhang L. Malignancy in dermatomyositis: a retrospective paired case-control study of 202 patients from Central China. Medicine (Baltimore). 2020;99(34):e21733. https://doi.org/10.1097/MD.0000000000021733. PMID: 32846794; PMCID: PMC7447459
9. Alterio D, Gerardi MA, Cella L, Spoto R, Zurlo V, Sabbatini A, Fodor C, D'Avino V, Conson M, Valoriani F, Ciardo D, Pacelli R, Ferrari A, Maisonneuve P, Preda L, Bruschini R, Cossu Rocca M, Rondi E, Colangione S, Palma G, Dicuonzo S, Orecchia R, Sanguineti G, Jereczek-Fossa BA. Radiation-induced acute dysphagia: prospective observational study on 42 head and neck cancer patients. Strahlenther Onkol. 2017;193(11):971–81. https://doi.org/10.1007/s00066-017-1206-x. English. Epub 2017 Sep 7. PMID: 28884310
10. Otter S, Schick U, Gulliford S, Lal P, Franceschini D, Newbold K, Nutting C, Harrington K, Bhide S. Evaluation of the risk of grade 3 oral and pharyngeal dysphagia using atlas-based method and multivariate analyses of individual patient dose distributions. Int J Radiat Oncol Biol Phys. 2015;93(3):507–15. https://doi.org/10.1016/j.ijrobp.2015.07.2263. Epub 2015 Jul 17. PMID: 26460992
11. Kramer S, Newcomb M, Hessler J, Siddiqui F. Prophylactic versus reactive PEG tube placement in head and neck cancer. Otolaryngol Head Neck Surg. 2014;150(3):407–12. https://doi.org/10.1177/0194599813517081. Epub 2013 Dec 31. PMI,D: 24381015

12. McClelland S 3rd, Andrews JZ, Chaudhry H, Teckie S, Goenka A. Prophylactic versus reactive gastrostomy tube placement in advanced head and neck cancer treated with definitive chemoradiotherapy: a systematic review. Oral Oncol. 2018;87:77–81. https://doi.org/10.1016/j.oraloncology.2018.10.028. Epub 2018 Oct 25. PMID: 30527247
13. Gunn GB, Garden AS, Ye R, Ausat N, Dahlstrom KR, Morrison WH, Fuller CD, Phan J, Reddy JP, Shah SJ, Mayo LL, Chun SG, Chronowski GM, Moreno AC, Myers JN, Hanna EY, Esmaeli B, Gillison ML, Ferrarotto R, Hutcheson KA, Chambers MS, Ginsberg LE, El-Naggar AK, Rosenthal DI, Zhu XR, Frank SJ. Proton therapy for head and neck cancer: a 12-year, single-institution experience. Int J Part Ther. 2021;8(1):108–18. https://doi.org/10.14338/IJPT-20-00065.1. PMID: 34285940; PMCID: PMC8270083
14. Strojan P, Hutcheson KA, Eisbruch A, Beitler JJ, Langendijk JA, Lee AWM, Corry J, Mendenhall WM, Smee R, Rinaldo A, Ferlito A. Treatment of late sequelae after radiotherapy for head and neck cancer. Cancer Treat Rev. 2017;59:79–92. https://doi.org/10.1016/j.ctrv.2017.07.003. Epub 2017 Jul 18. PMID: 28759822; PMCID: PMC5902026
15. Langendijk JA, Doornaert P, Verdonck-de Leeuw IM, Leemans CR, Aaronson NK, Slotman BJ. Impact of late treatment-related toxicity on quality of life among patients with head and neck cancer treated with radiotherapy. J Clin Oncol. 2008;26(22):3770–6. https://doi.org/10.1200/JCO.2007.14.6647. PMID: 18669465
16. Pavy JJ, Denekamp J, Letschert J, Littbrand B, Mornex F, Bernier J, Gonzales-Gonzales D, Horiot JC, Bolla M, Bartelink H, EORTC Late Effects Working Group. Late effects toxicity scoring: the SOMA scale. Int J Radiat Oncol Biol Phys. 1995;31(5):1043–7. https://doi.org/10.1016/0360-3016(95)00059-8. PMID: 7713775
17. Szczesniak MM, Maclean J, Zhang T, Graham PH, Cook IJ. Persistent dysphagia after head and neck radiotherapy: a common and under-reported complication with significant effect on non-cancer-related mortality. Clin Oncol (R Coll Radiol). 2014;26(11):697–703. https://doi.org/10.1016/j.clon.2014.08.009. Epub 2014 Sep 16. PMID: 25239671
18. Cohen EE, et al. American Cancer Society head and neck cancer survivorship care guideline. CA Cancer J Clin. 2016;66(3):203–39.
19. Abu-Ghanem S, et al. Endoscopic management of postradiation dysphagia in head and neck cancer patients: a systematic review. Ann Otol Rhinol Laryngol. 2019;128(8):767–73.
20. Committee, A.S.o.P, et al. The role of endoscopy in the evaluation and management of dysphagia. Gastrointest Endosc. 2014;79(2):191–201.
21. Ahlawat SK, Al-Kawas FH. Endoscopic management of upper esophageal strictures after treatment of head and neck malignancy. Gastrointest Endosc. 2008;68(1):19–24.
22. Everett SM. Endoscopic management of refractory benign oesophageal strictures. Ther Adv Gastrointest Endosc. 2019;12:2631774519862134. https://doi.org/10.1177/2631774519862134. PMID: 31460518; PMCID: PMC6702770
23. Kochman ML, McClave SA, Boyce HW. The refractory and the recurrent esophageal stricture: a definition. Gastrointest Endosc. 2005;62(3):474–5. https://doi.org/10.1016/j.gie.2005.04.050. PMID: 16111985
24. Palam S, Mohorek M, Rizvi S, Dua K. Clinical outcomes on weekly endoscopic dilations as the initial approach to manage patients with complex benign esophageal strictures: report on 488 dilations. Surg Endosc. 2022;36(9):7056–65. https://doi.org/10.1007/s00464-022-09248-0. Epub 2022 Apr 27. PMID: 35477807
25. Baerman E, Cruz CC, Black S, et al. Outcomes of endoscopic dilation for radiation therapy-related esophageal stricture. Curr Treat Options Gastro. 2025;23:5. https://doi.org/10.1007/s11938-025-00470-y.
26. Wu PI, Szczesniak MM, Maclean J, Choo L, Quon H, Graham PH, Zhang T, Cook IJ. Clinical utility of a functional lumen imaging probe in management of dysphagia following head and neck cancer therapies. Endoscopy. 2017;49(9):848–54. https://doi.org/10.1055/s-0043-110670. Epub 2017 May 31. PMID: 28564716.
27. Belafsky PC. Dilation of the upper esophageal sphincter. Foregut. 2024;4(4):487–96. https://doi.org/10.1177/26345161241282299.

28. Hirano I, Pandolfino JE, Boeckxstaens GE. Functional lumen imaging probe for the Management of Esophageal Disorders: expert review from the clinical practice updates committee of the AGA Institute. Clin Gastroenterol Hepatol. 2017;15(3):325–34. https://doi.org/10.1016/j.cgh.2016.10.022. PMID: 28212976; PMCID: PMC5757507
29. McMahon BP, Frøkjaer JB, Drewes AM, Gregersen H. A new measurement of oesophago-gastric junction competence. Neurogastroenterol Motil. 2004;16(5):543–6. https://doi.org/10.1111/j.1365-2982.2004.00540.x. PMID: 15500510
30. Richards DM, Naz SMD, Dai J, Triadafilopoulos G, Fuller CD, Barbon C, Shafi MA, Jones C, Hutcheson K. S668 FLIP distensibility index correlates with radiation dose in cancer patients with radiation exposure and dysphagia. Am J Gastroenterol. 2024;119(10S):S461–3. https://doi.org/10.14309/01.ajg.0001032040.02739.d7.
31. Kahn A, Halland M, Fleischer DE. Self-dilation of refractory benign esophageal strictures. Am J Gastroenterol. 2022;117(3):364–6. https://doi.org/10.14309/ajg.0000000000001589. PMID: 34913874
32. Zhang T, Maclean J, Szczesniak M, Bertrand PP, Quon H, Tsang RK, Wu PI, Graham P, Cook IJ. Esophageal dysmotility in patients following total laryngectomy. Otolaryngol Head Neck Surg. 2018;158(2):323–30. https://doi.org/10.1177/0194599817736507. Epub 2017 Dec 12. PMID: 29231090
33. Stoner PL, Fullerton AL, Freeman AM, Chheda NN, Estores DS. Endoscopic dilation of refractory postlaryngectomy strictures: a case series and literature review. Gastroenterol Res Pract. 2019;2019:8905615. https://doi.org/10.1155/2019/8905615. PMID: 31275367; PMCID: PMC6558613
34. Cortina LE, Wu MP, Meyer CD, Feng AL, Varvares MA, Richmon JD, Deschler DG, Lin DT. Predictors of multiple dilations and functional outcomes after total laryngectomy and laryngopharyngectomy. Head Neck. 2024;46(1):138–44. https://doi.org/10.1002/hed.27545. Epub 2023 Oct 31. PMID: 37908173
35. Harris RL, Grundy A, Odutoye T. Radiologically guided balloon dilatation of neopharyngeal strictures following total laryngectomy and pharyngolaryngectomy: 21 years' experience. J Laryngol Otol. 2010;124(2):175–9. https://doi.org/10.1017/S0022215109991320. Epub 2009 Oct 20. PMID: 19840423
36. Regan J, Walshe M, Timon C, McMahon BP. Endoflip® evaluation of pharyngo-oesophageal segment tone and swallowing in a clinical population: a total laryngectomy case series. Clin Otolaryngol. 2015;40(2):121–9. https://doi.org/10.1111/coa.12337. PMID: 25314664
37. Jayaraj M, et al. Safety and efficacy of combined antegrade and retrograde endoscopic dilation for complete esophageal obstruction: a systematic review and meta-analysis. Ann Gastroenterol. 2019;32(4):361–9.
38. Liu D, et al. Outcomes of combined Antegrade-retrograde dilations for radiation-induced esophageal strictures in head and neck cancer patients. Dysphagia. 2021;36:1040.
39. Koutroumpakis F, Richards D. What's with the lump in the throat? Globus, dysphagia, and the role of the upper esophageal sphincter in laryngopharyngeal reflux disease. Otolaryngol Clin N Am. 2025;S0030-6665(25):00005–2. https://doi.org/10.1016/j.otc.2025.01.005. Epub ahead of print. PMID: 40133104
40. Wang Y, Liang Q, Luo J, Miao H, Qin G, Bao Y. Laryngopharyngeal reflux in otolaryngology-head and neck surgery clinic: an epidemiological survey. Ear Nose Throat J. 2024:1455613241301601. https://doi.org/10.1177/01455613241301601. Epub ahead of print. PMID: 39567883
41. Lechien JR, Vaezi MF, Chan WW, Allen JE, Karkos PD, Saussez S, Altman KW, Amin MR, Ayad T, Barillari MR, Belafsky PC, Blumin JH, Johnston N, Bobin F, Broadhurst M, Ceccon FP, Calvo-Henriquez C, Eun YG, Chiesa-Estomba CM, Crevier-Buchman L, Clarke JO, Dapri G, Eckley CA, Finck C, Fisichella PM, Hamdan AL, Hans S, Huet K, Imamura R, Jobe BA, Hoppo T, Maron LP, Muls V, O'Rourke AK, Perazzo PS, Postma G, Prasad VMN, Remacle M, Sant'Anna GD, Sataloff RT, Savarino EV, Schindler A, Siupsinskiene N, Tseng PH, Zalvan CH, Zelenik K, Fraysse B, Bock JM, Akst LM, Carroll TL. The Dubai definition and diagnostic criteria of laryngopharyngeal reflux: the IFOS consensus. Laryngoscope. 2024;134(4):1614–24. https://doi.org/10.1002/lary.31134. Epub 2023 Nov 6. PMID: 37929860

11 Regional Disorders of Sensory-Motor Dysfunction: Esophagus

George Triadafilopoulos, David M. Richards, and Mehnaz A. Shafi

11.1 Esophagus

Gastroesophageal Reflux Disease (GERD) GERD is the most common cause of esophageal symptoms and mucosal injury, affecting about 10–20% of the population, albeit with significant geographical differences [1, 2]. Endoscopic evaluation of GERD symptoms involves an inspection for erosive esophagitis (according to the Los Angeles classification), diaphragmatic hiatus (Hill grade of flap valve), sliding hiatal hernia length, and inspection for Barrett's esophagus. Erosive reflux esophagitis (Los Angeles B or greater) and/or the presence of long-segment (≥3 cm) Barrett's esophagus, with Los Angeles C or D esophagitis constituting severe erosive disease (Fig. 11.1).

On endoscopy up to 80% of symptomatic patients will not have objective mucosal damage from reflux on endoscopy [3]. Such symptomatic patients may have overlap symptoms, simulating GERD, such as functional dyspepsia (acid indigestion), esophageal motility disorder (i.e., achalasia, or ineffective esophageal motility), or gastroparesis. In the absence of esophagitis on endoscopy, esophageal pH monitoring should be considered to prove pathologic esophageal acid exposure (defined as % esophageal pH < 4.0 > 6) and to classify the patient as having nonerosive reflux disease (NERD) or normal esophageal acid exposure (defined as % esophageal pH < 4.0 < 6). In the latter cases, when there is a high degree (>90%) of symptom correlation to acid events, patients are classified as having "hypersensitive" esophagus [4].

GERD is associated with impaired health-related quality of life, decreased productivity, and costs. Therefore, for the nearly nine million outpatient visits for

G. Triadafilopoulos (✉) · D. M. Richards · M. A. Shafi
Department of Gastroenterology, Hepatology and Nutrition, UT MD Anderson Cancer Center, Houston, TX, USA
e-mail: gtriadafilopoulo@mdanderson.org

G. Triadafilopoulos (ed.), *Onco-Neurogastroenterology*,
https://doi.org/10.1007/978-3-031-98848-6_11

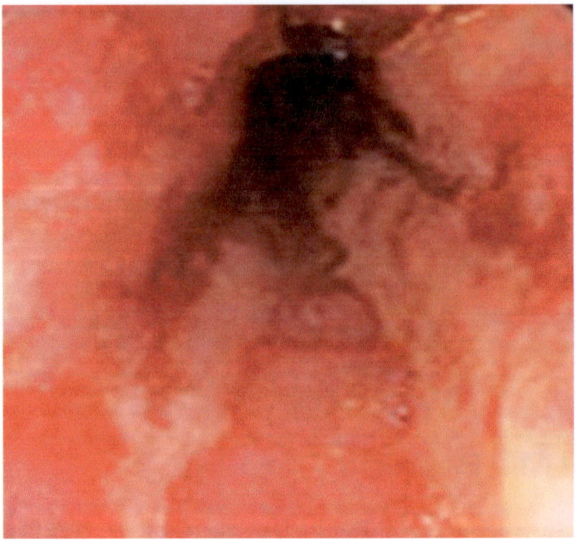

Fig. 11.1 Endoscopic appearance of LA grade C esophagitis, characterized by extensive ulcerations in the distal esophagus

GERD in the US per year, correct diagnosis, evaluation, and effective management of this chronic, relapsing disease that may alter quality of life and lead to serious complications (i.e., cancer) is imperative [5]. The typical symptoms of GERD are heartburn, esophageal chest pain, and regurgitation. Belching, hoarseness, chronic cough, and wheezing may be pathophysiologically, but not conclusively, related to reflux disease. The Lyon Consensus 2.0 provides a modern definition of actionable GERD, where evidence from esophageal testing supports revising, escalating, or personalizing GERD management for the symptomatic patient [6]. Clinical response to an empiric PPI trial alone is insufficient for a conclusive GERD diagnosis, since both heartburn and chest pain can arise from motor disorders [7]. Long duration of GERD symptoms predisposes patients to Barrett's esophagus (BE) and esophageal adenocarcinoma. GERD symptoms are also frequent in patients after oncologic surgery, such as Ivor-Lewis surgery or gastric resection. Recognizing, assessing, and managing GERD is a key mission for onco-neurogastroenterologists, mostly aiming at improving quality of life. The impact of such involvement on preventing cancer is unclear, mostly because of inadequate screening for Barrett's esophagus [8]. The increasing prevalence of obesity and central adiposity contributing to GERD symptoms and esophageal cancer will certainly justify more focused attention on this condition, beyond over the counter use of acid suppressive therapies [9]. Several novel endoscopic techniques have been introduced for the management of GERD, providing minimally invasive ways to eliminate pharmacologic acid inhibition and the need for antireflux surgery, minimizing short- and long-term adverse effects. The respective strengths and weaknesses of such therapies and their applicability to patients with GERD vis-à-vis other minimally invasive therapies, such as magnetic sphincter augmentation (LINX), are subjects of ongoing clinical research and debate [10]. Figure 11.2 outlines aspects of GERD management that would be best

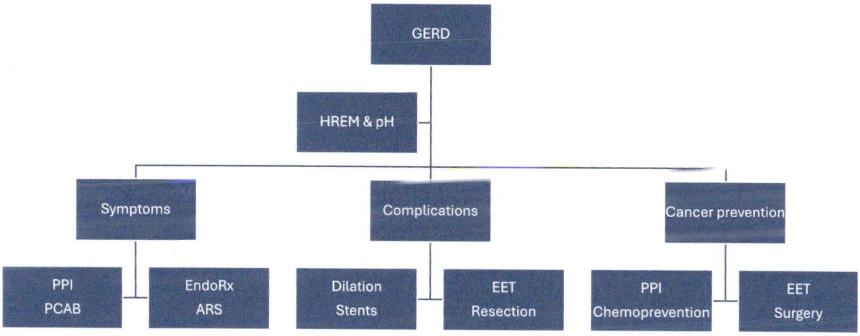

Fig. 11.2 Key aspects of GERD management. A significant overlap exists with Barrett's esophagus, a predisposing factor to esophageal adenocarcinoma, under the influence of acid and bile reflux

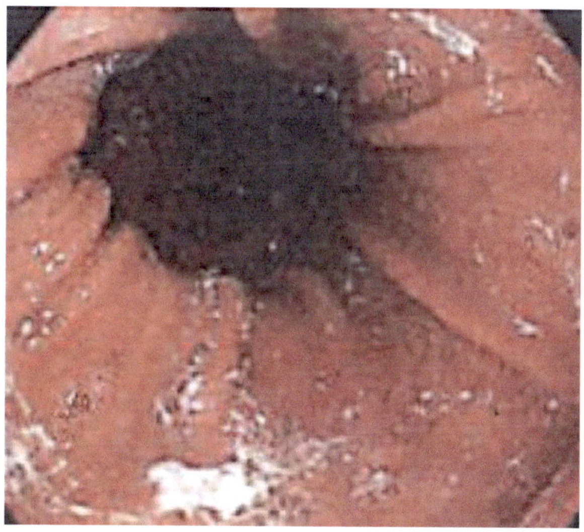

Fig. 11.3 Antegrade view of a large sliding (axial) hiatal hernia in a patient with refractory GERD. Note the gastric folds above a gaping hiatus, conducive to frequent and at times prolonged acid reflux episodes, particularly in the supine position and at night. She ultimately required laparoscopic hernia repair with partial fundoplication with symptomatic relief

coordinated through a specialized center, although specific clinical and cost outcome data are currently lacking. Key in this process is the availability of HREM and ambulatory esophageal pH monitoring.

The complementary use of both these modalities allows not only the exclusion of other conditions (i.e., esophageal achalasia, scleroderma) but also an appreciation of the magnitude and pathophysiologic significance of underlying functional esophageal impairment (i.e., ineffective esophageal motility, IEM), if any [11]. In practice, patients with symptoms suggestive of GERD, such as chest pain, heartburn, regurgitation, and dysphagia, are typically treated initially with a course of proton pump inhibitors (PPIs). The evaluation of patients who have either not responded at all or they have partially and inadequately responded to such therapy requires a more detailed history and may involve an endoscopy to rule out sliding hiatal hernia (Fig. 11.3) and esophageal biopsies (to rule out complications, such as Barrett's esophagus), followed by esophageal manometry, ambulatory esophageal pH monitoring, and gastric emptying scanning (to rule out underlying silent gastroparesis) [12].

Figure 11.2 also synthesizes the essential aspects of GERD management, based on properly characterized diagnosis, endoscopic, manometric, and histologic. Such characterization is then followed by an assessment of disease severity, an effort to predict and modify disease course, as well as consideration of the risk for neoplasia for each individual patient [13]. Classifying patients into low or high risk for complications facilitates the decision on the need, intensity, and duration of pharmacologic therapy and the decision for antireflux surgery (ARS). Further, treat-to-target medical, endoscopic, or surgical efforts, instituted early and tightly monitored, may improve long-term outcomes. Barium radiography, high-resolution manometry, and pH monitoring allow better prediction of disease evolution and may guide the need for surgery to control symptoms and curtail disease severity [14]. In patients with increased neoplasia risk (those with Barrett's esophagus), surveillance with biopsies or other biomarkers and endoscopic eradication therapy (EET) may need to be implemented [15]. Additionally, recently introduced new technologies, either diagnostic (optical coherence tomography, OCT) or therapeutic (radiofrequency ablation RFA or balloon cryotherapy (BC), magnetic sphincter augmentation MSA or LINX) are increasingly used [16, 17]. Diagnostic and prognostic tools, such as WATS-3D (wide-area transepithelial sampling with three-dimensional analysis), a specialized brush biopsy, and TissueCypher, a molecular test designed to predict the risk of progression from BE to cancer are poised to enhance our ability to control and monitor disease over time [18, 19].

Symptom control in GERD is accomplished using diet and lifestyle modifications, and most often pharmacologically using acid blockers, such as antacids and H2-receptor antagonists (H2RA), proton pump inhibitors (PPI) and more recently, potassium-competitive acid blockers (PCABs). If symptoms are inadequately controlled (refractory GERD), various endoscopic therapies, such radiofrequency (Stretta) or transoral incisionless fundoplication (TIF), or antireflux surgery (with hiatal hernia repair, as needed) may be tried (Fig. 11.4) [15, 20].

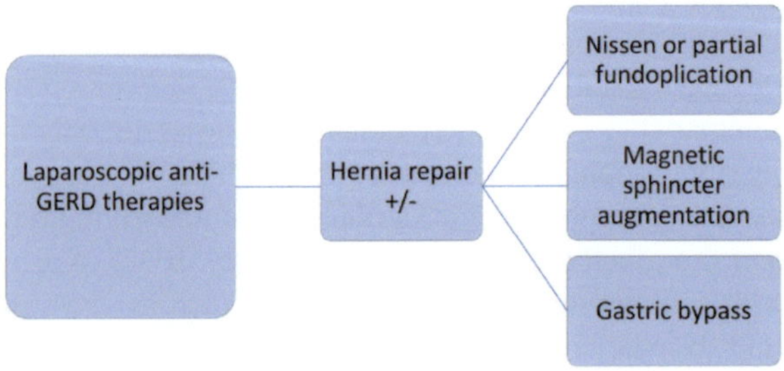

Fig. 11.4 Laparoscopic antireflux approaches to be considered in patients with refractory GERD. Decision-making needs to be highly individualized and carefully considered to avoid operative failures or recurrences. An exchange between the onco-neurogastroenterologist and the surgeon is essential to proper planning

Table 11.1 Common HREM abnormalities in patients with GERD

Variable	Value
LES length (*n* = >3 cm)	Short
LES resting pressure (*n* = 20–40 mmHg)	Normal or low
Median IRP (*n* = <15 mmHg)	Normal
LES-CD separation (*n* = <1 cm; no hiatal hernia)	Absent or present (hiatal hernia)
Intact esophageal body peristalsis (DCI >450)	Mostly (70%) present
Weak (DCI 100–450)	Present or absent
Failed (DCI <100)	Rarely present
Distal latency (DL) (*n* = >4.5 s)	Normal or low
Complete bolus clearance	Normal, impaired or absent

Complications, such as strictures, are typically managed endoscopically using serial bougies, or through the scope (TTS) balloon dilations and removable self-expanding stents (SEMS). Barrett's esophagus with dysplasia is increasingly managed by endoscopic eradication therapy (EET), using radiofrequency (HALO) or cryoballoon ablation (for flat mucosa), endoscopic mucosal resection (EMR), or endoscopic submucosal dissection (ESD) (for nodular mucosa), or a combination of ablation and resection techniques. Cancer prevention aims to effectively contain acid and bile reflux [21, 22], ideally together with chemoprevention using aspirin or cyclo-oxygenase inhibitors [23, 24] or using EET or resective surgery for high-grade dysplasia [25].

Table 11.1 depicts common HREM abnormalities in patients with GERD. Important parameters that denote more severe disease (including Barrett's esophagus) are short LESP, low LES resting pressure, sliding hiatal hernia, and impaired esophageal body contractility [26].

In all patients with gastroesophageal reflux symptoms, but more so in patients with cancer in whom the integrity of esophageal function might have been compromised by radiation or resection, one should consider the essential mechanisms—protective or conducive—to reflux. Obesity, sliding (axial) hiatal hernia, and/or prior bariatric surgery may also contribute. Figure 11.5 highlights the key parameters of esophagogastric junction physiology, and the thoraco-abdominal relations involved. The negative intrathoracic pressure as compared to the positive intrabdominal pressure creates a gradient favoring influx into the thorax of gastric contents, but this is inhibited by a competent lower esophageal sphincter pressure (LESP). In contrast, a sliding (axial) hiatal hernia facilitates such reflux by displacing or weakening the sphincter. Most patients with GERD, particularly those with nonerosive disease, suffer from increased frequency of transient lower esophageal sphincter relaxations (tLESRs), which are allowing short-lived acid reflux events to occur in the distal esophagus and give rise to symptoms.

Wireless, ambulatory esophageal pH measurement (Bravo pH) provides an objective tool for the diagnosis and management of GERD. The test is used to confirm pathological distal esophageal acid exposure in patients with reflux symptoms that fail to respond to acid suppressive therapy, to correlate reflux events and symptoms, and to validate the presence of pathologic esophageal acid exposure in patients considered as candidates for antireflux surgery [27]. In clinical practice, pH

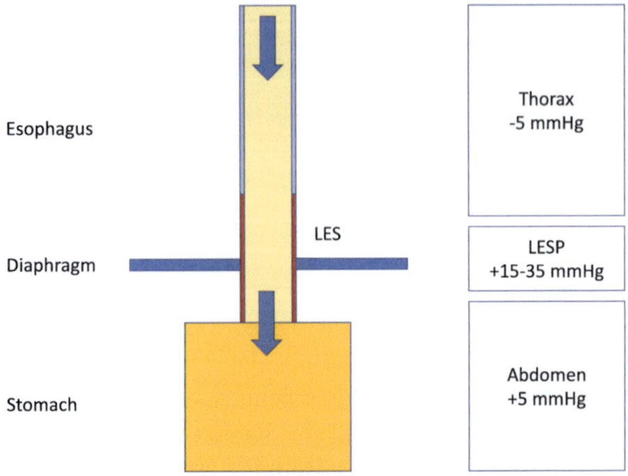

Fig. 11.5 Thoraco-abdominal relations protective to reflux. An intact LESP is essential

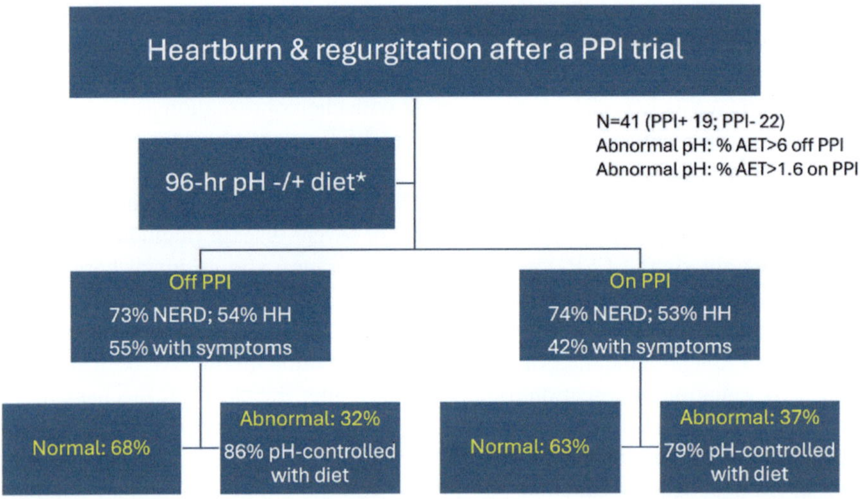

Fig. 11.6 Bravo pH outcomes in two cohorts of patients with ongoing heartburn and regurgitation after an empiric PPI trial who were tested off- and on-PPI. Both cohorts had ongoing esophageal pathologic acid exposure in >30% of cases, mostly (>80%) controlled with dietary restriction. PPI use reduced but did not eliminate reflux symptoms and had a marginally favorable impact on symptom perception (symptom association probability, SAP)

measurements can be very useful in assessing all such patients, establishing the diagnosis by pH criteria, and identifying who may truly benefit from long-term PPI use. Given emerging data regarding PPI adverse effects, increasing patient anxiety regarding treatment and financial implications, Bravo pH that objectively assesses distal esophageal acid reflux events and correlates them with reflux symptoms is clinically valuable. Figure 11.6 summarizes an assessment of the practical value of Bravo pH study in the diagnosis and management of patients presenting with refractory GERD either off- or on-PPI therapy and under dietary conditions that favor or

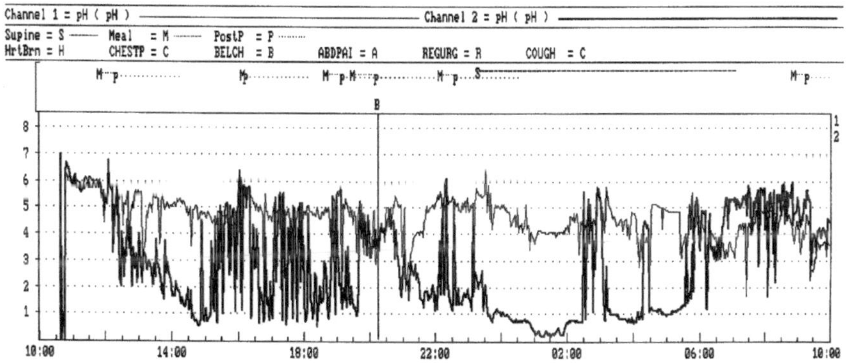

Fig. 11.7 Dual (esophageal and gastric) ambulatory 24-h pH monitoring study. This 48-year-old woman without symptoms while on PPI; 24-h pH study on omeprazole 40 mg bid. % time intra-esophageal pH < 4.0: 11; DeMeester score: 60.8; % time intra-gastric pH < 4.0: 44. Despite the lack of symptoms, she still has persistent pathologic intra-esophageal acid exposure that results from incomplete inhibition of acid secretion, particularly at night (gastric nocturnal acid break-through). The thin black line represents the intra-esophageal pH recording (sensor is located 5 cm above the esophagogastric junction); the thick black line depicts the intra-gastric pH (sensor is in the proximal, acid secretory portion of the stomach)

impede GER, using a standard, validated protocol [28]. Performing the pH study off-PPI, the most frequent approach, establishes the presence or not of pathologic esophageal acid exposure, further defining GERD and its magnitude by pH criteria. In contrast, a pH study performed on PPI assesses the adequacy or not of acid inhibition in patients who report symptoms while on therapy.

Abnormal intra-esophageal pH profile on PPI is frequent (up to 50%) in patients with BE who also tend to be free of symptoms while on PPI therapy.

Despite its short recording time (24 h) and the unpleasant experience it carries, the use of dual transnasal pH probe has the advantage of simultaneously recording both distal esophageal acid exposure and proximal intragastric pH. When performed on PPI therapy, the study provides a perspective on the degree of intragastric acidity over 24 h and the magnitude of PPI-induced hypochlorhydria (Fig. 11.7).

Barrett's Esophagus The diagnosis of Barrett's esophagus (BE), a common condition associated with GERD, is based on characteristic endoscopic findings (salmon-colored mucosa) (Fig. 11.8) that are confirmed by pathology showing specialized intestinal metaplasia (acid mucin-containing goblet cells). BE is endoscopically categorized into short-segment (≤3 cm, SSBE) or long-segment (>3 cm, LSBE). Since 2006, the Prague classification has been the standard for measuring the length of Barrett's esophagus. The lower measurement boundary is formed by the proximal cardial notch (upon moderate insufflation), and the two upper measurement boundaries are marked by the proximal limit of the circumferential Barrett's segment (C) and the longest tongue of Barrett's (M) [29]. BE is staged as non-dysplastic (no cancerous tissue present), low-grade dysplasia (minor cytologic

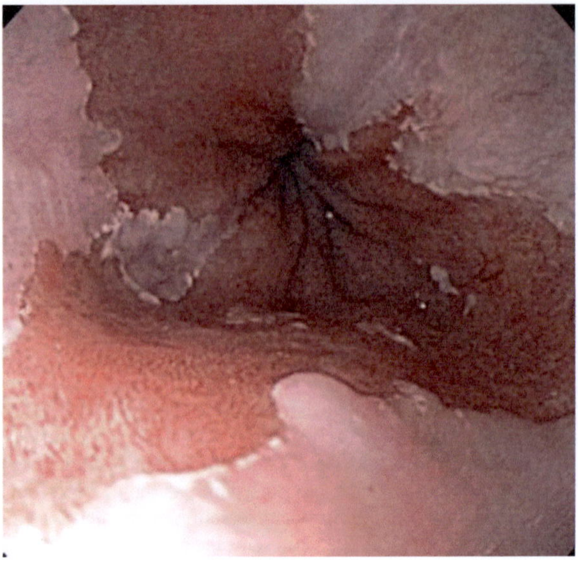

Fig. 11.8 Typical endoscopic appearance of short-segment Barrett's esophagus (SSBE) involving the distal esophagus. Mucosal projections of salmon-colored mucosa are extending upward from the esophagogastric junction to the squamous (pink) esophageal mucosa. There are no areas of nodularity to suggest dysplasia within the BE segment. The lack of erosions or inflammation within or around it will allow reliable histologic assessment of biopsies obtained

changes seen) and high-grade dysplasia (extensive cellular changes are found, but not yet cancer) and with intramucosal or invasive cancer. Patients with SSBE typically have a shorter history of GER symptoms or no symptoms and a lower incidence of dysplasia. Further, patients with SSBE have upright reflux, higher LES pressures, and better contractility than those with LSBE. In contrast, patients with LSBE have more severe, bi-positional and proximal reflux and a 15 times higher for esophageal adenocarcinoma. As such, patients with LSBE should be managed more aggressively and with more frequent surveillance.

BE is associated with altered esophageal sensation and motility, which impair symptom perception of acid reflux events and acid clearance due to frequently underlying ineffective esophageal motility (IEM). BE is the only known precursor to esophageal adenocarcinoma, a highly lethal cancer with an increasing incidence over the last five decades [30]. Yet, only 39% of screening-eligible patients undergo endoscopic screening, followed—as needed—by aggressive ablative and/or resective therapy and surveillance. Most of the examinations were triggered by refractory GERD symptoms rather than screening referrals [31]. This is why we advocate consideration of a tandem screening endoscopy for both BE and gastric cancer (GC), based on national guidelines, on all patients referred for screening or surveillance colonoscopy. Figure 11.9 depicts the % prevalence of intestinal metaplasia in various locations of the stomach and distal esophagus in a study of 317 individuals who did not originally volunteer any foregut symptoms, but they qualified for endoscopy based on questionnaires structured by national screening guidelines. In this study, classic BE was endoscopically discernable in only 2.2% of cases [32].

Implementation of precision therapy in BE (Fig. 11.10) is based on detailed demographic and phenotypic characterization allowing for maximization and

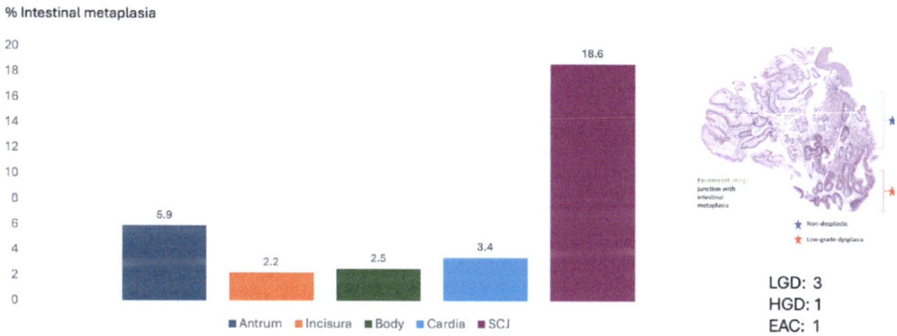

Fig. 11.9 Histologic % prevalence of foregut intestinal metaplasia, low-grade dysplasia (LGD), high-grade dysplasia (HGD), and esophageal adenocarcinoma (EAC)

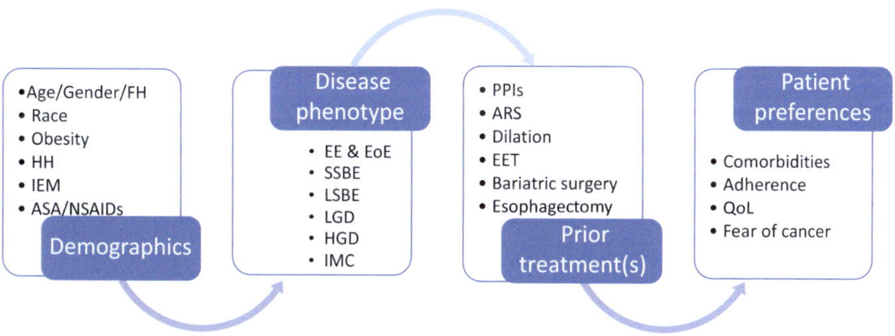

Fig. 11.10 Precision management of Barrett's esophagus

optimization of treatments based on individual features and patient preferences. Because of its multifaceted nature, BE is a key target for the onco-neurogastroenterologist. Erosive esophagitis (EE), at times with confluent esophageal ulcers, bleeding, and stricture formation, occur frequently in LSBE and independently increase the risk for BE fivefold. Aggressive treatment of EE, based on data obtained using HREM and esophageal pH monitoring, not only facilitates the endoscopic recognition and histologic assessment of dysplasia but favorably affects the natural history of the disease.

Several, sometimes overlapping, esophageal functional abnormalities may be seen in patients with BE. Characterizing esophageal motor physiology may help to risk-stratify patients, since reduced esophageal contractility is independently associated with dysplastic progression [33]. As compared with other GERD phenotypes, esophageal acid exposure, particularly supine, is significantly higher, and weakly acidic reflux and duodeno-gastroesophageal reflux are more common. The metaplastic epithelium reduces esophageal mucosal impedance, sometimes to the point that prevents detection of reflux episodes. Ineffective esophageal motility (IEM) and lower esophageal sphincter basal pressure hypotonicity are also more common in BE patients (Figs. 11.11 and 11.12). Underlying reduced chemoreceptor and

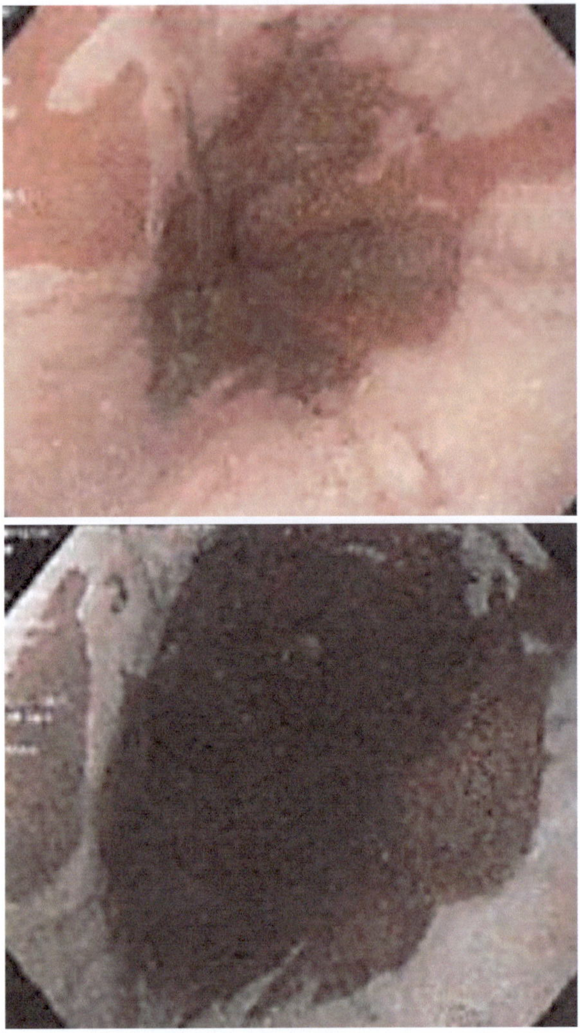

Fig. 11.11 Endoscopic images of a patient with GERD symptoms despite twice-daily PPI therapy, associated long-segment BE. (Top): White light endoscopy revealing circumferential BE, mucosal projections (tongues) of BE (salmon-colored) and interspersed islands (pink) of squamous mucosa. (Bottom): Narrowband imaging (NBI) of the distal esophagus in the same patient, used to better define areas of dysplasia in consideration of endoscopic eradication therapy (EET). In this case, the BE mucosa did not show any abnormalities suggestive of dysplasia

mechanoreceptor sensitivity to acid and balloon distention may explain the reduced or absent symptom perception in up to 50% of BE patients. Using a multimodal probe for mechanical, thermal, electrical, and chemical (acid) stimulation of the esophagus, BE patients demonstrate reduced sensory perception thresholds compared with normal controls. Thankfully, many BE patients regain esophageal sensitivity after successful endoscopic eradication therapy [34].

BE exemplifies the importance of the onco-neurogastroenterologist in long-term management (Fig. 11.13). Through their involvement at the precancer stage, not only aggressive endoscopic screening is emphasized at the population level [32, 35], but aggressive acid and bile reflux control is instituted aiming at symptom control and cancer chemoprevention [36]. Available options for an "active"

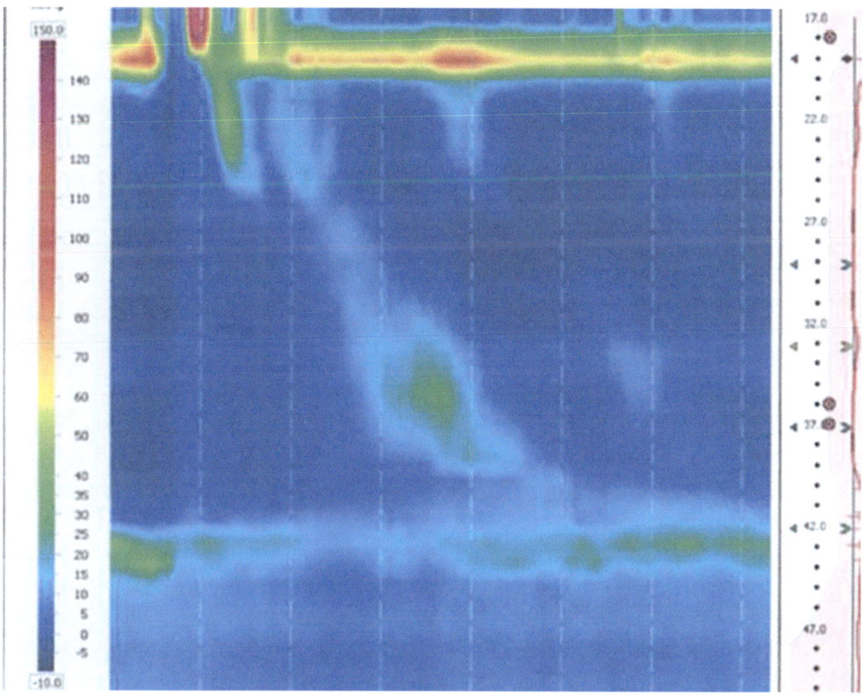

Fig. 11.12 High-resolution esophageal manometry revealing LES hypotonicity, hiatal hernia, and ineffective esophageal motility (DCI 350) in a patient with refractory heartburn and underlying long-segment BE

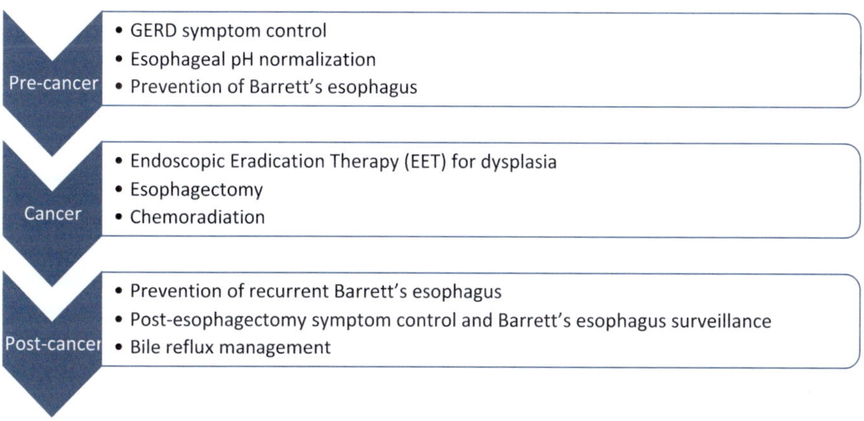

Fig. 11.13 Endpoints in the management of BE at the precancer (screening, therapy, and surveillance), cancer (EET, surgery), and post-cancer stages (prevention or recurrence and symptom control) of the discasc

Table 11.2 Available options for an "active" management of Barrett's esophagus. This is in contrast to the "passive" approach of periodic endoscopic surveillance aiming only at dysplasia detection, largely practiced

Active management of Barrett's esophagus	Options
Control of GERD symptoms	PPI qd
Healing of co-existing esophagitis	PPI bid
Prevention of recurrent esophagitis	PPI bid
Control of bile relfux	Fundoplication
Prevention of stricture formation	PPI bid; fundoplication
Regression/elimination of Barrett's surface	EET + PPI bid
Regression/elimination of dysplasia	EET + PPI bid
Chemoprevention of dysplasia and adenocarcinoma	PPI bid + ASA (or COX-2)

management of Barrett's esophagus are listed in Table 11.2. At the cancer stage, clinical outcomes are enhanced through pH and bile reflux optimization, using medical [37] or surgical (antireflux) measures [38], based on the underlying physiology. Post-cancer management aims at GERD symptom control and prevention of recurrence of Barrett's esophagus with routine endoscopic surveillance and acid and bile reflux optimization, driven by proper assessment of foregut motility [39].

Figure 11.14 depicts the evolution of GERD, starting from acid-induced esophageal injury, inflammation, induction of esophageal metaplasia (Barrett's esophagus), followed by evolution to low- and high-grade dysplasia and eventually esophageal adenocarcinoma, under the influence of luminal elements coming into direct contact with the mucosa (i.e., acid or bile), other factors (i.e., gender, race, obesity), and genetic alterations.

The progression of BE to dysplasia and adenocarcinoma is linked to increased and disordered proliferation that is related to several factors. Reduced esophageal acid sensitivity in BE allows ongoing, poorly recognized, and untreated reflux. In ex vivo organ culture experiments, cell proliferation is increased after exposure to short pulses of acid, while proliferation is reduced in BE specimens taken from patients with esophageal acid exposure normalized by antisecretory therapy. In long-term clinical studies, consistent and profound esophageal acid suppression using PPIs decreases cell proliferation, as assessed by proliferating cell nuclear antigen (PCNA) expression, while it increases differentiation as assessed by villin expression in BE. Increased cyclooxygenase-2 (COX-2) expression and activity at baseline and after pulses of acid or bile salts have also been noted in ex vivo studies. In clinical practice, PPIs relieve symptoms and induce partial regression to squamous epithelium, but abnormal esophageal acid exposure and the risk for dysplasia or adenocarcinoma persist in many patients. The combined treatment of esomeprazole 40 mg bid and aspirin 325 mg qd significantly decreased mucosal prostaglandin E2 content and all treatments containing esomeprazole significantly reduced proliferating cell nuclear antigen (PCNA) expression in patients with Barrett's esophagus (Fig. 11.15) [40].

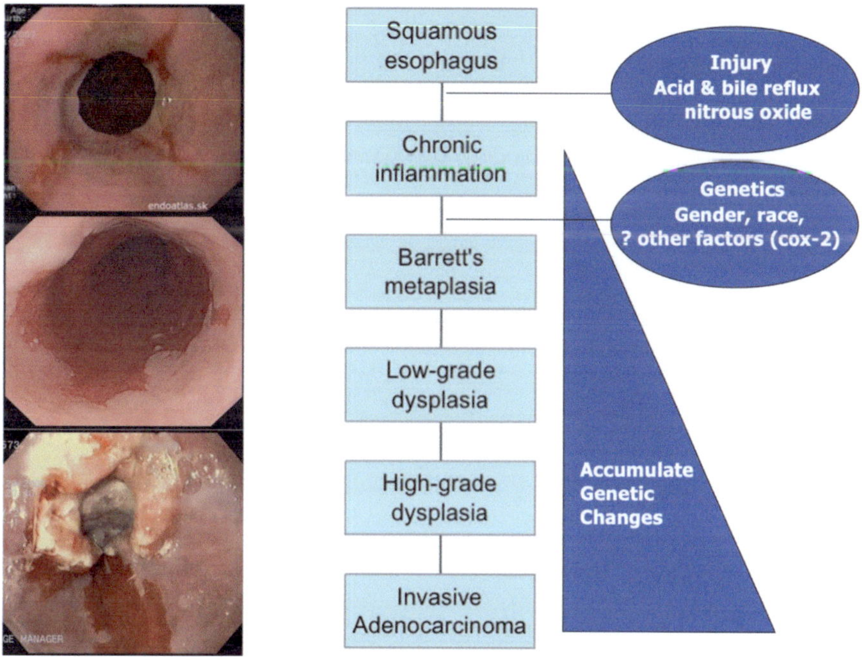

Fig. 11.14 Sequential evolution of GERD toward esophageal adenocarcinoma. Currently, ample opportunities for intervention exist along this path, if properly considered

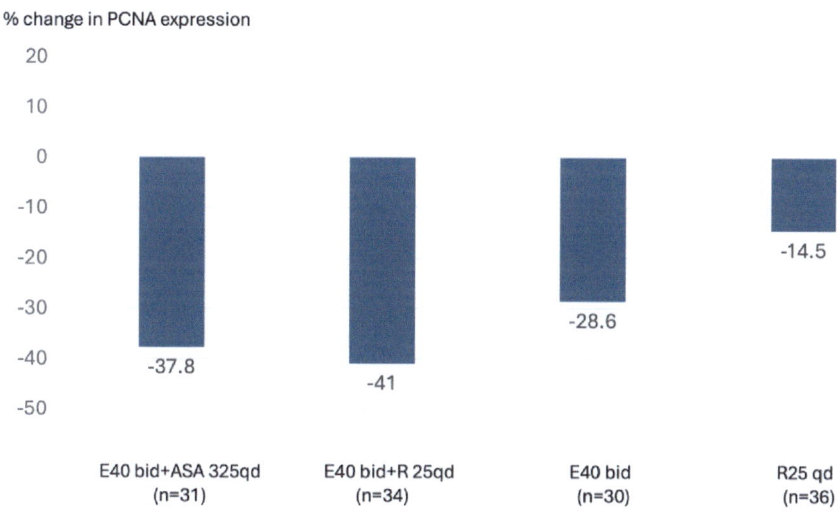

Fig. 11.15 PCNA expression in response to cyclooxygenase inhibition of PGE-2 release with and without high-dose acid suppression

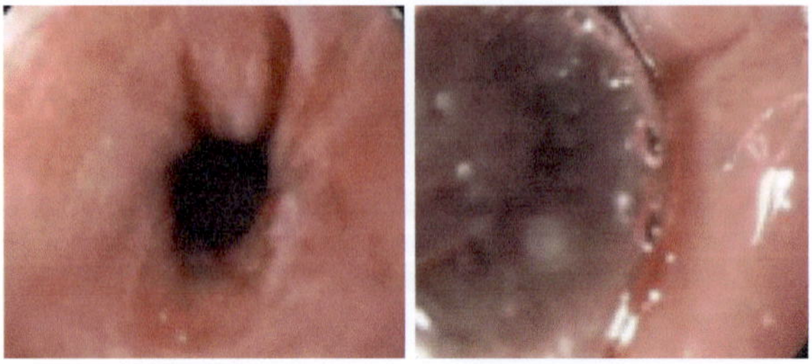

Fig. 11.16 Endoscopic appearance of a peptic esophageal stricture (left) and at the time of balloon (through-the-scope, TTS) dilation

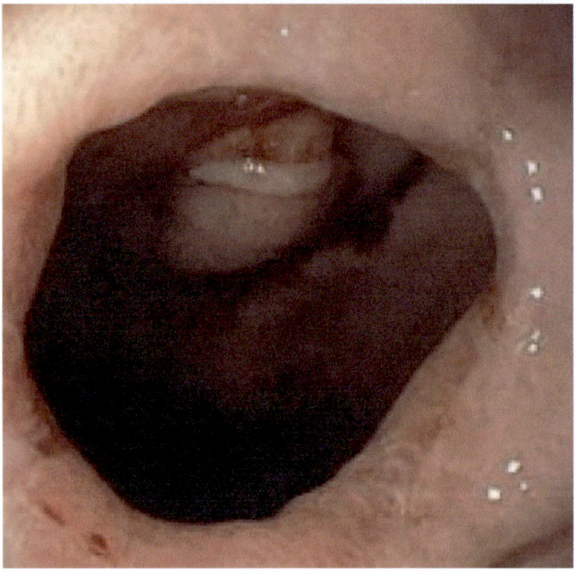

Fig. 11.17 Endoscopic appearance of an inflamed distal esophageal ring, proximal to a sliding hiatal hernia, that had led to food bolus impaction. The ring was dilated using a through the scope (TTS) to 15 mm, followed by oral omeprazole 20 mg daily, with long-lasting relief of solid food dysphagia

Esophageal Stricture Esophageal strictures may be malignant or benign. Most benign strictures result from long-standing GERD, and they are treated by endoscopic dilation combined with long-term proton pump inhibitors (Fig. 11.16). Differentiation from distal esophageal (Schatzki's) ring proximal to a sliding hiatal hernia may be challenging when the ring is inflamed from a recent episode of food impaction (Fig. 11.17). Regardless, endoscopic dilation, followed by PPI therapy to prevent recurrences, is needed in both conditions.

Increasingly, eosinophilic esophagitis is recognized, particularly in atopic individuals. Other causes for benign esophageal strictures are radiation therapy, caustic ingestion, esophageal surgical anastomosis, prior ablative therapy, or endoscopic resection, particularly endoscopic submucosal resection (ESD) or combined eradication therapy for Barrett's esophagus. Variceal ligation, epidermolysis bullosa, lichen planus, and pemphigus are rarely encountered. Based on their endoscopic or radiologic appearance, benign strictures can be classified as simple or complex. Simple esophageal strictures are smooth, short, and concentric and often allow the passage of the endoscope. Complex strictures are longer than 2 cm, angulated, irregular, with severely narrowed lumen compromising the passage of the endoscope, and are frequently associated with large hiatal hernia or esophageal diverticula. In patients with complex strictures, biopsies from the stricture to exclude malignancy are imperative. Strictures that are not successfully dilated to a diameter of 14 mm over five endoscopic sessions at 2-week intervals are defined as refractory. To reduce the chances for complications, simple esophageal strictures are dilated by no more than three push (bougie) dilators (typically over guidewire) of progressively larger diameter or no more than three incremental balloon inflation sizes during a single session. For narrow, long, and complex strictures, only one or two balloon dilations of 1 mm each should be performed per session [41]. Since complex strictures, particularly those associated with a large hiatal hernia, may be associated with underlying esophageal dysmotility, their refractoriness to dilation may be due to underlying muscle dysfunction. In most cases, dilation to 16 mm should be adequate to relieve dysphagia and higher levels of endoscopic dilation may carry unjustifiable risks for complications. Long-term therapy with proton pump inhibitors, typically twice daily, is needed to control ongoing acid reflux and prevent recurrences.

Immune Checkpoint Inhibitor (ICI) Esophagitis ICI therapy-related esophagitis is rare and often occurs in conjunction with nausea, emesis, and dysphagia. While the diagnosis is one of exclusion, the disease often remains mild, is rarely associated with complications, and can be managed with proton pump inhibitors or H2 receptor blockers. To what degree ICI esophagitis is related to underlying esophageal body dysmotility is unclear [42].

Achalasia and Cancer-Associated Achalasia (CAA) Achalasia is a well-characterized esophageal motility disorder with an incidence of approximately 1 per 100,000 persons per year and a prevalence of 10 per 100,000 persons. Secondary achalasia (pseudo-achalasia) is typically a benign (30%) or malignant (cancer-associated (70%) disorder resulting in clinical, radiographic, and manometric features indistinguishable from primary achalasia, characterized by incomplete relaxation of the lower esophageal sphincter and absence of peristalsis in the esophageal body (Fig. 11.18). There may be various mechanisms for secondary achalasia (i.e., infiltration, neuronal degradation, paraneoplastic), but its main distinguishing feature is the complete reversal after successful therapy of the underlying malignancy. Onco-neural antibodies, such as anti-Hu antibody (also known as antineuronal nuclear antibody-type 1, ANNA-1), anti-CV2/CRMP-5 antibodies, and anti-ganglionic AchR antibodies, are important in defining the diagnosis. True malignant pseudo-achalasia accounts for 3–4% of all achalasia cases and is characterized by onset in old age, shorter duration of dysphagia, and rapid and significant weight loss [43]. In a retrospective review, hematologic malignancies were the most common cancers associated with achalasia, seen in 25% of cases. Stage IV cancer was the presenting stage in 56% of solid tumors. Cancer preceded the achalasia in 95% patients with a median time interval of 56 months. Active cancer was present

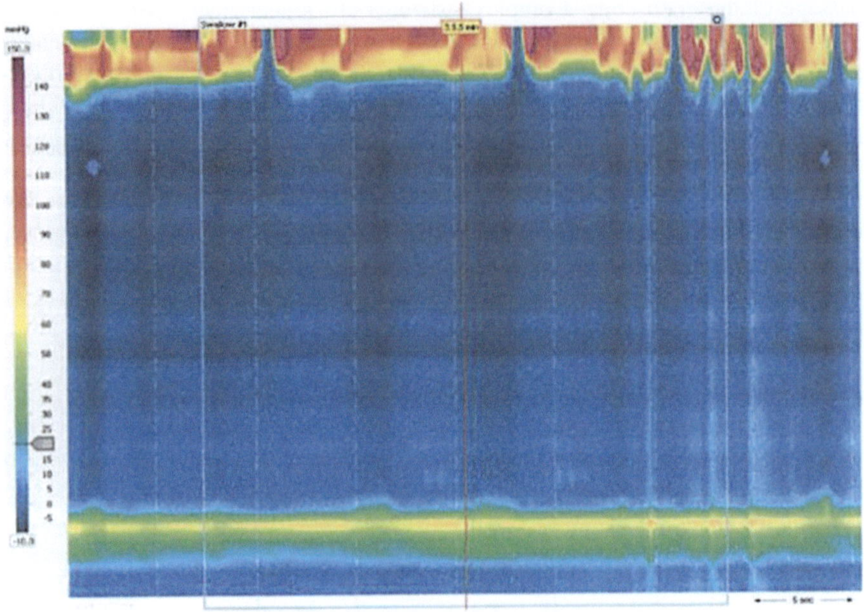

Fig. 11.18 High-resolution esophageal manometry revealing type I esophageal achalasia. There is absent esophageal body peristalsis and lack of LES relaxation upon swallowing

at the time of achalasia in 67.5% of cases [44]. Treatment options need to be tailored accordingly and vary from therapy of the underlying cancer to local therapies, such as BoTox of the EGJ or pneumatic dilation to POEM.

Long-standing idiopathic achalasia confers an increased risk of esophageal cancer, both squamous cell carcinoma (SCC) and esophageal adenocarcinoma (EAC), compared with the general population. The hypothesized pathophysiology for higher SCC risk in those with achalasia reflects a markedly delayed esophageal clearance of food and oropharyngeal secretions leading to stasis esophagitis, and for EAC, poor clearance of refluxed gastric contents (acid and bile). The diagnosis of esophageal cancer in patients with achalasia may be delayed because dysphagia is often attributed to recurring or deteriorating disease. Current society guidelines do not recommend routine endoscopic surveillance for esophageal carcinoma in patients with achalasia [45]. Nevertheless, alarm symptoms, such as weight loss or anemia, acute onset of dysphagia, food bolus impaction, or odynophagia (usually due to Candida infection or cancer), call for an endoscopy for both diagnosis and therapy. Figure 11.19 depicts a barium esophagogram revealing severe esophageal dilation and tortuosity in a patient with cancer-associated achalasia secondary to EAC. EndoFLIP is an increasingly used modality to assess the incomplete LES relaxation in achalasia before and after therapy (Fig. 11.20).

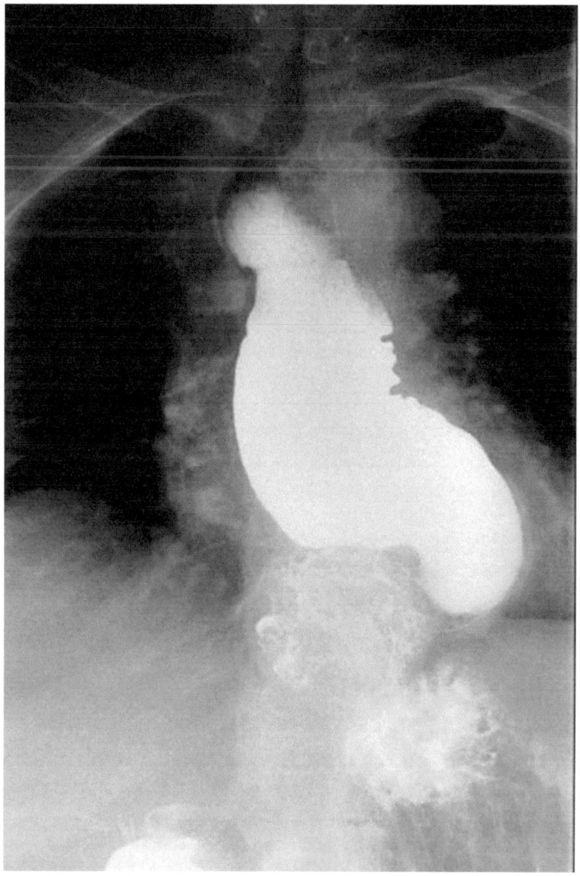

Fig. 11.19 Barium esophagogram revealing severe esophageal dilation and tortuosity in a patient with cancer-associated achalasia secondary to EAC

Ineffective Esophageal Motility (IEM) The etiology and clinical impact of ineffective esophageal motility (IEM) remain poorly understood. Unless gastroesophageal acid reflux (GERD) is identified, symptomatic patients with IEM are challenging to treat. According to the Chicago 4.0 classification, a conclusive diagnosis of IEM is manometric and requires more than 70% ineffective swallows or at least 50% failed peristalsis (Fig. 11.21) [46].

About one third of patients with GERD symptoms are found to have IEM when studied by HREM and 2/3 of them have abnormal esophageal acid exposure. GER symptoms are not discriminatory in patients with IEM with and without underlying pathologic acid reflux. IEM appears to be an early, primary event, eventually associated with pathologic acid exposure, particularly supine. Higher BMI is also associated with abnormal esophageal acid exposure in such patients. Clinical response to PPI depends on the presence of pathologic acid reflux. Those with IEM and normal acid exposure remain symptomatic and mostly resistant to therapy [47].

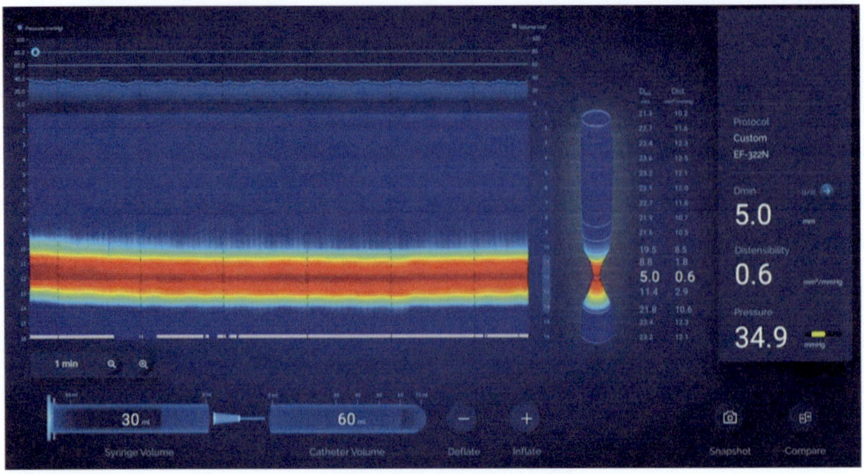

Fig. 11.20 EndoFLIP study showing absent contractility and low DI (0.6) in a patient with type II achalasia

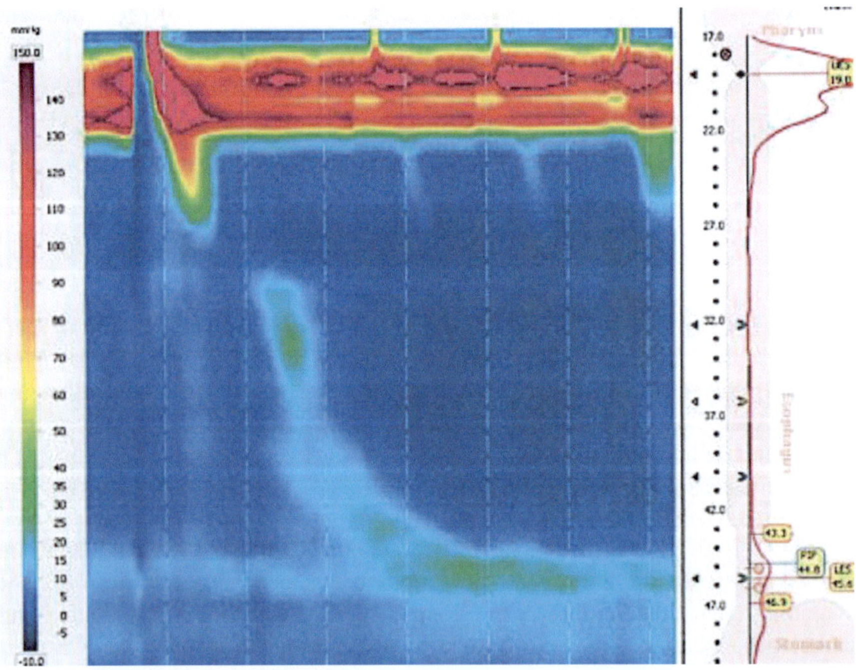

Fig. 11.21 HREM image of a patient with IEM (% failed contractions: 60; % weak 30; DCI 417)

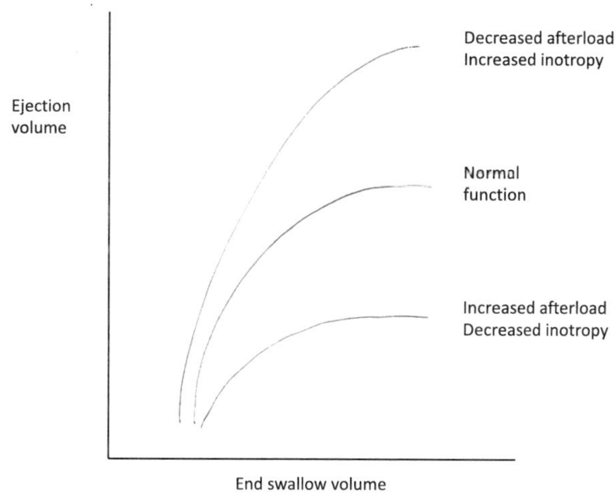

Fig. 11.22 Relationships among ejection volume, end swallowing volume (residual), and effective contractility (inotropy)

To better understand and treat IEM and other esophageal motility disorders (i.e., achalasia, IEM), one should conceptualize esophageal preload, afterload, and contractility. Preload is the initial stretching of the esophageal muscle prior to contraction. It is related to filling and accommodation. Afterload is the load against which the esophagus contracts to eject the bolus or refluxed material into the stomach. Afterload goes down when LES pressure decreases during relaxation. Contractility is the intrinsic strength of the esophageal muscle independent of preload, but a change in preload will affect the force of contraction (Laplace law). As we examine swallowing, end swallow volume is the volume of esophageal contents after bolus ejection. Inotropy is the impact of pharmacologic agents (inotropes) on the esophageal muscle, affecting the rate of fiber contraction. Positive inotropes increase and negative inotropes decrease esophageal contractility. Ejection volume is the amount (ml) ejected from the esophagus per swallow. Figure 11.22 highlights these relationships and helps guide therapy.

Dysmotility Following ESD Some patients complain of dysphagia after endoscopic submucosal dissection (ESD) for the treatment of superficial esophageal cancer, even without any endoscopically visible postoperative strictures. The circumferential mucosal defect ratio, endoscopic balloon dilation, and repeated ESD are predictors for impaired esophageal motility and dysphagia, presumably resulting from myenteric nerve plexus damage and/or direct electric damage to the proper muscle layer, leading to muscle atrophy [48].

Medication-Induced Esophageal Dysfunction Opioids, particularly oxycodone or hydrocodone, are frequently used by patients with cancer and they may be associated with type III achalasia, EGJOO, and DES, in turn causing dysphagia and regurgitation. Withdrawing the opioid—if feasible—and repeating the manometry study are ideal to see if the abnormality resolves. Invasive treatment options, such as POEM or surgical myotomy, should be avoided. If opioid withdrawal is not an option, consideration should be made toward changing to tramadol, a partial agonist. If symptoms persist, endoscopic botulinum toxin injection should be considered [49].

Medication-Induced Esophageal injury (Drug-Induced Esophagitis) If tablets are ingested with minimal amount of water and in a supine position or before sleep, the medication may stagnate within the esophagus and result in tissue mucosal damage. This may also occur if there is underlying impaired motility (i.e., IEM, achalasia). Potentially harmful agents include antibiotics, particularly tetracycline and doxycycline, oral bisphosphonates, NSAIDs, potassium chloride, and iron pills. Acetaminophen, warfarin, colchicine, ascorbic acid, antihypertensives, and antiarrhythmic agents may also induce esophagitis. By exerting a induce esophagitis by exerting a direct corrosive effect on the mucosa, and resulting in dysphagia, pain during swallowing, and persistent heartburn. To minimize the risk of esophageal injury, patients at risk should take these medications with ample water while sitting or standing [50].

Esophageal Dysmotility in Patients after Total Laryngectomy Esophageal dysmotility may affect deglutition or trachea-esophageal (TE) phonation after total laryngectomy. In patients with dysphagia after total laryngectomy 1–12 years prior, esophageal achalasia, EGJ outflow obstruction, diffuse esophageal spasm, and other peristaltic disorders may be seen. Although dysmotility is not associated with poor phonation, trachea-esophageal puncture (TEP) prosthesis leakage might be linked to poor esophageal clearance [51]. Endoscopic dilations of a flap or anastomotic stricture improve life of the TEP.

Of note, normal swallowing requires the close functional coordination of the mouth, pharynx, and esophagus, and if one of these components becomes functionally or structurally impaired, the others may be affected. A study combining video-fluoroscopy and HRM showed that oropharyngeal function is significantly altered in patients with esophageal motility disorders and dysphagia and, vice versa, esophageal motor dysfunction occurs in patients with oropharyngeal dysphagia. These changes may represent either a compensatory mechanism or concomitant involvement of the oropharynx or the esophagus by the underlying neuromotor disorder. Combined assessment by HRM and video-fluoroscopy of both the oropharyngeal and esophageal phases of swallowing may improve diagnosis and therapy in patients with nonobstructive dysphagia [52].

Radiation-Induced Esophageal Injury Endoscopy-negative dysphagia due to esophageal motor dysfunction, mostly ineffective esophageal motility (IEM), or achalasia, may be a late (>10 years) sequel of cervical or thoracic radiation therapy (RT) in patients with breast, lung, head, and neck cancer and Hodgkin's lymphoma [53].

Post-Esophagectomy Syndrome (PES) When the functional outcomes after Ivor-Lewis esophagectomy (ILE) with intrathoracic anastomosis were examined in patients with adenocarcinoma, squamous cell cancer, and high-grade Barrett's

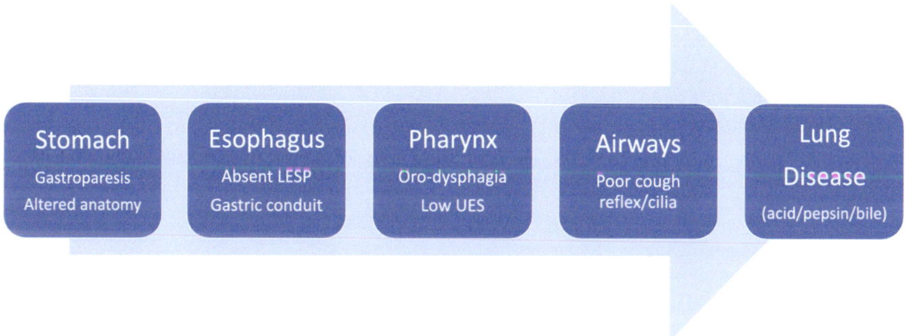

Fig. 11.23 Potential factors in PES that predispose to pulmonary aspiration

dysplasia, with and without preoperative chemoradiation (CRT), reflux (39%), delayed gastric emptying (37%), dumping (21.4%), and anastomotic stenosis (16%) were found. Postoperative reflux was associated with higher BMI, whereas dumping was predicted by female gender and age. Yet, quality of life was good in 82% of the patients [54]. Full evaluation is warranted in all PES cases to guide therapy tailored to the underlying abnormality (i.e., proton pump inhibitors, prokinetics, esophageal dilation, pyloric BoTox injection, or dilation). Figure 11.23 highlights the underlying mechanisms, through which pulmonary aspiration may occur as part of PES.

Despite the availability of sophisticated tools to further characterize PES, there is limited amount of information to help clinicians further understand specific aspects of its pathophysiology that contribute to overlapping, persistent, or alternating symptoms, QoL impairment, and its impact on morbidity/mortality. PES remains challenging to treat, refractory, and prone to iatrogenic errors and omissions. Further, medical and endoscopic management approaches have high potential for failure, because of the multitude of desired therapeutic outcomes (i.e., control of acid and bile reflux symptoms, reduction of nocturnal aspiration events and incidence of pneumonia, or improvement of dysphagia) [55].

Emetogenic Esophagitis Chemotherapy-induced nausea and vomiting (CINV) with associated emetogenic injury to the esophagus depends primarily on the agent used (Fig. 11.24). Intravenous cisplatin, doxorubicin, and cyclophosphamide are the most emetogenic agents.

Most chemotherapy regimens are not highly emetogenic, and effective prophylaxis is available. With an increasing number of molecular-targeted and immunological therapies, more agents with low and minimal emetogenic potentials are becoming available. Several guidelines of antiemetic therapy for chemotherapy recommend prescriptions based on the emetogenic risk of the chemotherapeutic agent

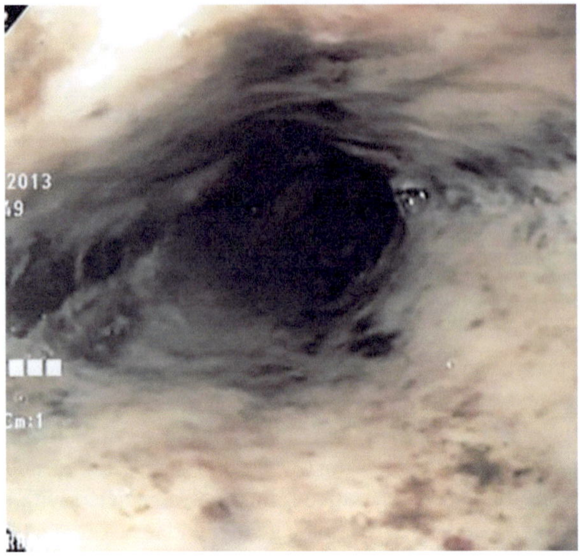

Fig. 11.24 Endoscopic image of the distal esophagus in a patient with severe nausea and vomiting during chemotherapy. There is extensive esophagitis (white areas) and necrosis (dark areas)

Table 11.3 Pharmacologic category and agents used in prevention and management of refractory chemotherapy-induced nausea and vomiting

Class	Agents
NK 1R antagonist	Aprepitant (oral or IV); fosaprpeitant; rolapitant (oral)
5-HT3 antagonists	Granisetron (oral, IV, SQ, transdermal); Ondasetron (oral, IV); palonosetron (oral, IV); dolasetron (oral); tropisetron (oral, IV); ramostron (IV)
Glucocorticoid	Dexamethasone (oral, IV)
5-HT2 and D2 receptor antagonist	Olanzapine (oral)

used [56]. In patients who are high emetic risk, Table 11.3 highlights the preferred classes of agents used in combination.

Eosinophilic Esophagitis Eosinophilic esophagitis (EoE) is a chronic disorder of the esophagus characterized by an eosinophil-predominant inflammation (≥15 eosinophils per high-powered field in at least one mucosal sample) and symptoms of esophageal dysfunction, particularly dysphagia. The condition may be suspected endoscopically by finding multiple rings or furrows mostly in the proximal and distal esophageal body (Fig. 11.25) or strictures, impeding the passage of the endoscope and requiring endoscopic dilation. Eosinophils can influence esophageal motility, leading to worsening dysphagia. In a systematic review to investigate esophageal motility in EoE, all types of manometric motor patterns could be found, but pan-esophageal pressurization was the most common. Some motility abnormalities may reverse after medical treatment [57].

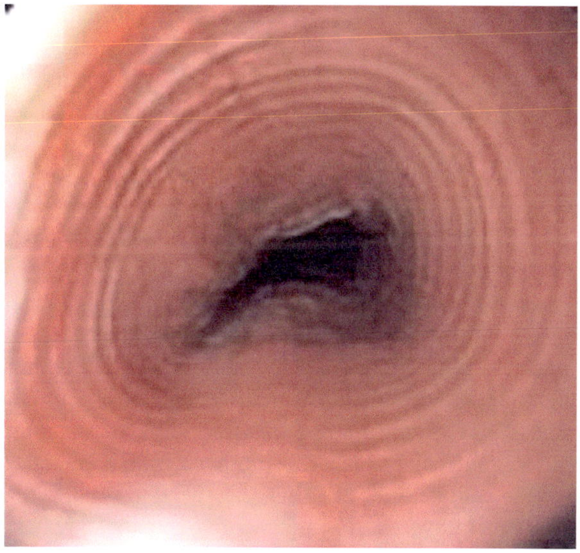

Fig. 11.25 Endoscopic image of eosinophilic esophagitis. Multiple rings are seen along the proximal and mid-esophagus

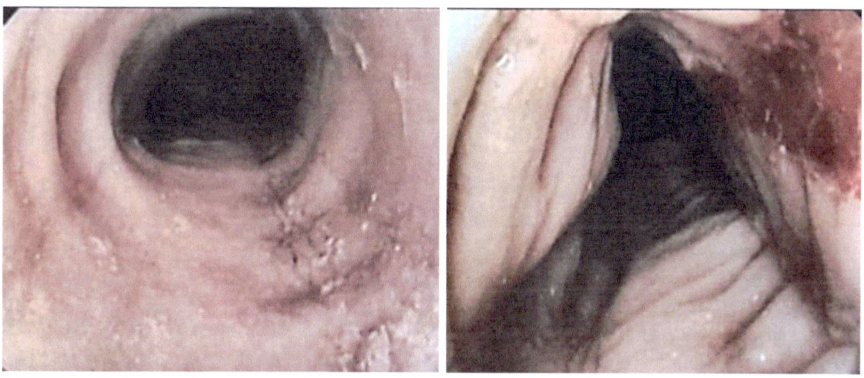

Fig. 11.26 Endoscopic appearance of EoE before (left) and after (right) dilation using Savary bougienage. Note the mucosal tear (between 1 and 3 o'clock position) that is common in such patients. It is essential to endoscopically assess the mucosal appearance before advancing to the next dilation level to avoid perforation

Up to 50% of patients presenting with food impaction have EoE. Because tearing and perforation can occur without perceived resistance when passing a dilator or the endoscope, esophageal dilation should be performed carefully. It is important to assess the mucosa histologically prior to proceeding with dilation in cases of food or foreign body impaction, to minimize the risk of complications such as bleeding and esophageal perforation (Fig. 11.26) [58].

Nonspecific motility disorders were common in patients with EoE, but major motility disorders are rare. In a meta-analysis of 425 EoE patients in 14 studies who underwent HREM, the pooled prevalence of any motility abnormality was 53%

(95% CI: 43%–63%), largely comprised of minor motility disorders, such as IEM and fragmented peristalsis. Major motility disorders were less common, with pooled prevalence of 2% (0%–7%), 10% (5%–16%), and 1% (0%–3%), for achalasia, esophagogastric-junction outflow obstruction, and hypercontractile disorders, respectively [59].

Mixed Esophageal Disease (MED) The increased utilization of diagnostic tools in esophageal disease has led to the recent recognition of overlapping, coexisting conditions causing esophageal symptoms. MED may be spontaneous (idiopathic), systemic, or post-interventional and may cause persistent or alternating symptoms. As such, MED may significantly impair QoL and impact the patients' morbidity and mortality. The condition may be a pre-stage, or aftermath, of significant disease complications and because of its multifaceted pathophysiology, it is challenging to treat, refractory, and prone to iatrogenic errors and omissions. Further, surgical or endoscopic management efforts have a high potential for failure. As clinicians manage the complexities of MED, they need to set differential therapeutic outcomes as their goals. Overall, this novel entity is inadequately studied, particularly in cancer patients [60].

References

1. Dent J, El-Serag HB, Wallander MA, Johansson S. Epidemiology of gastro-oesophageal reflux disease: a systematic review. Gut. 2005;54(5):710–7. https://doi.org/10.1136/gut.2004.051821. PMID: 15831922; PMCID: PMC1774487
2. Vakil N, van Zanten SV, Kahrilas P, Dent J, Jones R. Global Consensus Group. The Montreal definition and classification of gastroesophageal reflux disease: a global evidence-based consensus. Am J Gastroenterol. 2006;101(8):1900–20. https://doi.org/10.1111/j.1572-0241.2006.00630.x. quiz 1943. PMID: 16928254
3. Yadlapati R, Gyawali CP, Pandolfino JE, CGIT GERD Consensus Conference Participants. AGA clinical practice update on the personalized approach to the evaluation and management of GERD: expert review. Clin Gastroenterol Hepatol. 2022;20(5):984–994.e1. https://doi.org/10.1016/j.cgh.2022.01.025. Epub 2022 Feb 2. Erratum in: Clin Gastroenterol Hepatol. 2022;20(9):2156. doi: 10.1016/j.cgh.2022.05.005. PMID: 35123084; PMCID: PMC9838103
4. Saracco M, Savarino V, Bodini G, Saracco GM, Pellicano R. Gastroesophageal reflux disease: key messages for clinicians. Minerva Gastroenterol (Torino). 2021;67(4):390–403. https://doi.org/10.23736/S2724-5985.20.02783-X. Epub 2020 Oct 26. PMID: 33103406
5. Tack J, Becher A, Mulligan C, Johnson DA. Systematic review: the burden of disruptive gastro-oesophageal reflux disease on health-related quality of life. Aliment Pharmacol Ther. 2012;35(11):1257–66. https://doi.org/10.1111/j.1365-2036.2012.05086.x. Epub 2012 Apr 8. PMID: 22486579
6. Gyawali CP, Yadlapati R, Fass R, Katzka D, Pandolfino J, Savarino E, Sifrim D, Spechler S, Zerbib F, Fox MR, Bhatia S, de Bortoli N, Cho YK, Cisternas D, Chen CL, Cock C, Hani A, Remes Troche JM, Xiao Y, Vaezi MF, Roman S. Updates to the modern diagnosis of GERD: Lyon consensus 2.0. Gut. 2024;73(2):361–71.
7. Boeckxstaens G, El-Serag HB, Smout AJ, Kahrilas PJ. Symptomatic reflux disease: the present, the past and the future. Gut. 2014;63(7):1185–93.

8. Shaheen N, Falk G, Iyer P, et al. Diagnosis and management of Barrett's esophagus: an updated ACG guideline. Amer J Gastroenterol. 2022;117:559–87.
9. Cook MB, Thrift AP. Epidemiology of Barrett's esophagus and esophageal adenocarcinoma: implications for screening and surveillance. Gastrointest Endosc Clin N Am. 2021;31:1–26.
10. Triadafilopoulos G. Endoscopic options for gastroesophageal reflux: where are we now and what does the future hold? Curr Gastroenterol Rep. 2016;18:47.
11. Triadafilopoulos G, Azagury D. How can we deal with the GERD treatment gap? Ann N Y Acad Sci. 2016;1381(1):14–20. https://doi.org/10.1111/nyas.13104. Epub 2016 Jul 6. PMID: 27384084
12. Galindo G, Vassalle J, Marcus SN, Triadafilopoulos G. Multimodality evaluation of patients with gastroesophageal reflux disease symptoms who have failed empiric proton pump inhibitor therapy. Dis Esophagus. 2013;26(5):443–50. https://doi.org/10.1111/j.1442-2050.2012.01381.x. Epub 2012 Aug 2. PMID: 22862422
13. Souza RF. From reflux esophagitis to esophageal adenocarcinoma. Dig Dis. 2016;34(5):483–90. https://doi.org/10.1159/000445225. Epub 2016 Jun 22. PMID: 27331918; PMCID: PMC4936412
14. Levine MS, Carucci LR, DiSantis DJ, Einstein DM, Hawn MT, Martin-Harris B, Katzka DA, Morgan DE, Rubesin SE, Scholz FJ, Turner MA, Wolf EL, Canon CL. Consensus Statement of Society of Abdominal Radiology disease-focused panel on barium esophagography in gastroesophageal reflux disease. AJR Am J Roentgenol. 2016;207(5):1009–15. https://doi.org/10.2214/AJR.16.16323. Epub 2016 Aug 4. PMID: 27490234
15. Kolb JM, Wani S. Endoscopic eradication therapy for Barrett's oesophagus: state of the art. Curr Opin Gastroenterol. 2020;36(4):351–8. https://doi.org/10.1097/MOG.0000000000000650. PMID: 32487852; PMCID: PMC9275014
16. Mashimo H, Gordon SR, Singh SK. Advanced endoscopic imaging for detecting and guiding therapy of early neoplasias of the esophagus. Ann N Y Acad Sci. 2020;1482(1):61–76. https://doi.org/10.1111/nyas.14523. Epub 2020 Nov 12. PMID: 33184872; PMCID: PMC7780427
17. Fadel MG, Tarazi M, Dave M, Reddy M, Khan O, Fakih-Gomez N, Ashrafian H, Fehervari M. Magnetic sphincter augmentation in the management of gastro-esophageal reflux disease: a systematic review and meta-analysis. Int J Surg. 2024;110(10):6355–66. https://doi.org/10.1097/JS9.0000000000001558. PMID: 38729117; PMCID: PMC11487049
18. Codipilly DC, Krishna Chandar A, Wang KK, Katzka DA, Goldblum JR, Thota PN, Falk GW, Chak A, Iyer PG. Wide-area transepithelial sampling for dysplasia detection in Barrett's esophagus: a systematic review and meta-analysis. Gastrointest Endosc. 2022;95(1):51–59.e7. https://doi.org/10.1016/j.gie.2021.09.015. Epub 2021 Sep 17. PMID: 34543648; PMCID: PMC8671247
19. Souza RF, Spechler SJ. Advances in biomarkers for risk stratification in Barrett's esophagus. Gastrointest Endosc Clin N Am. 2021;31(1):105–15. https://doi.org/10.1016/j.giec.2020.08.007. Epub 2020 Oct 26. PMID: 33213790
20. Triadafilopoulos G. Endoscopic non-ablative radiofrequency treatment (Stretta) for gastroesophageal reflux disease (GERD). Curr Gastroenterol Rep. 2024;26(4):93–8. https://doi.org/10.1007/s11894-024-00917-9. Epub 2024 Feb 23. PMID: 38393432
21. Ouatu-Lascar R, Fitzgerald RC, Triadafilopoulos G. Differentiation and proliferation in Barrett's esophagus and the effects of acid suppression. Gastroenterology. 1999;117(2):327–35. https://doi.org/10.1053/gast.1999.0029900327. PMID: 10419913
22. Kaur BS, Ouatu-Lascar R, Omary MB, Triadafilopoulos G. Bile salts induce or blunt cell proliferation in Barrett's esophagus in an acid-dependent fashion. Am J Physiol Gastrointest Liver Physiol. 2000;278(6):G1000–9. https://doi.org/10.1152/ajpgi.2000.278.6.G1000. PMID: 10859231
23. Shirvani VN, Ouatu-Lascar R, Kaur BS, Omary MB, Triadafilopoulos G. Cyclooxygenase 2 expression in Barrett's esophagus and adenocarcinoma: ex vivo induction by bile salts and acid exposure. Gastroenterology. 2000;118(3):487–96. https://doi.org/10.1016/s0016-5085(00)70254-x. PMID: 10702199

24. Jankowski JAZ, de Caestecker J, Love SB, Reilly G, Watson P, Sanders S, Ang Y, Morris D, Bhandari P, Brooks C, Attwood S, Harrison R, Barr H, Moayyedi P, AspECT Trial Team. Esomeprazole and aspirin in Barrett's oesophagus (AspECT): a randomised factorial trial. Lancet. 2018;392(10145):400–8. https://doi.org/10.1016/S0140-6736(18)31388-6. Epub 2018 Jul 26
25. Badgery H, Read M, Winter NN, Taylor ACF, Hii MW. The role of esophagectomy in the management of Barrett's esophagus with high-grade dysplasia. Ann N Y Acad Sci. 2020;1481(1):72–89. https://doi.org/10.1111/nyas.14439. Epub 2020 Aug 18. PMID: 32812261
26. Yadlapati R. High-resolution esophageal manometry: interpretation in clinical practice. Curr Opin Gastroenterol. 2017;33(4):301–9. https://doi.org/10.1097/MOG.0000000000000369. PMID: 28426462; PMCID: PMC5568812
27. Gyawali CP, de Bortoli N, Clarke J, Marinelli C, Tolone S, Roman S, Savarino E. Indications and interpretation of esophageal function testing. Ann N Y Acad Sci. 2018;1434(1):239–53. https://doi.org/10.1111/nyas.13709. Epub 2018 May 12. PMID: 29754440
28. Triadafilopoulos G, Kamal A, Clarke JO. Value of 96-hour ambulatory esophageal pH monitoring in the assessment of patients with refractory acid reflux symptoms and their response to anti-reflux diet. Dis Esophagus. 2023;36(7):doac102. https://doi.org/10.1093/dote/doac102. PMID: 36567531
29. Sharma P, Dent J, Armstrong D, Bergman JJ, Gossner L, Hoshihara Y, Jankowski JA, Junghard O, Lundell L, Tytgat GN, Vieth M. The development and validation of an endoscopic grading system for Barrett's esophagus: the Prague C & M criteria. Gastroenterology. 2006;131:1392–9. Epub 2006 Aug 16
30. Shaheen NJ, Falk GW, Iyer PG, Souza RF, Yadlapati RH, Sauer BG, Wani S. Diagnosis and management of Barrett's esophagus: an updated ACG guideline. Am J Gastroenterol. 2022;117(4):559–87. https://doi.org/10.14309/ajg.0000000000001680. PMID: 35354777
31. Eluri S, Reddy S, Ketchem CC, Tappata M, Nettles HG, Watts AE, Cotton CC, Dellon ES, Shaheen NJ. Low prevalence of endoscopic screening for Barrett's esophagus in a screening-eligible primary care population. Am J Gastroenterol. 2022;117(11):1764–71. https://doi.org/10.14309/ajg.0000000000001935. Epub 2022 Aug 12. PMID: 35971219; PMCID: PMC9633338
32. Triadafilopoulos G. Prevalence of abnormalities at tandem endoscopy in patients referred for colorectal cancer screening/surveillance colonoscopy. Cancers (Basel). 2024;16(23):3998. https://doi.org/10.3390/cancers16233998. PMID: 39682185; PMCID: PMC11639759
33. Yadlapati R, Triggs J, Quader F, Eluri S, Bhatia S, Kaizer A, Pandolfino JE, Komanduri S, Gyawali P, Shaheen NJ, Menard-Katcher P, Wani S. Reduced esophageal contractility is associated with dysplasia progression in Barrett's esophagus: a multicenter cohort study. Dig Dis Sci. 2020;12;65(12):3631.
34. Fass R, Teramoto O, Kurin M, Khalessi A, Kitayama Y, Shibli F. Esophageal function abnormalities in patients with Barrett's esophagus. J Clin Gastroenterol. 2020;54(6):485–92.
35. Gerson LB, Shetler K, Triadafilopoulos G. Prevalence of Barrett's esophagus in asymptomatic individuals. Gastroenterology. 2002;123(2):461–7. https://doi.org/10.1053/gast.2002.34748. PMID: 12145799
36. Fitzgerald RC, Lascar R, Triadafilopoulos G. Review article: Barrett's oesophagus, dysplasia and pharmacologic acid suppression. Aliment Pharmacol Ther. 2001;15(3):269–76. https://doi.org/10.1046/j.1365-2036.2001.00939.x. PMID: 11207503
37. Akiyama J, Marcus SN, Triadafilopoulos G. Effective intra-esophageal acid control is associated with improved radiofrequency ablation outcomes in Barrett's esophagus. Dig Dis Sci. 2012;57(10):2625–32. https://doi.org/10.1007/s10620-012-2313-2. Epub 2012 Aug 10. PMID: 22878916
38. Allaix ME, Patti MG. Antireflux surgery for dysplastic Barrett. World J Surg. 2015;39(3):588–94. https://doi.org/10.1007/s00268-014-2632-x. PMID: 24806626

39. Wolfsen HC, Hemminger LL, DeVault KR. Recurrent Barrett's esophagus and adenocarcinoma after esophagectomy. BMC Gastroenterol. 2004;4:18. https://doi.org/10.1186/1471-230X-4-18. PMID: 15327696; PMCID: PMC516033
40. Triadafilopoulos G, Kaur B, Sood S, Traxler B, Levine D, Weston A. The effects of esomeprazole combined with aspirin or rofecoxib on prostaglandin E2 production in patients with Barrett's oesophagus. Aliment Pharmacol Ther. 2006;23(7):997–1005. https://doi.org/10.1111/j.1365-2036.2006.02847.x. PMID: 16573802
41. Hagel AF, Naegel A, Dauth W, Matzel K, Kessler HP, Farnbacher MJ, Hohenberger WM, Neurath MF, Raithel M. Perforation during esophageal dilatation: a 10-year experience. J Gastrointestin Liver Dis. 2013;22(4):385–9. PMID: 24369319
42. Panneerselvam K, Amin RN, Wei D, Tan D, Lum PJ, Zhang HC, Richards DM, Altan M, Grivas P, Thompson JA, Thomas AS, Wang Y. Clinicopathologic features, treatment response, and outcomes of immune checkpoint inhibitor-related esophagitis. J Natl Compr Cancer Netw. 2021;19(8):896–904.
43. Schizas D, Theochari NA, Katsaros I, Mylonas KS, Triantafyllou T, Michalinos A, Kamberoglou D, Tsekrekos A, Rouvelas I. Pseudoachalasia: a systematic review of the literature. Esophagus. 2020;17(3):216–22. https://doi.org/10.1007/s10388-020-00720-1. Epub 2020 Jan 27. PMID: 31989338
44. Naz S, Elhariri A, Richards DM, Triadafilopoulos G, Shafi MA. Clinical characteristics of cancer-associated achalasia (CAA): a 25-year review from a cancer hospital. ASCO Abstract. 2025;43
45. Low EE, Demb J, Shah SC, Liu L, Bustamante R, Yadlapati R, Gupta S. Risk of esophageal cancer in achalasia: a matched cohort study using the Nationwide veterans affairs achalasia cohort. Am J Gastroenterol. 2024;119(4):635–45. https://doi.org/10.14309/ajg.0000000000002591. Epub 2023 Nov 17. PMID: 37975607; PMCID: PMC10994742
46. Yadlapati R, Kahrilas PJ, Fox MR, Bredenoord AJ, Prakash Gyawali C, Roman S, Babaei A, Mittal RK, Rommel N, Savarino E, Sifrim D, Smout A, Vaezi MF, Zerbib F, Akiyama J, Bhatia S, Bor S, Carlson DA, Chen JW, Cisternas D, Cock C, Coss-Adame E, de Bortoli N, Defilippi C, Fass R, Ghoshal UC, Gonlachanvit S, Hani A, Hebbard GS, Wook Jung K, Katz P, Katzka DA, Khan A, Kohn GP, Lazarescu A, Lengliner J, Mittal SK, Omari T, Park MI, Penagini R, Pohl D, Richter JE, Serra J, Sweis R, Tack J, Tatum RP, Tutuian R, Vela MF, Wong RK, Wu JC, Xiao Y, Pandolfino JE. Esophageal motility disorders on high-resolution manometry: Chicago classification version 4.0©. Neurogastroenterol Motil. 2021;33(1):e14058. https://doi.org/10.1111/nmo.14058. Erratum in: Neurogastroenterol Motil. 2024 Feb;36(2):e14179. doi: 10.1111/nmo.14179. PMID: 33373111; PMCID: PMC8034247
47. Shetler KP, Bikhtii S, Triadafilopoulos G. Ineffective esophageal motility: clinical, manometric, and outcome characteristics in patients with and without abnormal esophageal acid exposure. Dis Esophagus. 2017;30(6):1–8. https://doi.org/10.1093/dote/dox012. PMID: 28475749
48. Takahashi K, Takeuchi M, Sato Y, Sato H, Mizuno K, Hashimoto S, Kobayashi M, Terai S. Evaluation of esophageal motility after endoscopic submucosal dissection for superficial esophageal cancer. Eur J Gastroenterol Hepatol. 2015;27(10):1187–92.
49. Zikos TA, Triadafilopoulos G, Clarke JO. Esophagogastric junction outflow obstruction: current approach to diagnosis and management. Curr Gastroenterol Rep. 2020;22(2):9. https://doi.org/10.1007/s11894-020-0743-0. PMID: 32020310
50. Iwamuro M, Kawano S, Otsuka M. Drug-induced mucosal alterations observed during esophagogastroduodenoscopy. World J Gastroenterol. 2024;30(16):2220–32. https://doi.org/10.3748/wjg.v30.i16.2220. PMID: 38690017; PMCID: PMC11056913
51. Zhang T, Maclean J, Szczesniak M, Bertrand PP, Quon H, Tsang RK, Wu PI, Graham P, Cook IJ. Esophageal dysmotility in patients following total laryngectomy. Otolaryngol Head Neck Surg. 2018;158(2):323–30. https://doi.org/10.1177/0194599817736507. Epub 2017 Dec 12. PMID: 29231090).
52. Triadafilopoulos G, Hallstone A, Nelson-Abbott H, et al. Oropharyngeal and esophageal interrelationships in patients with nonobstructive dysphagia. Digest Dis Sci. 1992;37:551–7.

53. Vitton V, Andrianjafy C, Luciano L, Gonzalez JM, Padovani L. Radio-induced esophageal motility disorders: an unrecognized diagnosis. Cancer Radiother. 2021;25(3):249–53. https://doi.org/10.1016/j.canrad.2020.09.006. Epub 2021 Jan 14. PMID: 33454192
54. Deldycke A, Van Daele E, Ceelen W, Van Nieuwenhove Y, Pattyn P. Functional outcome after Ivor Lewis esophagectomy for cancer. J Surg Oncol. 2016;113:24–8. https://doi.org/10.1002/jso.24084.
55. Edmondson J, Hunter J, Bakis G, O'Connor A, Wood S, Qureshi AP. Understanding post-esophagectomy complications and their management: the early complications. J Clin Med. 2023;12(24):7622. https://doi.org/10.3390/jcm12247622. PMID: 38137691; PMCID: PMC10743498
56. Okuyama A, Boku N, Higashi T. Real-world emetic risk of chemotherapy and the corresponding antiemetic therapy in Japan: a study based on a nationwide database. Cancer Rep (Hoboken). 2022;5(3):e1482. https://doi.org/10.1002/cnr2.1482. Epub 2021 Jun 27. PMID: 34176233; PMCID: PMC8955058
57. Visaggi P, Ghisa M, Barberio B, Marabotto E, de Bortoli N, Savarino E. Systematic review: esophageal motility patterns in patients with eosinophilic esophagitis. Dig Liver Dis. 2022;54(9):1143–52. https://doi.org/10.1016/j.dld.2022.01.003. Epub 2022 Jan 25. PMID: 35090825
58. Rajagopalan J, Triadafilopoulos G. Ring(s)-related esophageal meat bolus impaction: biopsy first, dilate later. Dis Esophagus. 2009;22(5):E14–6. https://doi.org/10.1111/j.1442-2050.2008.00894.x. Epub 2008 Nov 12. PMID: 19018847
59. Reddy SB, Ketchem CJ, Dougherty MK, Eluri S, Dellon ES. Association between eosinophilic esophagitis and esophageal dysmotility: a systematic review and meta-analysis. Neurogastroenterol Motil. 2023;35(2):e14475. https://doi.org/10.1111/nmo.14475. Epub 2022 Sep 27. PMID: 36168184
60. Triadafilopoulos G, Mashimo H, Tatum R, O'Clarke J, Hawn M. Mixed esophageal disease (MED): a new concept. Dig Dis Sci. 2023;68(9):3542–54. https://doi.org/10.1007/s10620-023-08008-x. Epub 2023 Jul 20. PMID: 37470896

Regional Disorders of Sensory-Motor Dysfunction: Stomach

12

George Triadafilopoulos and Mehnaz A. Shafi

12.1 Stomach

***H. pylori* Infection** *Helicobacter pylori* (HP) infection is one of the most frequent bacterial infections in humans, with approximately half of the global population being infected. HP may also be associated with gastric motility disorders, such as functional dyspepsia (FD) and delayed gastric emptying (DGE) [1]. Mostly, patients with chronic *H. pylori* gastritis can present with peptic ulcer disease or gastroduodenal complications of chronic infection, including gastric atrophy, intestinal metaplasia, gastric cancer, and mucosa-associated lymphoid tissue (MALT) lymphoma. It is unclear if chronic H. *pylori* infection causes epigastric abdominal pain in the absence of peptic ulcer disease, but it has been associated with functional dyspepsia. When signs or symptoms do occur with *H. pylori* infection, they are nonspecific, and they may include an ache or burning pain in the upper abdomen (dyspepsia) that may be worse when the stomach is empty, nausea, loss of appetite, frequent burping, bloating, or unintentional weight loss. As such, the infection needs to be considered in all patients presenting with such vague upper abdominal complaints and a careful endoscopic examination, using white-light and digital chromoendoscopy with systematic biopsies, using the Sydney protocol, needs to be undertaken. With the ubiquitous availability of over-the-counter proton pump inhibitors and their effectiveness in controlling dyspepsia and acid reflux, many patients fail to seek medical attention, or those who are under active cancer treatment tend to attribute their symptoms to such therapy. Hence, a low threshold is needed to proceed with formal evaluation, either with noninvasive testing for active infection (i.e., *H. pylori* stool antigen testing) or, preferably, an endoscopy. Endoscopy is normal in as many as 50% of patients with chronic *H. pylori* infection, not revealing gastritis or peptic

G. Triadafilopoulos (✉) · M. A. Shafi
Department of Gastroenterology, Hepatology and Nutrition, UT MD Anderson Cancer Center, Houston, TX, USA
e-mail: GTriadafilopoulo@mdanderson.org; mashafi@mdanderson.org

G. Triadafilopoulos (ed.), *Onco-Neurogastroenterology*,
https://doi.org/10.1007/978-3-031-98848-6_12

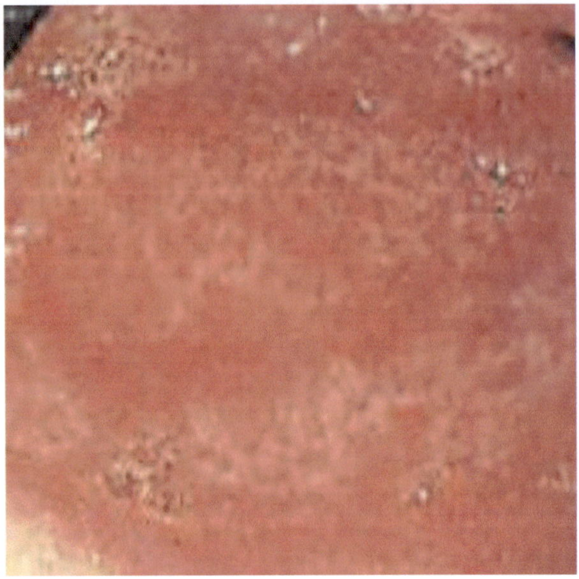

Fig. 12.1 Endoscopic image of the antrum in a patient with predominantly erythematous, nonerosive, *H. pylori* gastritis, without ulceration, who presented with nonspecific dyspepsia. On histology, there was no evidence of gastric intestinal metaplasia (GIM) or dysplasia. He was effectively treated with triple therapy against the infection that was eradicated

Table 12.1 Agents used in empiric therapy of *H. pylori* infection in the USA

Empiric anti-HP regimen	Specific agents
Bismuth subsalicylate quadruple therapy ×14 days	PeptoBismol®) 2 tablets or 2 capsules q.i.d. + tetracycline 500 mg + metronidazole 500 mg with meals q.i.d. + PPI, 30 min b.i.d. before meals and bedtime
Bismuth sulfate quadruple therapy (Pylera®) ×14 days	Combination tablets with meals + PPI, q.i.d. with meals and bedtime
Rifabutin triple therapy ×14 days	Esomeprazole 40 mg or rabeprazole 20 mg 30 min before meals b.i.d.+ Rifabutin 150 mg b.i.d. + amoxicillin 1 gm t.i.d. with or 30 min after meals

ulceration. Other patients may have nonspecific endoscopic features, such as significant erythema, friability, and nodularity (Fig. 12.1). Regardless of the mucosal appearance, systematic biopsies using the Sydney protocol are essential to confirm the infection and rule out gastric intestinal metaplasia (GIM), dysplasia, or early cancer. Regardless of symptoms, the infection will require eradication therapy (typically with combination regimens of proton pump inhibition and antibiotics) (Table 12.1), aimed at benign peptic ulcer and gastric cancer prevention [2]. For patients with early-stage *H. pylori*-positive gastric extra-nodal marginal zone lymphoma of mucosa-associated lymphoid tissue (MALT lymphoma), initial *H. pylori* eradication therapy depends on local antibiotic resistance patterns and patient's allergies [3].

In dyspeptic patients with *H. pylori* infection, the incidence of abdominal pain, epigastric burning sensation, abdominal distension, nausea, belching, and early satiety significantly improve with therapy [1]. In patients with uncomplicated ulcers

Table 12.2 Agents used for the therapy of *H. pylori* infection after susceptibility testing in the USA

Susceptibility-based therapy	Specific regimen
Clarithromycin triple therapy ×2 weeks	Clarithromycin 500 mg b.i.d + amoxicillin 1 gm b.i.d + PPI b.i.d with meals
Metronidazole triple therapy ×2 weeks	Metronidazole 500 mg b.i.d + amoxicillin 1 gm b.i.d + PPI b.i.d with meals
Levofloxacin triple therapy ×2 weeks	Levofloxacin 500 mg b.i.d + amoxicillin 1 gm b.i.d + PPI b.i.d with meals

PPI should be equivalent to 40 mg omeprazole bid (e.g., rabeprazole 40 b.i.d or esomeprazole 40 mg b.i.d.

Instead of PPI, the PCAB vonoprazan 20 mg b.i.d may also be used, but it is currently much more costly

due to *H. pylori* infection, triple therapy is adequate in inducing healing. In the absence of persistent or recurrent symptoms after therapy, there is no need for maintenance antisecretory therapy.

The treatment of *H. pylori* infection is constantly evolving, driven by the developing resistance of the bacterium to antibiotics, and can be empiric (Table 12.1), or in response to prior susceptibility testing, a strategy that has been found cost-effective. Such molecular testing can be obtained for all six relevant antibiotics. Currently in the USA, for clarithromycin-, metronidazole-, or levofloxacin-susceptible infections, when given in conjunction with high-potency PPI, the triple therapy (e.g., metronidazole + amoxicillin + esomeprazole) cure rates are higher than 90% (Table 12.2).

Autoimmune Gastritis Autoimmune gastritis (AIG) is a chronic inflammatory disorder affecting the acid-secreting compartment of the gastric mucosa, leading to progressive mucosal atrophy and hypo- and achlorhydria. The inflammation is restricted to the corpus and fundic glands of the stomach, sparing the antrum, in contrast to other conditions leading to atrophic gastritis (such as *Helicobacter pylori* infection) (Fig. 12.2). AIG is associated with anti-intrinsic factor antibodies (IFAs) and anti-parietal cell antibodies (PCAs), and it is caused by the destruction of parietal cells, secondary to the actions of PCAs, which recognize subunits of the proton pump, H+/K+ ATPase, which is unique to the parietal cells. Up to 30% of individuals with *H. pylori* infection display autoantibodies to the canaliculi of parietal cells, which disappear after eradication of infection [4]. Postprandial fullness, early satiety, non-acid reflux, nausea, and weight loss are the most common symptoms of AIG. Achlorhydria can impair gastric motility and might favor small intestinal bacterial overgrowth (SIBO). Pernicious (megaloblastic) anemia—due to vitamin B12 deficiency—is a classic feature, but combined B12 and iron deficiency may also be noted. AIG predisposes patients to develop both type 1 gastric neuroendocrine tumors (NET) and gastric adenocarcinoma. Persistently increased level of gastrin-17 is a risk factor for enterochromaffin cell hyperplasia, dysplasia, and type 1 gastric NET1. *H. pylori* should be eradicated whenever detected, as its eradication might decrease the risk of gastric adenocarcinoma. Premalignant alterations (i.e., gastric intestinal metaplasia (GIM), atrophy, and dysplasia) are the most important

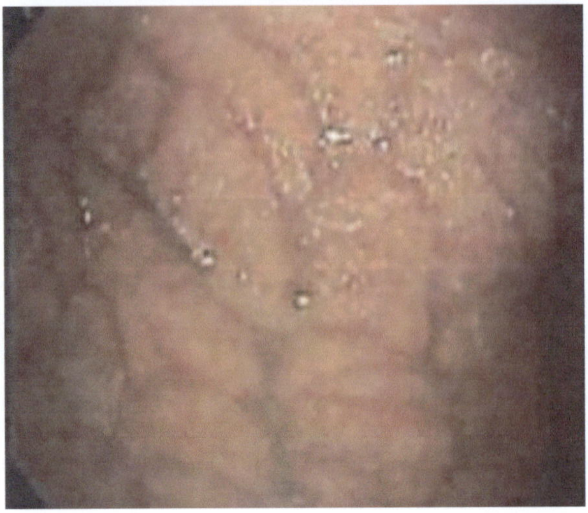

Fig. 12.2 Endoscopic images of the fundus and proximal body in a patient with autoimmune gastritis (AIG). The blood vessels are sparse amidst the atrophic mucosa. Urease testing for *H. pylori* was negative

determinants of gastric cancer risk. The multifocal pattern, described as extensive atrophic gastritis, has been associated with the highest risk of gastric cancer, as well as with the presence of gastric intestinal metaplasia. While worldwide autoimmune gastritis is significantly less common than *H. pylori*-induced gastritis, in Western nations the estimated prevalence of autoimmune gastritis may be as high as 2% of the population. Individuals with AIG are both at risk for gastric adenocarcinomas and neuroendocrine tumors driven by hypergastrinemia. Pernicious anemia may serve as a marker of particularly high risk, since it is both a late manifestation of disease and an indicator of severity. Endoscopic surveillance with histologic confirmation at an interval of 3–5 years is recommended. Micronutrient supplementation is key in the treatment of patients with AIG. Proton pump inhibitors should be discouraged. There is no anti-inflammatory, immunosuppressive, or biological therapy available for AIG. Oral iron, particularly in conjunction with vitamin C, is comparable in efficacy to intravenous iron in the treatment of iron deficiency anemia. Oral iron is better absorbed if taken on an empty stomach, but this may increase dyspeptic symptoms, abdominal pain, constipation, or diarrhea. Patients who fail to respond to oral supplementation after usually 2 months require parenteral iron therapy. In patients with newly diagnosed vitamin B12 deficiency, parenteral supplementation is recommended to attain rapid correction, particularly when neurological symptoms are present. For maintenance, oral supplementation with cyanocobalamin and parenteral administration can theoretically be equally effective, because oral vitamin B12 absorption takes place by simple diffusion through the intestinal wall, but only when high doses of the vitamin are given. Treatment of SIBO using antibiotics is useful in select cases.

Gastric Intestinal Metaplasia (GIM) In low-incidence nations such as the USA, screening of the general population for gastric cancer is unlikely to be cost-effective. Hence, gastric intestinal metaplasia (GIM) is typically found at endoscopy performed for the evaluation of dyspepsia. In addition to targeted biopsies from

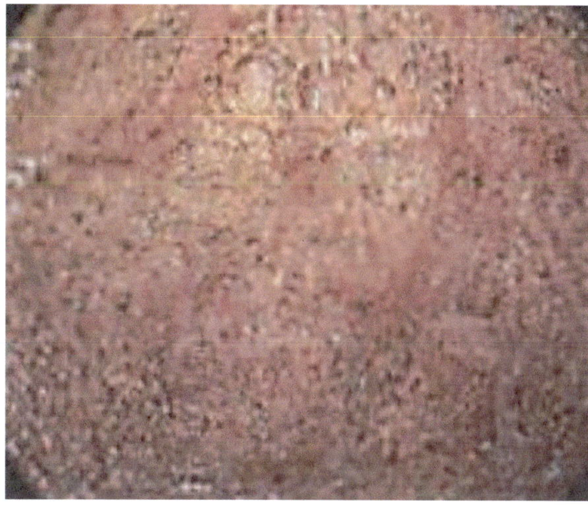

Fig. 12.3 Endoscopic image of extensive atrophy and gastric intestinal metaplasia secondary to long-standing *H. pylori* infection in a patient presenting with troublesome dyspepsia who did not respond to empiric acid suppression therapy

suspicious areas, one-to-two biopsies should be taken from each of five sites (the greater and lesser curvature of antrum, the incisura angularis, and the greater and lesser curvature of the corpus and the cardia) to map the extent of mucosal changes for risk stratification [5]. Narrowband imaging (NBI) has been shown to be superior to standard, "white-light" endoscopy for the detection of GIM by revealing regular ridges or tubule-villous-mucosa and blue-whitish patchy areas that have been termed "light blue crests." The prevalence of GIM is estimated around 5–7%, although it may be significantly greater in high-risk populations, such as racial/ethnic minority groups, immigrants from high-risk countries, and those with a family history of gastric cancer (GC). However, once GIM has developed, individuals are at risk of subsequent gastric cancer, regardless of race or ethnicity. The annual progression rate from GIM to GC is estimated to be 0.1% per year, though certain subtypes of IM are considered to have a higher risk of progression. Individuals with incomplete IM (which resembles the colonic epithelium and lacks a brush border) have a higher progression rate compared to those with complete IM (which resembles small intestinal epithelium, with a brush border and goblet cells) (Fig. 12.3). The risk of GC has also been demonstrated to be higher among individuals with extensive IM, defined as IM in both the antrum and corpus [6].

To examine the prevalence of foregut endoscopic and histologic precancerous abnormalities in patients undergoing endoscopy, a rigorous protocol, involving white-light and NBI chromoendoscopy, in conjunction with meticulous histologic assessment using the Sydney classification, the Seattle biopsy protocol, and histologic assessment of the squamocolumnar junction (SCJ) and the duodenum is advised. This approach, when applied on patients who qualify for an endoscopy based on the number of criteria that are met by national guidelines (Fig. 12.4), can yield gastric intestinal metaplasia or intestinal metaplasia of the squamocolumnar junction and serve as tool for both gastric and esophageal cancer screening during

Screening criteria for BE	Yes (1); No (0)	Screening criteria for GC	Yes (1); No (0)
Chronic heartburn & regurgitation		First degree relative with GC	
Male		First-generation immigrants from high Hp prevalence regions	
Age > 50		African Americans, Alaskan Natives, American Indians, Asian Americans, and Hispanic Americans.	
White		Age > 60 with dyspepsia* symptoms	
Tobacco			
Obesity (BMI>30)			
Total	**EGD if score > 4**		**EGD if score > 1**

*Dyspepsia: A persistent or recurrent pain or discomfort in the upper abdomen

Fig. 12.4 Clinical criteria used *justify* screening for Barrett's esophagus (BE) and gastric cancer (GC) during an index endoscopy

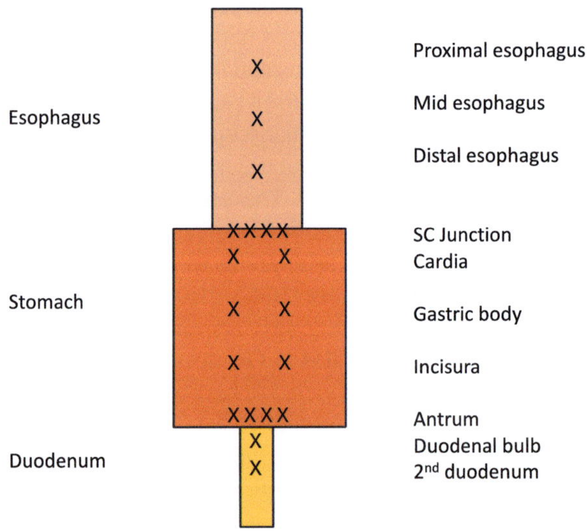

Fig. 12.5 Diagram of a detailed protocol sampling the stomach and the esophagus for precancerous changes

one index endoscopy. Using this approach, a recent study of 317 patients, initially referred for screening or surveillance colonoscopy but responded positively to screening questionnaires for BE and GC screening, found intestinal metaplasia in 27%, dysplasia in 2%, and foregut cancer in 0.9% [7].

Figure 12.5 highlights the details of the histologic protocol used in that study, aiming to identify precancerous for both gastric (body and cardia) and esophageal cancer with one examination. Studies have revealed the gradual molecular and phenotypic transition from a gastric to intestinal phenotype (IM) in the esophagus and stomach. Because BE-IM and GIM can predispose to cancer, this new understanding of a common developmental trajectory leads to a more unified approach to detection and treatment [8].

Malignancy-Associated Gastroparesis (MAG) Gastroparesis, presenting with anorexia, postprandial fulness and early satiety, nausea, vomiting, epigastric abdominal pain, and profound weight loss may occur in several malignancies, such as esophageal, esophagogastric junction (EGJ), gastric, pancreatic, gallbladder, and lung, but its exact prevalence is unknown. MAG can result from either malignant ENS infiltration, from paraneoplastic dysmotility with autoantibody-mediated destruction of the ICC, or of the myenteric plexus [9]. MAG may also occur after radiation therapy or result from a coexisting condition, such as diabetes. Gastric and small intestinal mechanical obstruction should be excluded by upper endoscopy or preferably, by MR enterography. After excluding obstruction, the gastric emptying delay should be quantified and monitored, using gastric emptying scintigraphy (GES) or a wireless motility capsule (WMC). The latter study will also assess small bowel and colonic transit. Adequate hydration and nutritional support using small frequent meals, preferably liquid, prokinetics, and antiemetics, are the initial treatment steps. For refractory MAG, a neurostimulation device (Enterra, Medtronic, Minneapolis, MN) can be placed temporarily by endoscopy, or permanently by surgery, and lead to symptom improvement despite marginal changes in gastric emptying [10]. Simultaneous "dual" Enterra implantation and surgical pyloroplasty may significantly improve symptoms, expedite gastric emptying, facilitate weight gain, mitigate malnutrition, and reduce duration of hospitalization [11].

Extranodal marginal zone B-cell lymphoma (ENMZL) of mucosa-associated lymphoid tissue (MALT), a rare subtype of B-cell lymphoma, is typically associated with *Helicobacter pylori* infection of the stomach [12]. Approximately 75% of *H. pylori*-positive gastric ENMZL cases achieve complete remission (CR) with *H. pylori* eradication therapy. Patients with gastric ENMZL may be asymptomatic or present with epigastric pain, anorexia, weight loss, or occult blood loss. Small intestinal lesions often manifest as diarrhea, abdominal pain, or malabsorption. Classic B symptoms like fever, night sweats, and weight loss are rare in gastric ENMZL.

Postoperative Gastroparesis After vagotomy, the fundus does not relax normally after meals, resulting in rapid antral filling. Vagotomy may also cause gastric dysrhythmias, decreased antral contractility, and poorly coordinated gastroduodenal activity; a pyloroplasty may be needed in symptomatic patients. Similarly, resection of the lower esophagus for esophageal cancer (Ivor-Lewis esophagectomy) transects the vagus nerves and drastically reduces the fundic reservoir. Pyloric Botox, G-POEM, or surgical pyloroplasty may be needed to control chronic nausea, postprandial pain, and vomiting. Antrectomy associated with either Billroth I or II anastomosis or Roux-en-Y gastrojejunostomy for gastric neoplasia also causes neuromuscular gastric dysfunction due to lack of proper postprandial food mixing, grinding, and emptying. Specifically, even in the absence of anastomotic stenosis, Roux-en-Y gastroenterostomy may cause functional postprandial pain, bloating, and nausea, due to delayed gastric emptying. After vagotomy and antrectomy, patients may also develop dumping syndrome. Gastroparesis, due to vagal nerve injury and impaired fundic relaxation, and manifesting with early satiety, bloating, and nausea, may result from prior fundoplication performed for refractory GERD, with or without Barrett's esophagus, and sliding hiatal hernia repair [9].

There are two aspects to gastroparesis after pylorus preserving pancreatoduodenectomy (PPPD). The first is early gastric stasis that may be attributed to the absence of phase III activity of the migrating motor complex. Phase III of the MMC is a short band (8 min) of vigorous contractions of maximal amplitude called an "activity front," and it is considered to play a role in transporting gastric juice into the duodenum. The second aspect is postprandial delayed gastric emptying that is caused by the effects of the impaired hormonal, intrinsic, and/or extrinsic neural controls of gastric motility. Delayed gastric emptying scan leads to postprandial fullness with nausea and vomiting. This delayed gastric emptying may persist for as long as 6 months postoperatively, before eventual recovery. The presence of pancreatic cancer itself may cause gastroparesis, in the absence of gastroduodenal invasion or obstruction [13].

In a retrospective study of 196 consecutive patients who underwent pancreaticoduodenectomy, delayed gastric emptying (DGE) occurred in 71 patients (36.2%). A pancreatic fistula and intra-abdominal fluid collection significantly and independently correlated with DGE rates, as was a body mass index ≥25 kg/m^2 [14].

GERD-Related Gastroparesis Twenty to 30% of patients with typical GERD have additional early satiety, postprandial fullness, and nausea, due to delayed gastric emptying. In some patients, nausea represents a subtle, atypical symptom, and it improves after aggressive acid suppression therapy with PPI. Symptoms associated with gastroparesis may improve and gastric dysrhythmias revert to normal 3-cpm gastric myoelectrical activity (GMA) after treatment of the lower esophageal sphincter with radiofrequency ablation (RFA) using the Stretta procedure. Lower esophageal sphincter abnormalities, including increased numbers of transient lower esophageal sphincter relaxations (tLESRs), may contribute to inefficient gastric emptying and gastric dysrhythmias. Patients with GERD also tend to retain solids and liquids in the proximal stomach and in turn stimulate excessive transient lower esophageal sphincter relaxations. RFA treatment at the lower esophageal sphincter region (Stretta) or fundoplication in patients with heartburn and dyspepsia may improve heartburn, gastric emptying rates, and gastric dysrhythmias [15]. Endoscopic pyloric botulinum toxin injection alleviates both symptoms of GERD and gastroparesis [16]. Manometrically, lack of phase III of the migratory motor complex (MMC) in the gastric tube causes GER symptoms post-esophagectomy. Further, pyloric Botox prevents delayed gastric emptying after esophagectomy. G-POEM is also a minimally invasive therapy with long-term effectiveness and safety in treating postsurgical gastroparesis [17].

Glucagon-Like Peptide-1 Receptor Agonists (GLP-1RAs)-Gastroparesis Glucagon-like peptide-1 receptor agonists (GLP-1RAs) have revolutionized the care of patients with metabolic disease, decreasing hyperglycemia and enhancing satiety. GLP-1, a naturally secreted polypeptide, acts on the GLP-1R in multiple organs, including the pancreas and stomach, prolonging gastric emptying time. The perioperative use of GLP-1RA has raised safety concerns due to delayed gastric emptying causing residual gastric contents and potentially leading to pulmonary aspiration on the day of the procedure, despite fasting. Further, GLP-1RAs may induce nausea, vomiting, abdominal pain, and constipation, which may complicate the diagnosis and treatment of preoperative and postoperative disease states that share these symptoms [18].

Gastric Emptying after ESD for Gastric Cancer Using scintigraphy, gastric emptying may be delayed at 1 and 8 weeks after ESD, compared to before. The changes in the Tlag and T1/2 values from before ESD to 1 week after ESD are greater for proximal than for distal stomach lesions ($P = 0.028$, $P < 0.001$) [19]. Delayed gastric emptying (DGE) with food retention after gastric ESD is associated with lesions located in the lesser curvature of the upper stomach, submucosal invasion of the lesion, age > 80 years, and post-ESD bleeding, but it is temporary in most cases [20].

Immunotherapy-Associated Gastroparesis Use of immune checkpoint inhibitors (ICI) has been associated with delayed gastric emptying on gastric scintigraphy [21]. Of note, ICI-related gastroparesis may coexist with other causes (i.e., diabetes, narcotic-induced, etc.) in these patients with cancer undergoing therapy, and full consideration and treatment of all possible etiologies should be given.

Duodenogastric Bile Reflux Although there are no clear recommendations regarding the type of reconstruction after subtotal distal gastrectomy [22], Roux-en-Y reconstruction may be superior to Billroth II reconstruction, since it may prevent duodenogastric bile reflux gastritis and provide a better quality of life for patients [23]. Yet, in some patients, Roux-en-Y reconstruction may lead to Roux stasis syndrome, with delayed gastric emptying, postprandial pain, nausea, and vomiting [24]. Roux stasis may occur despite construction of Braun anastomosis, which is intended to mitigate reflux, dumping syndrome, or postprandial distress [25].

References

1. Zhang CL, Geng CH, Yang ZW, Li YL, Tong LQ, Gao P, Gao YQ. Changes in patients' symptoms and gastric emptying after Helicobacter pylori treatment. World J Gastroenterol. 2016;22(18):4585–93. https://doi.org/10.3748/wjg.v22.i18.4585. PMID: 27182168; PMCID: PMC4858640.
2. Moss SF, Shah SC, Tan MC, El-Serag HB. Evolving concepts in *Helicobacter pylori* management. Gastroenterology. 2024;166(2):267–83.
3. Stathis A, Chini C, Bertoni F, Proserpio I, Capella C, Mazzucchelli L, Pedrinis E, Cavalli F, Pinotti G, Zucca E. Long-term outcome following Helicobacter pylori eradication in a retrospective study of 105 patients with localized gastric marginal zone B-cell lymphoma of MALT type. Ann Oncol. 2009;20(6):1086–93. https://doi.org/10.1093/annonc/mdn760. Epub 2009 Feb 4. PMID: 19193705.

4. Lenti MV, Rugge M, Lahner E, Miceli E, Toh BH, Genta RM, De Block C, Hershko C, Di Sabatino A. Autoimmune gastritis. Nat Rev Dis Primers. 2020;6(1):56.
5. Fansiwala K, Lewis MS, Pisegna JR. Gastritis: pathophysiology and clinical management. Am J Gastroenterol. 2025;120(1):5–8. https://doi.org/10.14309/ajg.0000000000003216. Epub 2024 Nov 21. PMID: 39569875; PMCID: PMC11695143.
6. Huang RJ, Laszkowska M, In H, Hwang JH, Epplein M. Controlling gastric cancer in a world of heterogeneous risk. Gastroenterology. 2023;164(5):736–51.
7. Triadafilopoulos G. Prevalence of abnormalities at tandem endoscopy in patients referred for colorectal cancer screening/surveillance colonoscopy. Cancers (Basel). 2024;16(23):3998. https://doi.org/10.3390/cancers16233998. PMID: 39682185; PMCID: PMC11639759.
8. Nowicki-Osuch K, Zhuang L, Cheung TS, Black EL, Masqué-Soler N, Devonshire G, Redmond AM, Freeman A, di Pietro M, Pilonis N, Januszewicz W, O'Donovan M, Tavaré S, Shields JD, Fitzgerald RC. Single-cell RNA sequencing unifies developmental programs of esophageal and gastric intestinal metaplasia. Cancer Discov. 2023;13(6):1346–63. https://doi.org/10.1158/2159-8290.CD-22-0824. PMID: 36929873; PMCID: PMC10236154.
9. Shafi MA, Pasricha PJ. Post-surgical and obstructive gastroparesis. Curr Gastroenterol Rep. 2007;9(4):280–5. https://doi.org/10.1007/s11894-007-0031-2.
10. Shanker A, Bashashati M, Rezaie A. Gastric electrical stimulation for treatment of refractory gastroparesis: the current approach to management. Curr Gastroenterol Rep. 2021;23(2):2. https://doi.org/10.1007/s11894-020-00803-0. PMID: 33483775; PMCID: PMC7822763.
11. Davis BR, Sarosiek I, Bashashati M, Alvarado B, McCallum RW. The long-term efficacy and safety of Pyloroplasty combined with gastric electrical stimulation therapy in gastroparesis. J Gastrointest Surg. 2017;21(2):222–7. https://doi.org/10.1007/s11605-016-3327-4. Epub 2016 Nov 28. PMID: 27896652.
12. Wotherspoon AC, Ortiz-Hidalgo C, Falzon MR, et al. *Helicobacter pylori*-associated gastritis and primary B-cell gastric lymphoma. Lancet. 1991;338:1175–6.
13. Tanaka M. Gastroparesis after a pylorus-preserving pancreato-duodenectomy. Surg Today. 2005;35(5):345–50. https://doi.org/10.1007/s00595-004-2961-8.
14. Liu QY, Li L, Xia HT, Zhang WZ, Cai SW, Lu SC. Risk factors of delayed gastric emptying following pancreaticoduodenectomy. ANZ J Surg. 2016;86(1–2):69–73. https://doi.org/10.1111/ans.12850. Epub 2014 Oct 13. PMID: 25312402.
15. Noar MD, Noar E. Gastroparesis associated with gastroesophageal reflux disease and corresponding reflux symptoms may be corrected by radiofrequency ablation of the cardia and esophagogastric junction. Surg Endosc. 2008;22(11):2440–4. https://doi.org/10.1007/s00464-008-9873-4. Epub 2008 Apr 24. PMID: 18437485.
16. Mirbagheri SA, Sadeghi A, Amouie M, Mansouri S, Forootan M, Rashidi A, Abouzari M. Pyloric injection of botulinum toxin for the treatment of refractory GERD accompanied with gastroparesis: a preliminary report. Dig Dis Sci. 2008;53(10):2621–6. https://doi.org/10.1007/s10620-007-0187-5. Epub 2008 Feb 7. PMID: 18256933.
17. Tan J, Shrestha SM, Wei M, Wang P, Shi J, Lu Y, Gao Q, Lu T, Zhou J, Shi R. Feasibility, safety, and long-term efficacy of gastric peroral endoscopic myotomy (G-POEM) for post-surgical gastroparesis: a single-center and retrospective study of a prospective database. Surg Endosc. 2021;35(7):3459–70. https://doi.org/10.1007/s00464-020-07793-0. Epub 2020 Sep 3. PMID: 32880749; PMCID: PMC8195960.
18. Kindel TL, Wang AY, Wadhwa A, Schulman AR, Sharaiha RZ, Kroh M, Ghanem OM, Levy S, Joshi GP, LaMasters TL. American Gastroenterological Association; American Society for Metabolic and Bariatric Surgery; American Society of Anesthesiologists; International Society of Perioperative Care of Patients with Obesity; Society of American Gastrointestinal and Endoscopic Surgeons. Multisociety clinical practice guidance for the safe use of glucagon-like peptide-1 receptor agonists in the perioperative period. Surg Obes Relat Dis. 2024;20(12):1183–6. https://doi.org/10.1016/j.soard.2024.08.033. Epub 2024 Oct 29
19. Watanabe K, Hikichi T, Sato M, Nakamura J, Obara K, Ohira H. Change in gastric emptying eight weeks after endoscopic submucosal dissection in patients with early gastric cancer.

Endosc Int Open. 2016;4(5):E597–602. https://doi.org/10.1055/s-0042-105202. Epub 2016 Apr 21. PMID: 27227121; PMCID: PMC4874802
20. Yoshizaki T, Obata D, Aoki Y, Okamoto N, Hashimura H, Kano C, Matsushita M, Kanamori A, Matsumoto K, Tsujimae M, Momose K, Eguchi T, Okuyama S, Yamashita H, Fujita M, Okada A. Endoscopic submucosal dissection for early gastric cancer on the lesser curvature in upper third of the stomach is a risk factor for postoperative delayed gastric emptying. Surg Endosc. 2018;32(8):3622–9. https://doi.org/10.1007/s00464-018-6091-6. Epub 2018 Feb 7. PMID: 29417229.
21. Atieh J, Sack J, Thomas R, Rahma OE, Camilleri M, Grover S. Gastroparesis following immune checkpoint inhibitor therapy: a case series. Dig Dis Sci. 2021;66(6):1974–80. https://doi.org/10.1007/s10620-020-06440-x. Epub 2020 Aug 7. Erratum in: Dig Dis Sci. 2020 Aug 7: PMID: 32594464; PMCID: PMC7867661.
22. So JB, Rao J, Wong AS, Chan YH, Pang NQ, Tay AYL, Yung MY, Su Z, Phua JNS, Shabbir A, Ng EKW. Roux-en-Y or Billroth II reconstruction after radical distal gastrectomy for gastric cancer: a multicenter randomized controlled trial. Ann Surg. 2018;267:236–42.
23. Cai Z, Zhou Y, Wang C, Yin Y, Shen C, Yin X, Chen Z, Zhang B. Optimal reconstruction methods after distal gastrectomy for gastric cancer: a systematic review and network meta-analysis. Medicine (Baltimore). 2018;97:e10823.
24. Otsuka R, Natsume T, Maruyama T, Tanaka H, Matsuzaki H. Antecolic reconstruction is a predictor of the occurrence of roux stasis syndrome after distal gastrectomy. J Gastrointest Surg. 2015;19:821–4.
25. Hwang HK, Lee SH, Han DH, Choi SH, Kang CM, Lee WJ. Impact of Braun anastomosis on reducing delayed gastric emptying following pancreaticoduodenectomy: a prospective, randomized controlled trial. J Hepatobiliary Pancreat Sci. 2016;23:364–72.

13 Regional Disorders of Sensory-Motor Dysfunction: Biliary-Pancreas

George Triadafilopoulos

13.1 Biliary-Pancreas

Pancreatic Neuroendocrine Tumors (NETs) Pancreatic neuroendocrine tumors (NETs) are made of fast-growing cells in the pancreas that produce hormones [1]. Previously called islet cell tumors, NETs are distinct from pancreatic adenocarcinomas, making up less than 5% of new pancreatic cancers [2]. NETs are subdivided into functional and non-functional. Functional NETs release high amounts of hormones producing clinically significant symptoms, depending on the type of hormone they overproduce. The most common type, the insulinomas, makes excess insulin causing hypoglycemia, with dizziness, fatigue, sweating, and hunger. Because of this, these tumors are frequently diagnosed early, while they are small, and they can often be surgically cured. Gastrinomas make excess gastrin and stomach acid, resulting in severe gastroesophageal acid reflux and peptic ulcers with abdominal pain and diarrhea. Glucagonomas make excess glucagon, leading to hyperglycemia, with fatigue, frequent urination, dry mouth, and unusual rashes on the face, abdomen, and legs. Somatostatinomas are very rare and produce excess somatostatin, in turn controlling the levels of several other hormones and resulting in symptoms of hyperglycemia, diarrhea, and weight loss. Similarly, VIPomas make excess vasoactive intestinal peptide (VIP), which controls several digestive functions, leading to secretory, large-volume diarrhea, muscle cramps, dehydration, weakness, and weight loss. Non-functional NETs are more common, but they do not produce high levels of hormones to cause severe symptoms, yet they may cause diarrhea, abdominal pain, and weight loss. Hence, these tumors often grow quite large before being diagnosed. The exact cause of pancreatic NETs is not known. These tumors are occasionally associated with genetic syndromes, such as multiple

G. Triadafilopoulos (✉)
Department of Gastroenterology, Hepatology and Nutrition, UT MD Anderson Cancer Center, Houston, TX, USA
e-mail: GTriadafilopoulo@mdanderson.org

G. Triadafilopoulos (ed.), *Onco-Neurogastroenterology*,
https://doi.org/10.1007/978-3-031-98848-6_13

endocrine neoplasia type 1 (MEN1), Von Hippel-Lindau (VHL), and neurofibromatosis (NF). The diagnosis of NETs is based on blood tests for the various released hormones and chromogranin A, a protein that is released even in non-functional pancreatic NETs. CT imaging of the pancreas is mostly used for tumor localization. Somatostatin receptor imaging using octreotate, which attaches to most pancreatic NETs, is mostly used for staging [3].

Localized pancreatic NETs are best treated surgically. Liver surgery can be used to remove liver metastases. Hormone therapy, using octreotide or lanreotide, can be used when surgery is not possible, and it is aiming at slowing a tumor's growth and spread but also to reduce the level of hormones produced by functional pancreatic NETs. Chemotherapy is used to stop tumor growth and to shrink larger tumors. Based on a patient's tolerability, temozolomide with capecitabine and fluorouracil (5-FU) with doxorubicin and streptozocin are typically given in combination. Targeted therapies, such as belzutifan, everolimus, and sunitinib, may be also used in select cases. Peptide receptor radionuclide therapy (PRRT) is used to treat somatostatin receptor-positive pancreatic NETs, through an intravenous delivery of a radioactive drug called lutetium Lu 177 dotatate. This drug delivers radiation by attaching to the tumor directly. Liver-directed therapy performed by interventional radiologists injects radioactive beads into the blood vessels, feeding the liver tumors. Rarely, observation may also be used as a treatment strategy for slow-growing tumors [4]. The onco-neuro-gastroenterologist is frequently involved in the care of patients with pancreatic NETs working together with surgery, medical and radiation oncology, and interventional radiology, aiding the management of the various symptoms encountered.

Sphincter of Oddi Dysfunction (SOD) Opioid analgesics, commonly used in oncology, are associated with a variety of gastrointestinal adverse effects (opioid-induced bowel dysfunction), including spasm/dysfunction of the sphincter of Oddi associated with episodes of severe abdominal pain, which may have the clinical features of either biliary colic or acute pancreatitis, which may occur either spontaneously or as a result of endoscopic intervention [5]. A high index of suspicion for this diagnosis is needed. Confirm, dynamic HIDA biliary imaging (with special sphincter of Oddi protocol) or secretin-stimulated MRCP. Treatment may involve antispasmodics (i.e., hyoscyamine sublingually), endoscopic ampullary Botox injection, ampullary balloon dilation, or sphincterotomy. Unfortunately, the effectiveness of endoscopic approaches has been questioned, and a thorough assessment of the risk-to-benefit ratio needs to be individualized [6].

Pancreatic Insufficiency Pancreatic insufficiency presents in two forms, which at times coexist: endocrine and exocrine insufficiency. The former reflects inadequate insulin release to meet the metabolic demands, and it is associated with subclinical or overt diabetes mellitus, and the latter is associated with inadequate pancreatic enzyme release. Both depend on the adequacy of functional pancreatic mass, and they may be encountered in chronic pancreatitis or pancreatic cancer or be the result of resective

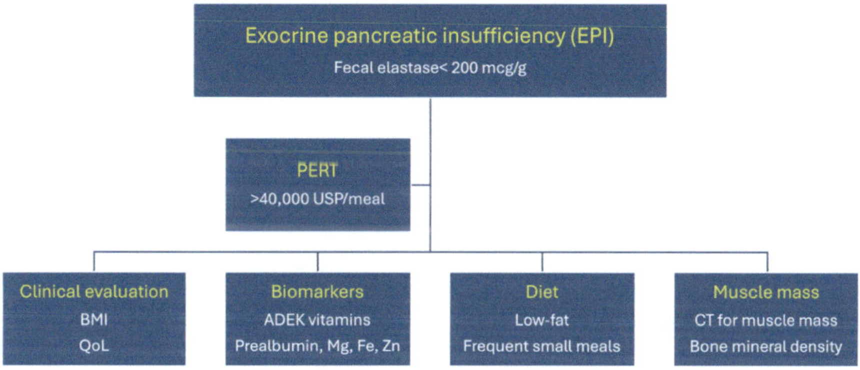

Fig. 13.1 Key parameters in the diagnosis, clinical evaluation, and management of exocrine pancreatic insufficiency. In cancer survivors, all these parameters should be considered regularly (yearly) to avoid deficiencies and complication

surgery, such as Whipple procedure for pancreatic head cancer or distal pancreatectomy for cancer of the body and tail of the pancreas. The condition may be asymptomatic, detectable on blood or stool testing, or it may be associated with chronic abdominal discomfort, bloating, diarrhea, and steatorrhea that leads to weight loss. The diagnosis is made when fecal elastase is ≤200 μg/g (<100 μg/g reflects severe disease). A trial of pancreatic enzymes at necessary doses is needed for symptom control (Fig. 13.1).

References

1. Ghabra S, Ramamoorthy B, Andrews SG, Sadowski SM. Surgical management and long-term evaluation of pancreatic neuroendocrine tumors. Surg Clin North Am. 2024;104(4):891–908. https://doi.org/10.1016/j.suc.2024.02.019. Epub 2024 Apr 4. PMID: 38944507; PMCID: PMC11214659
2. Chauhan A, Chan K, Halfdanarson TR, Bellizzi AM, Rindi G, O'Toole D, Ge PS, Jain D, Dasari A, Anaya DA, Bergsland E, Mittra E, Wei AC, Hope TA, Kendi AT, Thomas SM, Flem S, Brierley J, Asare EA, Washington K, Shi C. Critical updates in neuroendocrine tumors: version 9 American Joint Committee on Cancer staging system for gastroenteropancreatic neuroendocrine tumors. CA Cancer J Clin. 2024;74(4):359–67. https://doi.org/10.3322/caac.21840. Epub 2024 Apr 29. PMID: 38685134.
3. Tobias J, Keutgen XM. Diagnostics and imaging for pancreatic neuroendocrine tumors. Surg Clin North Am. 2024;104(4):883–90. https://doi.org/10.1016/j.suc.2024.02.015. Epub 2024 Mar 23. PMID: 38944506.
4. Kartik A, Armstrong VL, Stucky CC, Wasif N, Fong ZV. Contemporary approaches to the surgical management of pancreatic neuroendocrine tumors. Cancers (Basel). 2024;16(8):1501. https://doi.org/10.3390/cancers16081501. PMID: 38672582; PMCID: PMC11048062.
5. Wu SD, Zhang ZH, Jin JZ, Kong J, Wang W, Zhang Q, Li DY, Wang MF. Effects of narcotic analgesic drugs on human Oddi's sphincter motility. World J Gastroenterol. 2004;10(19):2901–4.
6. Cotton PB, Elta GH, Carter CR, Pasricha PJ, Corazziari ES, Rome IV. Gallbladder and sphincter of Oddi disorders. Gastroenterology. 2016;19:S0016-5085(16)00224-9. https://doi.org/10.1053/j.gastro.2016.02.033. Epub ahead of print. PMID: 27144629.

Regional Disorders of Sensory-Motor Dysfunction: Small Intestine

14

George Triadafilopoulos, Mehnaz A. Shafi, and Lavanya Viswanathan

14.1 Small Intestine

Small Intestinal NETs Similar to the pancreatic ones, some NETs that are located in the small bowel may produce biogenic amines and peptide hormones, which cause clinical syndromes, e.g., the carcinoid syndrome (i.e., flushing, diarrhea) due to unmetabolized overproduced serotonin, hypoglycemic syndrome in case of insulinoma, or Zollinger-Ellison syndrome (i.e., acid hypersecretion, diarrhea) due to gastrinoma. Driven by other studies, such as computed tomography (CT), magnetic resonance imaging (MRI), and positron emission tomography/computed tomography (PET/CT), or EUS with directed biopsies, allows endoscopic and histopathologic classification supplemented with immunohistochemistry, which is based on Ki67 expression and may classify NETs into low-grade (Ki67 $\leq 2\%$), intermediate (Ki67 3–20%), and high-grade (Ki67 $> 20\%$) and further guide decision-making [1].

Zollinger-Ellison Syndrome Zollinger-Ellison syndrome (ZES) is caused by secretion of gastrin by duodenal or pancreatic neuroendocrine tumors (gastrinomas). Most patients have duodenal gastrinomas, predominantly in the first part of the duodenum [2]. Due to the trophic action of gastrin on parietal cells and enterochromaffin-like (ECL) cells, excessive gastrin secretion from a gastrinoma results in high gastric acid output that cannot be fully reabsorbed, overwhelming the neutralizing capacity of pancreatic bicarbonate secretion, leading to a low intestinal luminal pH, which in turn inactivates pancreatic enzymes, alters fat emulsification by bile acids, and damages the intestinal epithelial surface and results in steatorrhea

G. Triadafilopoulos (✉) · M. A. Shafi · L. Viswanathan
Department of Gastroenterology, Hepatology and Nutrition, UT MD Anderson Cancer Center, Houston, TX, USA
e-mail: GTriadafilopoulo@mdanderson.org

G. Triadafilopoulos (ed.), *Onco-Neurogastroenterology*,
https://doi.org/10.1007/978-3-031-98848-6_14

(Fig. 14.1). Further, high serum gastrin concentrations inhibit sodium and water absorption by the small intestine (secretory diarrhea) [3].

Dumping Syndrome Occurring after esophagectomy, gastrectomy with Roux-en-Y gastric bypass, or antireflux surgery (ARS), dumping syndrome is characterized by postprandial discomfort, cramping, and diarrhea, together with sympathetic hyperactivity, either early (within 15 min of eating) or late, associated with hypoglycemia and autonomic symptoms (1–3 h after eating), and it is related to rapid transit of glucose to the intestine, increased gastrointestinal peptide secretion including GLP-1, excess insulin release, and subsequent hypoglycemia (Fig. 14.2) [4].

Dietary modification, acarbose, octreotide, and diazoxide can be used as treatments. Over time (years), many patients adjust and may require no treatment [5]. Figure 14.3 shows a barium contrast study outlining a normal esophago-jejunal anastomosis after distal esophagectomy for cancer. Figure 14.4 depicts an antegrade endoscopic view of a normal esophago-jejunostomy after a total gastrectomy for gastric cancer.

Celiac Disease Patients with various malabsorptive syndromes, including those with celiac disease (CD), have lower fasting and postprandial antral and duodenal motility indices than healthy subjects, and intravenous octreotide induces migratory motor complex (MMC) [6]. After treatment of celiac sprue with gluten-free diet, chronic diarrhea persists in 17% of patients, and diagnostic studies are warranted. In such refractory cases, non-adherence, microscopic colitis, exocrine pancreatic insufficiency, lactose or fructose malabsorption, fecal incontinence, and irritable

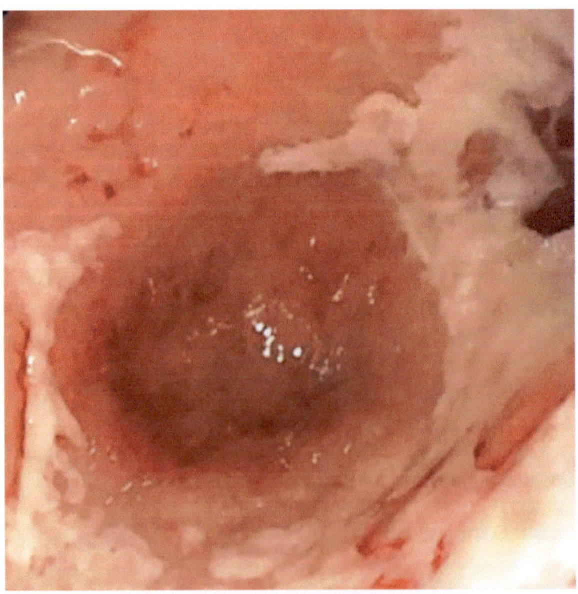

Fig. 14.1 Endoscopic appearance of the duodenal bulb in a patient with ZES and hypergastrinemia. There are extensive and confluent ulcerations and stricturing of the duodenum (top right corner of the image)

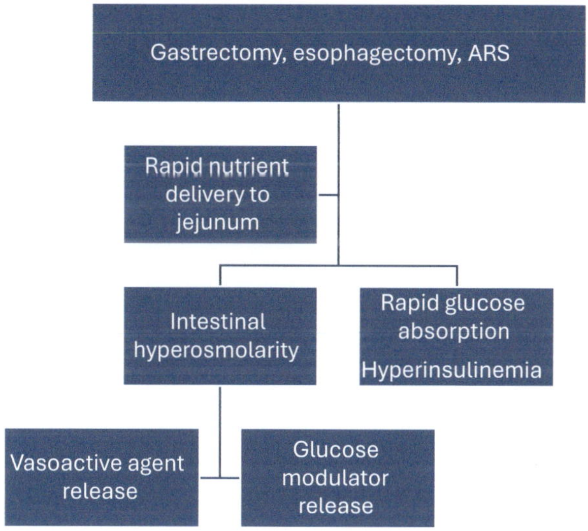

Fig. 14.2 Highlights of the pathophysiology of dumping syndrome

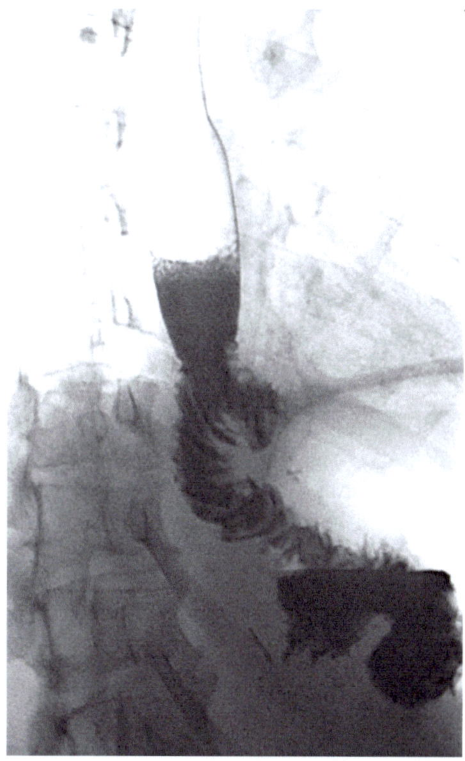

Fig. 14.3 Barium contrast study of a normal end-to-side esophago-jejunal anastomosis

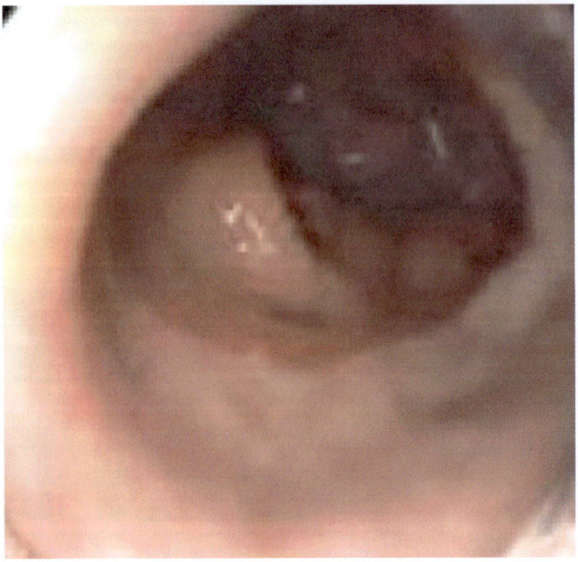

Fig. 14.4 Antegrade endoscopic view of a normal esophago-jejunostomy after a total gastrectomy

bowel syndrome are possible benign causes [7]. Celiac disease is associated with intestinal lymphoma and other cancers, such as adenocarcinoma of the small intestine, pharynx, and esophagus. Enteropathy-associated T-cell lymphoma (EATL) is a rare form of high-grade, T-cell non-Hodgkin lymphoma (NHL) of the proximal small intestine that arises in patients with either previously or concomitantly diagnosed CD. Strict gluten-free diet protects from cancer development, especially if started early [8]. Patient presentation can be highly variable, ranging from an asymptomatic state, to iron deficiency with or without anemia, to abnormal liver function tests, to more dramatic presentations, with diarrhea; flatulence; foul-smelling, floating stools due to steatorrhea; and signs of malabsorption, such as weight loss, anemia, vitamin deficiencies, and osteopenia from deficiency of vitamin D and calcium. The severity of histologic small bowel changes does not necessarily correlate with the severity of clinical presentation, and high index of suspicion is needed. Refractory disease, defined by the persistence of symptoms despite adherence to a strict gluten-free diet, calls for thorough evaluation to exclude EATL, adenocarcinoma, collagenous sprue, microscopic colitis, or autoimmune enteropathy.

Non-celiac Gluten Sensitivity Non-celiac gluten sensitivity (NCGS) is a syndrome of uncertain pathogenesis in which intestinal and extra-intestinal symptoms occur after gluten/wheat ingestion in subjects where the diagnosis of both celiac disease (CD) and IgE-mediated wheat allergy (WA) has been excluded. NCGWS may present with abdominal pain, bloating, reflux, and irregular bowel movements, at times associated with fatigue, headaches, "foggy mind," and dermatitis. Given the significant overlap in symptoms with irritable bowel syndrome (IBS), NCGWS relies on exclusion of CD and wheat allergy, patient's responsiveness to a gluten-free diet (GFD), and a double-blind, placebo-controlled gluten/wheat rechallenge, according to the "Salerno experts' criteria." Treatment consists of non-strict GFD that resolves both intestinal and extra-intestinal symptoms [9].

Immune Checkpoint Inhibitor (ICI)-Associated Celiac Disease This is a variant of ICI- duodenitis clinically and histologically, with diarrhea and abdominal pain after a median of 1.6 months on ICI therapy but shares the serological features and response to gluten withdrawal with classic celiac disease. Immunophenotyping of intraepithelial lymphocytes (IELs) in both conditions shows similar CD3, CD8, $\gamma\delta$ T-cell subsets, and PD-L1 populations, all of which differ quantitatively from classic celiac disease. Treatment strategies differ, with ICI-associated celiac disease improving with gluten-free diet alone, whereas ICI-duodenitis requires systemic immunosuppression [10].

Small Intestinal Intussusception Intussusception is a rare form of bowel obstruction in adults, which is defined as the telescoping of a proximal segment of the gastrointestinal tract, into the lumen of the adjacent distal segment (Fig. 14.5). It may occur intermittently, causing symptoms of partial or complete bowel obstruction (crampy abdominal pain, abdominal distention, nausea and vomiting), or subclinically (detected serendipitously on imaging) [11]. About 10% of small bowel intussusceptions in adults are idiopathic; if subtle and intermittent, intussusception may contribute to small intestinal bacterial overgrowth due to intermittent stasis of intestinal contents (Fig. 14.6) [12].

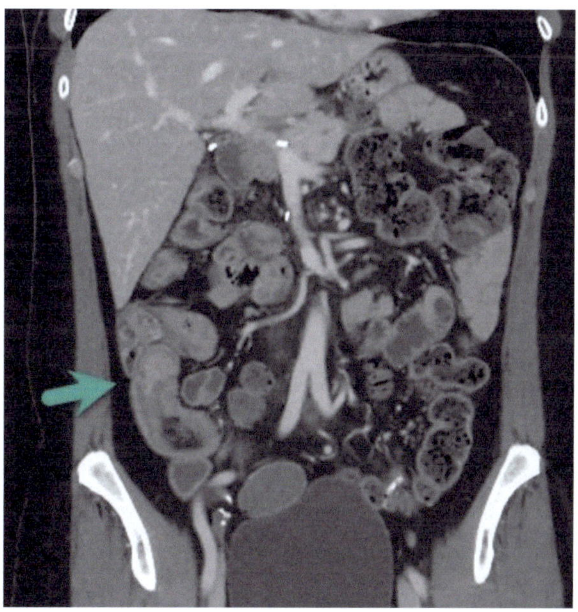

Fig. 14.5 Abdominal CT imaging revealing ileocolonic intussusception due to an ileal tubulovillous adenoma

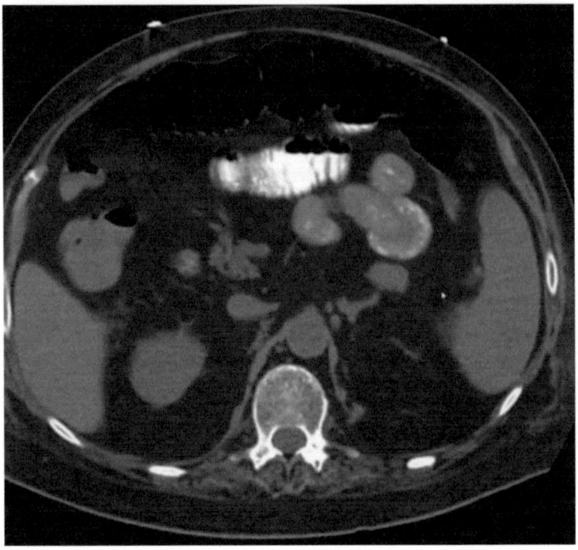

Fig. 14.6 Abdominal CT imaging revealing intermittent ileal intussusception. Because of intermittent abdominal pain and recurrent SIBO, she underwent laparoscopy that revealed no abnormalities

Small Intestinal Bacterial Overgrowth (SIBO) Since many patients with cancer are older, have altered surgical anatomy, and have received abdomino-pelvic radiation or they take narcotics for pain, there is altered motility leading to stasis and small bowel bacterial overgrowth (SIBO) that may need periodic treatment with antibiotics. SIBO is also common in post-gastrectomy patients and associated with postprandial fullness, borborygmi, dumping, and late hypoglycemia [13].

Symptoms of SIBO include postprandial abdominal bloating/distention, nonspecific abdominal discomfort, diarrhea, flatulence, or nonspecific dyspepsia. Such patients may also have altered sensation, and it is hard to recognize the symptoms, which are variable and intermittent. SIBO may present with nonspecific symptoms that may vary depending upon the severity of involvement but also the underlying primary disease that is causing bacterial overgrowth. The symptoms may be due to nutrient malabsorption, altered gut permeability, gut inflammation, and/or immune activation. Subjects with SIBO may also be asymptomatic. Physical examination findings in SIBO are nonspecific. Endoscopically, the small intestine is normal (Fig. 14.7). Abdominal CT imaging may reveal segmental small bowel dilation and stasis (Fig. 14.8).

Traditionally, small intestinal bacterial overgrowth (SIBO) is defined as the growth of bacteria $\geq 10^5$ colony-forming unit (CFU)/mL or ≥103 CFU/mL (particularly if coliforms are present) on a quantitative culture of upper gut aspirate. Glucose or lactulose breath tests are non-invasive, but they have poor sensitivity and specificity [14]. SIBO can be high or low threshold, depending upon the bacterial counts, and its microbiological spectrum may vary depending on the underlying etiology. Many pre- or co-existing gastrointestinal conditions are associated with SIBO, including IBS, IBD, celiac disease, small bowel diverticulosis, intestinal strictures or fistulas, radiation enteropathy, pancreatitis, and chronic liver disease. Further, other

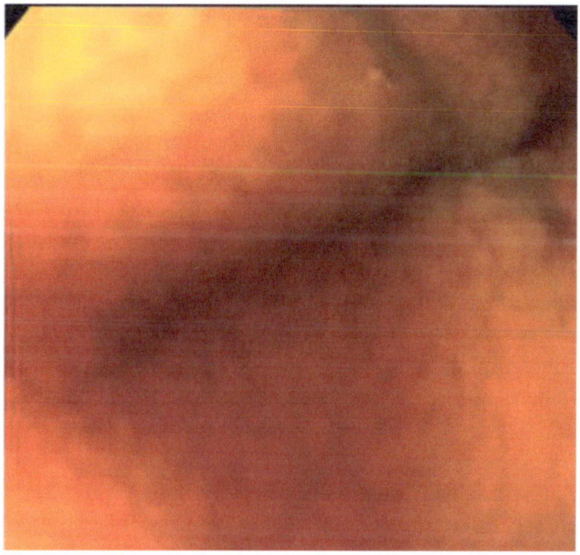

Fig. 14.7 Endoscopic appearance of normal terminal ileum in the context of SIBO

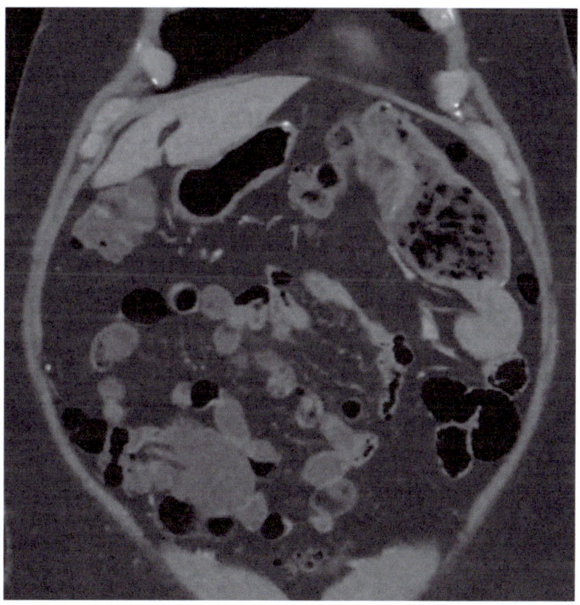

Fig. 14.8 Abdominal CT imaging revealing segmental small bowel dilation and fecal stasis in the jejunum, resulting from surgical adhesions. Patient experienced recurrent episodes of SIBO, requiring repetitive courses of rifaximin. Note the bowel loop dilation containing fecal matter

non-gastrointestinal conditions, such progressive systemic sclerosis, diabetes, hypothyroidism, obesity, Parkinson's disease, multiple sclerosis, or end-stage renal failure, may be associated with SIBO. The frequency of SIBO in these associated disorders is highly variable, sometimes reaching 90%. Achlorhydria or pharmacologically induced hypochlorhydria, poorly coordinated antegrade small bowel peristalsis or lack of phase III of migratory motor complex (MMC), poor integrity and/

or function of the ileocecal valve, altered intestinal mucosal immunity, and lack of protection by beneficial commensal flora may result in the development of SIBO. Drugs frequently used by patients with cancer, such as proton pump inhibitors (PPI), non-steroidal anti-inflammatory drugs (NSAIDs), opioids, anticholinergics, antidiarrheals, and tricyclic antidepressants, also play a key role. Due to the invasive nature of gut aspiration and the need for elaborate culture support, the lactulose breath test (LBT) for hydrogen and methane production is mostly used. Small intestinal biopsies are nonspecific. Treatment involves correction of the underlying cause (if possible), treatment with rifaximin and/or neomycin, and correction of any related nutritional deficiencies. Doxycycline, amoxicillin-clavulanic acid, ciprofloxacin, metronidazole, norfloxacin, tetracycline, or trimethoprim-sulfamethoxazole. Elemental diets are sometimes tried but their long-term feasibility and impact are uncertain. Recurrences are common, and treatment with repeat courses of different and—at times—rotating antibiotics and the use of probiotics are suggested, as needed.

Intestinal Methanogen Overgrowth (IMO) Clinically indistinguishable from SIBO, this is a separate clinical entity where methanogenic archaea have overgrown resulting in gastrointestinal symptoms. IMO is attributed to anaerobic organisms from the domain archaea, rather than bacteria [15]. IMO is diagnosed by $CH4 \geq 10$ ppm at any point of the 120-min breath test, and it typically presents with constipation, alternating bowel habits, postprandial abdominal bloating/distention, and brain fog (Fig. 14.9). In contrast to SIBO, IMO requires treatment with rifaximin plus neomycin or metronidazole or ciprofloxacin plus metronidazole for 2 weeks.

Small Intestinal Fungal Overgrowth (SIFO) Not uncommon in patients with cancer and immunosuppression, post-colectomy, and steroid or antibiotics users,

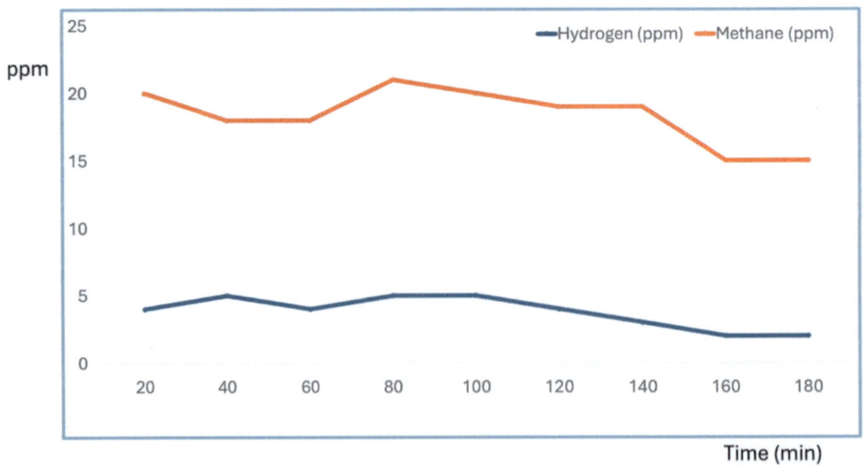

Fig. 14.9 Lactose breath test positive for IMO (red line) and negative for SIBO (blue line)

SIFO is characterized by excessive number of fungal organisms, mainly *Candida* species, in the small bowel and presents with abdominal bloating and distention, nonspecific abdominal discomfort, diarrhea, flatulence, and belching. The diagnosis is based on small bowel aspiration with quantitative cultures yielding $\geq 10^3$ CFU/mL, and it requires treatment with fluconazole for 3 weeks [16].

Disaccharidase Deficiencies These deficiencies include the lactase, sucrase, maltase, and isomaltase enzymes, which are produced by the intestinal brush border, and may result in abdominal pain, gas, bloating, and diarrhea by interfering with the breakdown and absorption of carbohydrates. Patients deficient in all four of these disaccharidases are considered as having "pan-disaccharidase" deficiency, a phenotype causing more weight loss. Diagnosis is based on duodenal biopsies and breath testing. Dietary restriction and enzyme replacement therapy are effective treatments. Patients who do not respond to traditional treatment strategies for DBGI may benefit from testing for disaccharidase deficiency [17].

Bile Acid Malabsorption (BAM) Because the terminal ileum is the major site of bile acid reabsorption, when a short ileal resection <100 cm is performed, increased hepatic synthesis of bile acids (BA) minimizes the effect on bile acid metabolism, and patients may develop watery diarrhea. An ileal resection greater than 100 cm can result in severe bile acid malabsorption and steatorrhea. Excess bile acids can cause GI symptoms because they enhance mucosal permeability, induce water and electrolyte secretion, and accelerate colonic transit. Common symptoms of bile acid malabsorption include watery diarrhea, steatorrhea, urgency, and abdominal cramping. Symptomatic response to bile acid sequestrants is the practical preferred method to confirm the diagnosis. Importantly, SIBO is a common cause of BAM because deconjugation of bile acids is mediated by bile salt hydrolase enzymes, which are widely expressed by the gut microbiota. Since patients with IBD are at higher risk for SIBO, SIBO should be ruled out [18].

Roux-en-Y Limb Motility after Total Gastrectomy Roux-en-Y stasis syndrome is a troublesome sequel after gastrectomy for proximal gastric cancer. Using HRM, peristaltic waves may be noted at the Roux-en-Y limb (RYL) in 37% of the patients. Overall, esophageal motility is normal after total gastrectomy with Roux-en-Y reconstruction, motor activity is always detectable at the proximal RYL, but peristalsis is abnormal and not necessarily symptomatic in most patients [19].

Blind Loop Syndrome Blind loop syndrome (BLS) is an uncommon malabsorptive disorder that results from postoperative alterations, such as adhesions from Billroth II, Roux-en-Y, Whipple procedure, underlying dysmotility, and inflammatory small bowel disease, such as Crohn's disease or radiation enteritis [20]. Bacterial overgrowth results of relative stagnation of the small intestine stasis enables the proliferation of species like *Bacteroides*, *E. coli*, *Streptococcus*, and *Lactobacillus* in abnormally high concentrations. Consequently, this overgrowth affects digestion and absorption, resulting in malnutrition, B12 deficiency, and steatorrhea [21].

Immune Checkpoint Inhibitor (ICI) Toxicity Immune checkpoint inhibitor (ICI) blockade has revolutionized the management, outcomes, and survival rates in advanced malignancies. However, the use of these immunotherapeutic agents comes with the risk of gastrointestinal adverse events that may vary in severity from mild to severe, life-threatening clinical presentations. Patients often present with diarrhea (increased stool frequency) or colitis (abdominal pain, rectal bleeding, or the presence of mucus in stools) sometimes along with radiologic evidence of colonic inflammation [22]. Involvement of the stomach and proximal small bowel is rare and may present clinically with abdominal pain, intractable nausea, and emesis. In mild cases, when endoscopy is relatively unremarkable, histologic changes show gastric intraepithelial neutrophilic infiltration and, at times, small duodenal villous blunting, lymphoplasmacytic lamina propria expansion, and plasma cell infiltration [23]. Mild symptoms are effectively managed with proton pump inhibitors or H2 receptor blockers.

Postoperative Ileus Postoperative ileus (POI) is a common condition occurring after abdominal surgery and reflects a slowing or complete cessation of bowel motility [24]. POI affects 10–25% of patients after abdominal surgery [25]. Pathophysiologically, there are at least two phases in POI, an early "neurogenic" phase involving neural pathways and a later "inflammatory" phase [26]. The two most consistently effective pharmacological treatments for reducing POI after abdominal surgery are prokinetics such as 5HT3 receptor antagonists (metoclopramide), selective 5HT4 receptor agonists (prucalopride), and ghrelin receptor agonists (ulimorelin) and opioid antagonists, since morphine and other opioid analgesics inhibit acetylcholine from the mesenteric plexus, thereby increasing colonic muscle tone and reducing propulsive activity. Both alvimopan and methylnaltrexone are the main peripheral opioid antagonists used [27].

Paraneoplastic Chronic Watery Diarrhea Diarrhea as a paraneoplastic manifestation of metastatic thymoma has been described in the form of autoimmune enteropathy, a rare disease characterized by villous atrophy of the small bowel, persistent diarrhea, and the presence of autoantibodies [28]. that may include infection (e.g., *Clostridium difficile*), radiotherapy (e.g., radiation enteritis), systemic cytotoxic therapy (e.g., 5-fluorouracil, irinotecan, capecitabine), immunomodulatory agents, surgical resection, and underlying cancer (e.g., pancreatic tumors, carcinoid tumor). Chronic intestinal pseudo-obstruction (SIPO) is most closely associated with small cell lung cancer. The mechanism of action is not clear. Treatment of the underlying malignancy may reverse the symptoms. Octreotide has been used to treat this successfully as well as therapies directed at the underlying etiology [29].

Narcotic Bowel Syndrome Narcotic bowel syndrome is characterized by chronic abdominal pain, nausea, vomiting, weight loss, and features of intestinal pseudo-obstruction, associated with prolonged abuse of narcotic analgesics; the symptoms resolved rapidly in all patients when narcotic administration was stopped [30]. Acute colonic pseudo-obstruction may also occur. Such patients are managed conservatively with bowel rest, but some may need treatment with either intravenous neostigmine, colonoscopy for colonic decompression alone, neostigmine followed by colonic decompression, or neostigmine followed by exploratory laparotomy [31].

Acute and Chronic Radiation Enteritis Patients receiving radiation therapy to the abdomen and pelvis for the treatment of gynecologic, genitourinary, gastrointestinal, and other malignancies are at risk of developing acute and chronic intestinal injury. Patients will experience GI symptoms up to 90% of the time after radiation to the abdomen and pelvis, and this may lead to permanent change in their bowel habits. Within the 90%, 3–10% of patients will develop radiation-induced bowel injury with signs of dysmotility, strictures, and/or fistulae. Thirty percent of such patients may require surgery that is associated with a 10–20% mortality rate. Due to the damage caused by the tumor or radiotherapy and chemotherapy, the integrity of the intestinal mucosa barrier is severely impaired. Radiotherapy and chemotherapy commonly reduce the functionality of cellular and humoral immune systems, contributing to inadequate nutritional intake, secondary infection, and alterations in the gut microbiota [32]. Common symptoms of radiation-induced bowel injury include diarrhea, abdominal pain, bloating, fecal incontinence, bleeding per rectum, and weight loss. The acute phase of symptoms usually occurs within 3 months of radiotherapy and resolves within 3 months. The chronic phase of symptoms typically occurs 6 months to years later and is defined by chronic inflammation, fibrosis, vasculitis, ischemia, and gut dysmotility. Treatment is supportive mostly to control of symptoms and prevention of infection and in providing adequate nutritional support. Diarrhea caused by chronic radiation enteritis is associated with more rapid intestinal transit and a high prevalence of bile acid and lactose malabsorption. Loperamide-N-oxide slows small intestinal transit, increases bile acid absorption, and is an effective treatment [33].

Chemotherapy- and/or Radiation-Induced Nausea and Vomiting Nausea and vomiting occur most commonly during chemotherapy, radiation, or both, and they significantly impact the patients' quality of life (QoL) and treatment compliance. The symptoms are frequently mediated by activation of serotonin type 3 receptors in the gastrointestinal tract. Risk factors depend on the types of chemotherapy drugs and their respective doses, the schedules and route of administration, and the patients' age, sex, and prior alcohol use. The various types of nausea and vomiting (i.e., acute, delayed, anticipatory, breakthrough, and refractory) require different treatment regimens, which often include 5HT3 receptor antagonists, NK1 receptor antagonists, and corticosteroids and often remain a challenge typically requiring combination strategies [34].

Autonomic Neuropathy Autonomic neuropathy frequently presents with dysmotility of the stomach, small bowel, and colon, such as gastroparesis, intestinal pseudo-obstruction, cardiac dysrhythmias, and postural hypotension, dry mouth, erectile dysfunction, anhidrosis, and sphincter dysfunction manifesting as nausea, bloating, diarrhea, constipation, and abdominal pain associated with several tumors, including SCLC, pancreas, testis, carcinoid tumors, and lymphoma. Serum anti-Hu and anti-CV2/CRMP5 antibodies may be positive. Postural orthostatic tachycardia syndrome (POTS) is an autonomic disorder that affects multiple organs, including the gastrointestinal system. POTS is more frequent in women (female to male ratio 4.5:1), and most cases occur between ages 15 and 25 [35]. The pathophysiology of POTS is multifactorial and includes impaired sympathetic vasoconstriction, hyper-adrenergic states, hypovolemia, and physical deconditioning. The condition is defined as an elevation of the heart rate of at least 30 beats per minute (bpm) within 10 min after standing upright or a heart rate ≥ 120 bpm after standing in the absence of orthostatic hypotension. In addition, patients may display symptoms of cerebral hypoperfusion (lightheadedness, blurred vision, cognitive difficulties, weakness) and sympathetic hyperactivity (palpitations, chest pain, and tremulousness). These patients often have multiple gastrointestinal complaints with a severe impact on their quality of life. Gastrointestinal dysmotility in POTS remains poorly understood and difficult to manage [36, 37].

The evaluation and management of POTS should be multidisciplinary, including cardiac evaluation to exclude other causes of inappropriate sinus tachycardia, autonomic reflex testing (i.e., tilt table test), and measurement of supine and standing plasma catecholamine levels. Management includes avoidance of exacerbating factors (i.e., heat exposure, physical exertion, heavy meals, prolonged recumbency), medications (diuretics, vasodilators, sympathomimetics), maintenance of intravascular volume with increased water and sodium intake, physical reconditioning, and pharmacotherapy (fludrocortisone, midodrine, beta-blockers, and/or pyridostigmine). The added benefit of pyridostigmine is that it may potentiate muscarinic receptor activation in the gut and may improve gastric emptying and constipation. Additionally, as a cholinesterase inhibitor, it may potentiate vagal effects [38].

Chronic Intestinal Pseudo-Obstruction (CIPO) Chronic intestinal pseudo-obstruction results in symptoms of bowel obstruction in the absence of mechanical causes. Peritoneal carcinomatosis is a common cause of CIPO, and it is best detected by CT imaging (Fig. 14.10). Clinical manifestations may include nausea, vomiting, abdominal distension, abdominal pain, constipation, malnutrition, and/or other symptoms, such as periods of diarrhea after bacterial overgrowth. Intractable abdominal pain is the most common symptom. Abdominal pain caused by CIPO is visceral, usually ill-defined, and poorly localized or peri-umbilical, due to mechanical stretching, distension, contraction, or torsion, thereby stimulating visceral nociceptors. Because of the severity of pain, narcotics are used, adding complexity to its management. The diagnosis is ideally but rarely made using high-resolution small intestinal manometry that classifies the condition as intestinal neuropathy (bursts of unpropagated activity) and myopathy (reduced amplitude during phase III of MMC) and excludes partial intestinal occlusion (short bursts of postprandial contractions every 1–2 min) [39]. Analgesics used in patients with CIPO include non-opioid (acetaminophen, non-steroidal anti-inflammatory drugs) and opioid drugs.

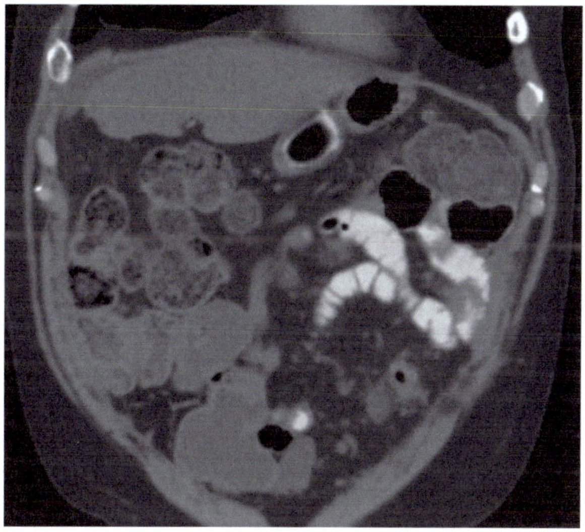

Fig. 14.10 Multifocal peritoneal stranding due to diffuse carcinomatosis from rectal cancer

Antidepressant and anticonvulsant drugs are also widely used. If pain is poorly controlled by morphine or side effects are dominant, Butrans might be an option. A variety of prokinetic agents are also used, as needed.

Acute Intestinal Graft-Versus-Host Disease (GVHD) Well-orchestrated transcriptional programs in intestinal epithelial cells (IECs) are essential for maintenance of optimal mucosal barrier functions. Several bacterial products are associated with gut barrier integrity in the context of GVHD [40]. For example, intragastric administration of butyrate to allogeneic recipients improved IEC junctional integrity and led to decreased GVHD. *Clostridia* commensals are known butyrate producers, and administration of a microbial cocktail including 17 strains of *Clostridiales* elevated intraluminal butyrate concentrations and decreased GVHD clinical scores. This could explain why selective antibiotic use may be associated with reduced GVHD-related mortality [41] and supports the use of fecal microbiota transplants for the treatment of GVHD [42]. Given the clear associations of microbial constituents and GVHD outcomes, manipulation of the enteric flora or associated metabolites represents promising approaches for clinical prevention and treatment of GVHD [43].

Afferent Loop Syndrome (ALS) This is a rare syndrome of acute or chronic mechanical obstruction of the afferent loop that occurs after gastrectomy with gastrojejunostomy, in which two exit limbs known as afferent and efferent loop are created. ALS is mostly benign, occurring after distal gastrectomy with Billroth II reconstruction, Roux-en-Y reconstruction, or pancreaticoduodenectomy with conventional loop and Roux-en-Y anastomosis, or may be malignant, associated with locoregional tumor recurrence obstructing the afferent loop at the anastomotic site or gastric remnant. The afferent loop, also called "A-limb" or biliopancreatic limb, consists of the duodenum and proximal jejunum that transfers bile, pancreatic, and other proximal intestinal secretions toward the gastrojejunostomy [44].

Acute ALS presents with sudden severe upper abdominal pain and vomiting, at times like acute pancreatitis or ascending cholangitis. If focal abdominal tenderness and guarding are noted, a concern about intestinal viability should be raised prompting urgent surgery. Chronic ALS is more difficult to diagnose. Patients report pressure-like, cramping epigastric pain or peri-umbilical discomfort that develops 15–30 min after a meal and lasts for several hours. Some patients only report postprandial epigastric fullness and nausea and may develop sitophobia and weight loss. Sudden, projectile, large-volume bilious vomiting is common. Typically, symptoms are relieved after vomiting due to the sudden decompression of the partially obstructed bowel loop. Steatorrhea, diarrhea, vitamin B12 deficiency, and malnutrition may result from chronic SIBO. Physical examination may reveal upper abdominal distension; mass in the upper abdomen, representing an obstructed afferent loop; hypotension, tachycardia, or peritonitis and shock in acute ALS; or pancreatitis and ascending cholangitis depending on the patency of prior biliary or pancreato-enteric anastomosis.

Contrast-enhanced abdominal CT provides information about the area and cause of obstruction, and it assesses for intestinal ischemia, perforation, pancreatitis, or inflammatory biliary changes. CT may show a dilated afferent loop that runs across the midline, the keyboard sign (projection of valvulae conniventes into the lumen), bowel wall thickening, an obstructing lesion at the anastomosis, or pancreaticobiliary tract dilation. It also assesses for lymphadenopathy, ascites, peritoneal enhancement, and metastatic lesions in malignant ALS. Magnetic resonance cholangiopancreatography (MRCP) or secretin-enhanced MRCP can be helpful to assess hepaticojejunostomy and pancreaticojejunostomy anastomotic strictures [45]. Biliary (HIDA) scintigraphy is also useful in chronic ALS, tracing bile flow into the obstructed bowel loop.

Surgery is usually the key treatment for ALS, and it may include adhesiolysis, bypass surgery, or excision with a reconstruction of obstructive malignant lesions. More recently, endoscopic approaches for afferent loop syndrome may involve the afferent loop, the bile duct, and the pancreatic duct. Treatment of malignant afferent loop syndrome is by endoscopic ultrasound (EUS)-guided transgastric drainage using lumen-apposing stent followed by a double pigtail stent [46]. Endoscopic therapy using lumen-apposing stent (LAMS) is increasingly a treatment option in benign ALS, and it remains crucial in malignancy-related ALS. Volvulus, adhesion, and internal herniation typically require surgical intervention [47].

Systemic Mastocytosis Systemic mastocytosis (SM) is a rare myeloid neoplasm characterized by variable infiltration and multifocal accumulation of neoplastic mast cells (MC) in bone marrow (BM), skin, and visceral organs. The major diagnostic criterion for the disease is the presence of MC aggregates (defined as 15 or more MCs) in BM or other organs, including the gastrointestinal tract. MC mediator release leads to various gastrointestinal symptoms, such as food intolerance, nausea, vomiting, abdominal cramping, and diarrhea, ultimately causing malabsorption and weight loss [48].

Intestinal Failure (IF) and Short Bowel Syndrome (SBS) Intestinal failure (IF) is defined as the gastrointestinal functional state that is inadequate to maintain a patient's nutrition and hydration without intravenous or enteral supplementation. Based on its duration, IF may be acute or chronic, with an intervening adaptation phase. Short bowel syndrome (SBS) describes IF that is caused by reduced small intestinal absorptive area, mostly due to extensive resection. Anatomically, SBS implies residual small bowel length <200 cm, with or without colon. Functional SBS sometimes describes patients with a residual small bowel >200 cm, but with impaired function due to severely impaired motility (fast or slow), altered sensation with poor accommodation, or inflammation (i.e., IBD). Intestinal adaptation is the process that follows intestinal resection, whereby the remaining bowel undergoes morphologic and functional changes that increase its absorptive capacity. Although overall, nearly one third of SBS cases are due to Crohn's disease, mesenteric ischemia, surgical complications, and radiation enteritis account for most cases in patients with cancer [49]. Because of the variable small bowel length and the remarkable ability of the bowel to functionally compensate over time, the clinical presentation of SBS only modestly correlates with the length of the resected intestine. SBS in patients with cancer results from extensive surgical resection or disease-associated loss of absorption (i.e., intestinal failure resulting from severe intestinal dysmotility) and is characterized by the inability to maintain protein-energy, fluid, electrolyte, or micronutrient balances when on a normal diet [50].

The symptoms associated with bowel resection depend upon the altered physiology of the remaining small bowel, as shown in Table 14.1, which may include diarrhea, steatorrhea (greasy, foul-smelling stools), fatigue, weight loss, malnutrition, and peripheral edema. Extensive small bowel resections also trigger gastric hypergastrinemia and acid hypersecretion, particularly if the duodenum and jejunum have been resected, in turn leading to high stool (or ostomy) output for up to 12 months postoperatively, and it requires vigorous fluid replacement and acid blocker use.

Due to its extent, resection of the entire ileum and colon with end-jejunostomy generally has the worst prognosis. Resection of variable length of jejunum, the entire ileum, ileocecal valve, and part of the colon with jejuno-colic anastomosis has variable prognosis, depending on the length of the remaining jejunum. In contrast, partial resection of the ileum with retention of the ileocecal valve and the colon with jejuno-ileocolonic anastomosis has the best prognosis. Management must be individualized, based on the phase of the disease (Fig. 14.11), success or failure of prior therapies, underlying comorbidities, and overall cancer prognosis. The onco-neurogastroenterologist should work together with the surgeons and oncologists for an elaborate multidisciplinary decision-making and management. This is particularly applicable in patients with extensive peritoneal carcinomatosis with CIPO, leading to functional SBS and IF.

Table 14.1 Intestinal sites of nutrient absorption causing impaired physiology in SBS

Organ	Impaired physiology
Duodenum	Absorption of calcium, iron, folate, amino acids, peptides, fat, and ADEK vitamins
Jejunum	Water-soluble vitamins and zinc absorption
Ileum	Bile acids and B12 absorption
Colon	Potassium and short-chain fatty acid absorption
Any of the above	Absorption of sodium and water

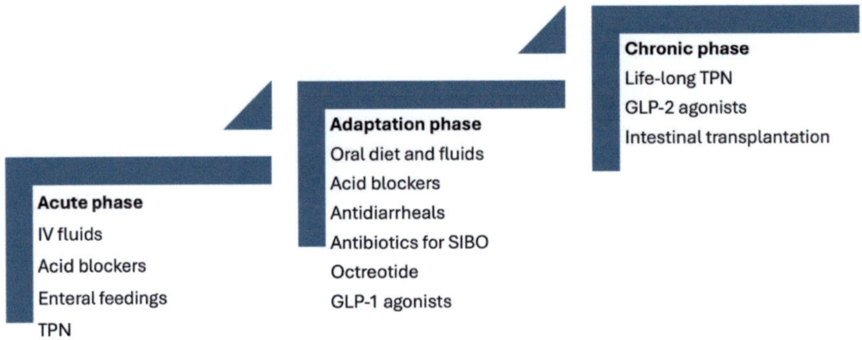

Fig. 14.11 Select therapy options for intestinal failure depending on its phase. Combinations of various therapeutic options have an additive effect

In cancer patients, arterial or venous thrombotic events, either as a consequence of the disease or resulting from oncologic therapy, may contribute to SBS. Because ischemia has a nonspecific clinical presentation, early diagnosis and treatment are difficult, contributing to a high early mortality. Successful introduction of inpatient and eventually long-term, home-based parenteral nutrition and monitoring by an onco-neurogastroenterologist are essential. As nutritional state is restored, such patients may resume their oncologic management, as needed [51].

Salvage surgery for patients with highly advanced or relapsed epithelial ovarian cancer may be complicated by bowel obstruction requiring extensive resection, in turn resulting in SBS, and requiring long-life total parenteral nutrition. Because of high mortality and low survival rates, such surgeries should be performed after careful consideration of the individual patient characteristics and only in a multidisciplinary setting with adequate infrastructure and home care support. In the absence of acute abdomen or intestinal perforation, conservative management is preferable in most cases [52].

Crohn's Disease of the Small Bowel Crohn's disease (CD) is a chronic inflammatory bowel disease (IBD) that frequently affects the small bowel. Individuals diagnosed with CD are at an increased risk of developing bowel cancer mostly adenocarcinoma, neuroendocrine tumors, and sarcomas, compared to the general population. The key risk factors for cancer in CD are male sex, disease duration, previous surgical intervention, perianal disease, and chronic inflammation. Recent guidelines do not recommend surveillance for cancer in patients with CD [53].

Commonly affecting the terminal ileum and proximal colon, CD inflammation is often discontinuous and patchy, segmental, and transmural. Identification of characteristic findings on ileocolonoscopy, imaging, and histology remains the diagnostic gold standard. Symptoms, such as diarrhea, abdominal pain, weight loss, and fatigue, can be variable, insidious, and dependent on location, disease phenotype, and severity. Mild CD often simulates irritable bowel syndrome (IBS). In patients with stricturing disease, postprandial abdominal pain, bloating, nausea, or vomiting might be presenting features. Creeping fat, the wrapping of mesenteric fat around the bowel wall, is a typical feature of CD and is associated with stricture formation and obstruction (Fig. 14.12) [54]. CD muscularis propria cells produce an extracellular matrix scaffold, which is in direct spatial and functional contact with the immediately overlaid creeping fat. Among other proteins, the scaffold contains fibronectin that is singularly upregulated by transforming growth factor-β1, driving the migration of the preadipocytes out of the mesenteric fat. Blockade of α5β1 on the preadipocyte surface inhibits such migration out of mesenteric fat and on 3D decellularized intestinal tissue extracellular matrix [55].

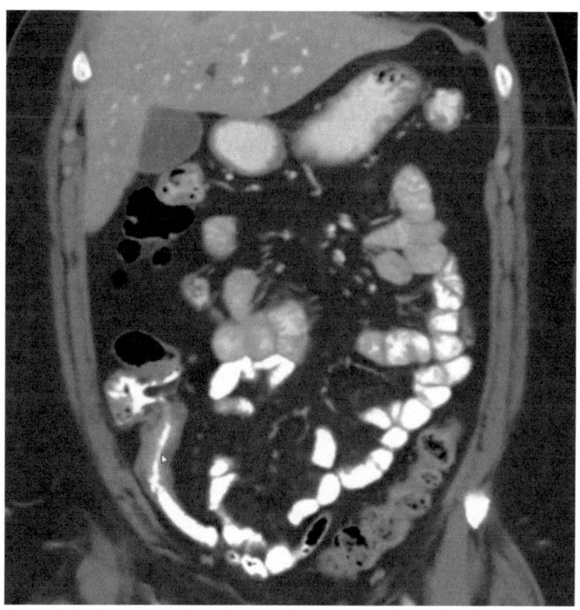

Fig. 14.12 Abdominal CT imaging showing active terminal ileitis, with mucosal thickening, creeping fat infiltration, and stricture formation for 11 cm upstream from the ileocecal valve (arrow)

References

1. Pobłocki J, Jasińska A, Syrenicz A, Andrysiak-Mamos E, Szczuko M. The neuroendocrine neoplasms of the digestive tract: diagnosis, treatment and nutrition. Nutrients. 2020;12(5):1437. https://doi.org/10.3390/nu12051437. PMID: 32429294; PMCID: PMC7284837.
2. Metz DC, Cadiot G, Poitras P, Ito T, Jensen RT. Diagnosis of Zollinger-Ellison syndrome in the era of PPIs, faulty gastrin assays, sensitive imaging and limited access to acid secretory testing. Int J Endocr Oncol. 2017;4(4):167–85.
3. Berna MJ, Hoffmann KM, Serrano J, Gibril F, Jensen RT. Serum gastrin in Zollinger-Ellison syndrome: I. Prospective study of fasting serum gastrin in 309 patients from the National Institutes of Health and comparison with 2229 cases from the literature. Medicine (Baltimore). 2006;85(6):295–330.
4. Tack J, Raymenants K, Van de Bruaene C, Scarpellini E. Dumping syndrome: update on pathophysiology, diagnosis, and management. Neurogastroenterol Motil. 2024;37:e14962.
5. Rogowitz E, Patti ME, Lawler HM. Time to dump late dumping syndrome terminology. Obes Surg. 2019;29(9):2985–6. https://doi.org/10.1007/s11695-019-04033-w. PMID: 31227985; PMCID: PMC7008495.
6. Das K, Sachdeva S, Misra A, Ghoshal UC. Malabsorption syndrome due to various causes is associated with antroduodenal hypomotility. Indian J Gastroenterol. 2006;25(2):58–61.
7. Fine KD, Meyer RL, Lee EL. The prevalence and causes of chronic diarrhea in patients with celiac sprue treated with a gluten-free diet. Gastroenterology. 1997;112(6):1830–8. https://doi.org/10.1053/gast.1997.v112.pm9178673. Erratum in: Gastroenterology 1998;114(2):424–5.
8. Catassi C, Bearzi I, Holmes GK. Association of celiac disease and intestinal lymphomas and other cancers. Gastroenterology. 2005;128(4 Suppl 1):S79–86. https://doi.org/10.1053/j.gastro.2005.02.027.
9. Manza F, Lungaro L, Costanzini A, Caputo F, Carroccio A, Mansueto P, Seidita A, Raju SA, Volta U, De Giorgio R, Sanders DS, Caio G. Non-celiac gluten/wheat sensitivity-state of the art: a five-year narrative review. Nutrients. 2025;17(2):220. https://doi.org/10.3390/nu17020220. PMID: 39861350; PMCID: PMC11767908.
10. Badran YR, Shih A, Leet D, Mooradian MJ, Coromilas A, Chen J, Kem M, Zheng H, Borowsky J, Misdraji J, Mino-Kenudson M, Dougan M. Immune checkpoint inhibitor-associated celiac disease. J Immunother Cancer. 2020;8(1):e000958. https://doi.org/10.1136/jitc-2020-000958. Erratum in: J Immunother Cancer. 2020 Jul;8(2):e000958corr1.
11. Potts J, Al Samaraee A, El-Hakeem A. Small bowel intussusception in adults. Ann R Coll Surg Engl. 2014;96(1):11–4. https://doi.org/10.1308/003588414X13824511650579. PMID: 24417823; PMCID: PMC5137662.
12. Wang LT, Wu CC, Yu JC, Hsiao CW, Hsu CC, Jao SW. Clinical entity and treatment strategies for adult intussusceptions: 20 years' experience. Dis Colon Rectum. 2007;50(11):1941–9. https://doi.org/10.1007/s10350-007-9048-8. Epub 2007 Sep 11. PMID: 17846839.
13. Paik CN, Choi MG, Lim CH, Park JM, Chung WC, Lee KM, Jun KH, Song KY, Jeon HM, Chin HM, Park CH, Chung IS. The role of small intestinal bacterial overgrowth in postgastrectomy patients. Neurogastroenterol Motil. 2011;23(5):e191–6. https://doi.org/10.1111/j.1365-2982.2011.01686.x. Epub 2011 Feb 16. PMID: 21324050.
14. Ghoshal UC, Sachdeva S, Ghoshal U, Misra A, Puri AS, Pratap N, Shah A, Rahman MM, Gwee KA, Tan VPY, Ahmed T, Lee YY, Ramakrishna BS, Talukdar R, Rana SV, Sinha SK, Chen M, Kim N, Holtmann G. Asian-Pacific consensus on small intestinal bacterial overgrowth in gastrointestinal disorders: an initiative of the Indian Neurogastroenterology and Motility Association. Indian J Gastroenterol. 2022;41(5):483–507. https://doi.org/10.1007/s12664-022-01292-x. Epub 2022 Oct 10. PMID: 36214973; PMCID: PMC9549446.
15. Pimentel M, Saad RJ, Long MD, Rao SSC. ACG clinical guideline: small intestinal bacterial overgrowth. Am J Gastroenterol. 2020;115:165–78.
16. Erdogan A, Rao SS. Small intestinal fungal overgrowth. Curr Gastroenterol Rep. 2015;17:16.

17. Viswanathan L, Rao SS. Intestinal disaccharidase deficiency in adults: evaluation and treatment. Curr Gastroenterol Rep. 2023;25(6):134–9. https://doi.org/10.1007/s11894-023-00870-z. Epub 2023 May 18. PMID: 37199899; PMCID: PMC10226910.
18. Min YW, Rezaie A, Pimentel M. Bile acid and gut microbiota in irritable bowel syndrome. J Neurogastroenterol Motil. 2022;28:549–61.
19. Herbella FA, Silva LC, Vicentine FP, Patti MG. Roux-en-Y limb motility after total gastrectomy. J Gastrointest Surg. 2014;18(5):906–10. https://doi.org/10.1007/s11605-014-2473-9 Epub 2014 Feb 5. PMID: 24496746.
20. Card WI. Blind loop syndrome. Proc R Soc Med. 1959;52(1):28–31.
21. Khoshini R, Dai SC, Lezcano S, Pimentel M. A systematic review of diagnostic tests for small intestinal bacterial overgrowth. Dig Dis Sci. 2008;53(6):1443–54.
22. Postow MA. Managing immune checkpoint-blocking antibody side effects. In: American Society of Clinical Oncology Educational Book; 2015. p. 76–83. https://doi.org/10.14694/EdBook_AM.2015.35.76.
23. Tang T, Abu-Sbeih H, Luo W, Lum P, Qiao W, Bresalier RS, Richards DM, Wang Y. Upper gastrointestinal symptoms and associated endoscopic and histological features in patients receiving immune checkpoint inhibitors. Scand J Gastroenterol. 2019;54(5):538–45.
24. Venara A, Meillat H, Cotte E, Ouaissi M, Duchalais E, Mor-Martinez C, Wolthuis A, Regimbeau JM, Ostermann S, Hamel JF, Joris J, Slim K. GRACE collaborative group for ileus study. Incidence and risk factors for severity of postoperative ileus after colorectal surgery: a prospective registry data analysis. World J Surg. 2020;44(3):957–66. https://doi.org/10.1007/s00268-019-05278-3. Erratum in: World J Surg. 2020 Apr;44(4):1331.
25. Chapman SJ, Pericleous A, Downey C, Jayne DG. Postoperative ileus following major colorectal surgery. Br J Surg. 2018;105:797–810.
26. Boeckxstaens GE, de Jonge WJ. Neuroimmune mechanisms in postoperative ileus. Gut. 2009;58(9):1300–11. https://doi.org/10.1136/gut.2008.169250. Erratum in: Gut. 2010;59(1):140.
27. Buscail E, Planchamp T, Le Cosquer G, Bouchet M, Thevenin J, Carrere N, Muscari F, Abbo O, Maulat C, Weyl A, Duffas JP, Philis A, Ghouti L, Canivet C, Motta JP, Vergnolle N, Deraison C, Shourick J. Postoperative ileus after digestive surgery: network meta-analysis of pharmacological intervention. Br J Clin Pharmacol. 2024;90(1):107–26.
28. Wei MT, Scapa J, Bingham D, Triadafilopoulos G. Gut dysthymia: paraneoplastic chronic watery diarrhea. Dig Dis Sci. 2020;65(8):2217–20. https://doi.org/10.1007/s10620-020-06058-z.
29. Sorhaug S, Steinshamn SL, Waldum HL. Octreotide treatment for paraneoplastic intestinal pseudo-obstruction complicating SCLC. Lung Cancer. 2005;48(1):137–40.
30. Choung RS, Locke GR 3rd, Zinsmeister AR, Schleck CD, Talley NJ. Opioid bowel dysfunction and narcotic bowel syndrome: a population-based study. Am J Gastroenterol. 2009;104(5):1199–204. https://doi.org/10.1038/ajg.2009.71. Epub 2009 Apr 14. PMID: 19367263; PMCID: PMC3209714
31. Haj M, Haj M, Rockey DC. Ogilvie's syndrome: management and outcomes. Medicine (Baltimore). 2018;97(27):e11187. https://doi.org/10.1097/MD.0000000000011187. PMID: 29979381; PMCID: PMC6076157.
32. Kumagai T, Rahman F, Smith AM. The microbiome and radiation induced-bowel injury: evidence for potential mechanistic role in disease pathogenesis. Nutrients. 2018;10(10):1405.
33. Yeoh EK, Horowitz M, Russo A, Muecke T, Robb T, Chatterton BE. Gastrointestinal function in chronic radiation enteritis–effects of loperamide-N-oxide. Gut. 1993;34(4):476–82. https://doi.org/10.1136/gut.34.4.476. PMID: 8491393; PMCID: PMC1374306.
34. Gupta K, Walton R, Kataria SP. Chemotherapy-induced nausea and vomiting: pathogenesis, recommendations, and new trends. Cancer Treat Res Commun. 2021;26:100278. https://doi.org/10.1016/j.ctarc.2020.100278. Epub 2020 Dec 11. PMID: 33360668.
35. Benarroch EE. Postural tachycardia syndrome: a heterogeneous and multifactorial disorder. Mayo Clin Proc. 2012;87:1214–25.

36. Babra D, Youn S, Devendra S. Postural orthostatic tachycardia syndrome (POTS) occurring during treatment for breast cancer. BMJ Case Rep. 2021;14(8):e242472. https://doi.org/10.1136/bcr-2021-242472. PMID: 34353826; PMCID: PMC8344319
37. Zhou W, Zikos TA, Clarke JO, Nguyen LA, Triadafilopoulos G, Neshatian L. Regional gastrointestinal transit and contractility patterns vary in postural orthostatic tachycardia syndrome (POTS). Dig Dis Sci. 2021;66(12):4406–13. https://doi.org/10.1007/s10620-020-06808-z. Epub 2021 Jan 11. PMID: 33428036.
38. Loavenbruck A, Iturrino J, Singer W, Sletten DM, Low PA, Zinsmeister AR, et al. Disturbances of gastrointestinal transit and autonomic functions in postural orthostatic tachycardia syndrome. Neurogastroenterol Motil. 2015;27:92–8.
39. Zenzeri L, Tambucci R, Quitadamo P, Giorgio V, De Giorgio R, Di Nardo G. Update on chronic intestinal pseudo-obstruction. Curr Opin Gastroenterol. 2020;36(3):230–7. https://doi.org/10.1097/MOG.0000000000000630.
40. Jansen SA, Nieuwenhuis EES, Hanash AM, Lindemans CA. Challenges and opportunities targeting mechanisms of epithelial injury and recovery in acute intestinal graft-versus-host disease. Mucosal Immunol. 2022;15(4):605–19. https://doi.org/10.1038/s41385-022-00527-6. Epub 2022 Jun 2. PMID: 35654837; PMCID: PMC9259481
41. Weber D, et al. Rifaximin preserves intestinal microbiota balance in patients undergoing allogeneic stem cell transplantation. Bone Marrow Transplant. 2016;51:1087–92.
42. van Lier YF, et al. Donor fecal microbiota transplantation ameliorates intestinal graft-versus-host disease in allogeneic hematopoietic cell transplant recipients. Sci Transl Med. 2020;12:eaaz8926.
43. DeFilipp Z, et al. Third-party fecal microbiota transplantation following Allo-HCT reconstitutes microbiome diversity. Blood Adv. 2018;2:745–53.
44. Termsinsuk P, Chantarojanasiri T, Pausawasdi N. Diagnosis and treatment of the afferent loop syndrome. Clin J Gastroenterol. 2020;13(5):660–8. https://doi.org/10.1007/s12328-020-01170-z. Epub 2020 Jul 8. PMID: 32638230.
45. Ramos-Andrade D, Andrade L, Ruivo C, et al. Imaging the postoperative patient: long-term complications of gastrointestinal surgery. Insights Imaging. 2016;7:7–20.
46. Kida A, Kido H, Matsuo T, et al. Usefulness of endoscopic metal stent placement for malignant afferent loop obstruction. Surg Endosc. 2020;34:2103–12.
47. Toliopoulos P, Manière T, Désilets E. Treatment of neoplastic afferent limb syndrome by endoscopic gastrojejunostomy with a lumen-apposing metal stent. VideoGIE. 2018;3:61–2.
48. Lübke J, Naumann N, Hoffmann O, et al. A clinical, morphological and molecular study of 70 patients with gastrointestinal involvement in systemic mastocytosis. Sci Rep. 2024;14:702. https://doi.org/10.1038/s41598-023-49749-z.
49. Pironi L, Steiger E, Joly F, Jeppesen PB, Wanten G, Sasdelli AS, Chambrier C, Aimasso U, Mundi MS, Szczepanek K, Jukes A, Theilla M, Kunecki M, Daniels J, Serlie M, Poullenot F, Cooper SC, Rasmussen HH, Compher C, Seguy D, Crivelli A, Santarpia L, Guglielmi FW, Kozjek NR, Schneider SM, Ellegard L, Thibault R, Matras P, Matysiak K, Van Gossum A, Forbes A, Wyer N, Taus M, Virgili NM, O'Callaghan M, Chapman B, Osland E, Cuerda C, Udvarhelyi G, Jones L, Won Lee AD, Masconale L, Orlandoni P, Spaggiari C, Díez MB, Doitchinova-Simeonova M, Serralde-Zúñiga AE, Olveira G, Krznaric Z, Czako L, Kekstas G, Sanz-Paris A, Jáuregui MEP, Murillo AZ, Schafer E, Arends J, Suárez-Llanos JP, Youssef NN, Brillanti G, Nardi E, Lal S, Home Artificial Nutrition and Chronic Intestinal Failure Special Interest Group of ESPEN; European Society for Clinical Nutrition and Metabolism. Characteristics of adult patients with chronic intestinal failure due to short bowel syndrome: an international multicenter survey. Clin Nutr ESPEN. 2021;45:433–41. https://doi.org/10.1016/j.clnesp.2021.07.004. Epub 2021 Jul 28. PMID: 34620351.
50. O'Keefe SJ, Buchman AL, Fishbein TM, Jeejeebhoy KN, Jeppesen PB, Shaffer J. Short bowel syndrome and intestinal failure: consensus definitions and overview. Clin Gastroenterol Hepatol. 2006;4(1):6–10. https://doi.org/10.1016/j.cgh.2005.10.002.
51. Perpar A, Brecelj E, Kozjek NR, Anderluh F, Oblak I, Vidmar MS, Velenik V. Mesenteric ischemia after capecitabine treatment in rectal cancer and resultant short bowel syndrome is not an

absolute contraindication for radical oncological treatment. Radiol Oncol. 2015;49(2):181–4. https://doi.org/10.2478/raon-2014-0024. PMID: 26029030; PMCID: PMC4387995.
52. Fotopoulou C, Braicu EI, Kwee SL, Kuhberg M, Richter R, Pietzner K, Feldheiser A, Bahra M, Schmidt SC, Sehouli J. Salvage surgery due to bowel obstruction in advanced or relapsed ovarian cancer resulting in short bowel syndrome and long-life total parenteral nutrition: surgical and clinical outcome. Int J Gynecol Cancer. 2013;23(8):1495–500. https://doi.org/10.1097/IGC.0b013e31829f81ca.
53. Faggiani I, D'Amico F, Furfaro F, Zilli A, Parigi TL, Cicerone C, Fiorino G, Peyrin-Biroulet L, Danese S, Allocca M. Small bowel cancer in Crohn's disease. Cancers (Basel). 2024;16(16):2901. https://doi.org/10.3390/cancers16162901. PMID: 39199671; PMCID: PMC11352503.
54. Dolinger M, Torres J, Vermeire S. Crohn's disease. Lancet. 2024;403(10432):1177–91. https://doi.org/10.1016/S0140-6736(23)02586-2. Epub 2024 Mar 1. PMID: 38437854.
55. Mao R, Doyon G, Gordon IO, Li J, Lin S, Wang J, Le THN, Elias M, Kurada S, Southern B, Olman M, Chen M, Zhao S, Dejanovic D, Chandra J, Mukherjee PK, West G, Van Wagoner DR, Fiocchi C, Rieder F. Activated intestinal muscle cells promote preadipocyte migration: a novel mechanism for creeping fat formation in Crohn's disease. Gut. 2022;71(1):55–67. https://doi.org/10.1136/gutjnl-2020-323719. Epub 2021 Jan 19. PMID: 33468536; PMCID: PMC8286985.

Regional Disorders of Sensory-Motor Dysfunction: Colon and Anorectum

15

George Triadafilopoulos and Lavanya Viswanathan

15.1 Colon and Anorectum

Irritable Bowel Syndrome (IBS) A causal association of constipation and IBS with other digestive tract cancers remains inconclusive [1]. However, significant, chronic gastrointestinal symptoms, often attributable to IBS, after the end of cancer treatments may occur, and they are often underreported by patients. Commonly used GI questionnaires generally fail to investigate key issues that are distressing to patients, such as severe flatulence [2]. The prevalence, severity, and type of chronic GI issues vary depending on cancer type and treatment, estimated to occur in 15–66% of survivors. However, given that patients may underreport their GI symptoms and the challenges with measurement and reporting of symptoms, the type, severity and duration of post-cancer treatment GI symptoms remains unclear.

Many studies report higher levels of anxiety, depression, and cognitive issues among adult cancer survivors, and some of these symptoms are also experienced by patients with IBS [3]. For instance, patients with IBS frequently present with comorbid GI and psychosocial symptoms, such as abdominal pain, bloating, constipation and/or diarrhea, anxiety, and depression [4]. The pattern of symptoms among patients with IBS and cancer survivors suggests similar underlying physiological mechanisms, such as gut dysbiosis and dysregulation of the neuroimmune system (Fig. 15.1) [5].

Current algorithms for the management of IBS focus on the exclusion of alarm features and empiric therapeutic trials with medications directed at constipation, diarrhea, or abdominal pain. More recently, actionable biomarkers for IBS have been proposed, involving the assessment of rectal evacuation disorder

G. Triadafilopoulos (✉) · L. Viswanathan
Department of Gastroenterology, Hepatology and Nutrition, UT MD Anderson Cancer Center, Houston, TX, USA
e-mail: GTriadafilopoulo@mdanderson.org; LViswanathan@mdanderson.org

G. Triadafilopoulos (ed.), *Onco-Neurogastroenterology*,
https://doi.org/10.1007/978-3-031-98848-6_15

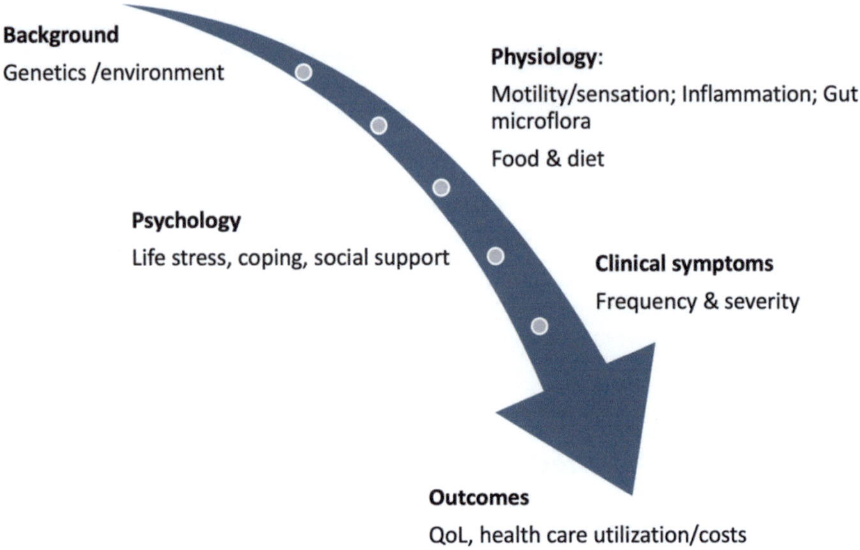

Fig. 15.1 Factors involved in the pathogenesis of IBS and its clinical presentation and outcomes

(dyssynergia), abnormal gut transit, bile acid diarrhea, disaccharidase deficiencies, reactions to food, hypersensitivity/hypervigilance, and altered gut microbiome. These in turn offer target-directed treatments [6].

Chronic depression may increase the risk of cancer. However, a recent nationwide propensity-matched analysis revealed comparable prevalence and risk of CRC in young depressed patients with *or* without IBS [7].

IBS responds to treatments using central neuromodulators, which enhance the synaptic transmission of 5-hydroxytryptamine, noradrenaline, and dopamine, desensitizing their postsynaptic receptors. Central neuromodulators act on receptors along the brain-gut axis, so they are useful in treating psychiatric comorbidities, modifying gut motility, and improving central downregulation of visceral signals. The first-line treatment for pain management in IBS is using tricyclic antidepressants (TCAs) or alternatively using serotonin and noradrenaline reuptake inhibitors (SNRIs). Selective serotonin reuptake inhibitors (SSRIs) are not useful in the treatment of abdominal pain. When choosing a neuromodulator, it is important to inquire about bowel habits since SSRIs may cause diarrhea, while TCAs may cause constipation. Clinical response may take 6–8 weeks, but long-term treatment (usually 6–12 months) is needed to prevent relapses. Enhanced therapy may help when the therapeutic effect of the first agent is inadequate, or it is associated with side effects. It is better to reduce the dose of the first agent before adding a second agent. When tapering central neuromodulators, the dose should be reduced slowly over at least 4 weeks [8].

Carbohydrate Malabsorption When malabsorbed carbohydrates reach the colon, they are fermented by colonic bacteria, producing short-chain fatty acids and gas, lowering colonic pH. Depending on the balance between the production and

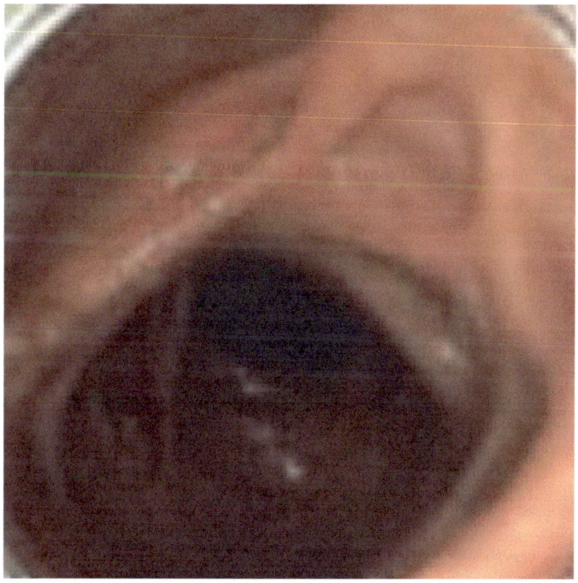

Fig. 15.2 Scarring and associated colonic pseudodiverticulosis resulting from chronic inactive ulcerative colitis

elimination of these fermentation products, diarrhea and/or flatulence may occur. A diet low in "fermentable, oligo-, di-, and monosaccharides and polyols" (FODMAPs) is frequently an effective treatment [9, 10].

Ulcerative Colitis It is well established that patients with ulcerative colitis (UC) should be periodically screened for colorectal cancer. New or recurrent symptoms (i.e., diarrhea, constipation, or fecal incontinence) or disease refractoriness to treatment regimens that were previously effective in achieving remission should prompt urgent, appropriate, and adequate investigations to rule out colorectal cancer [11]. Despite achieving remission, persistent gastrointestinal symptoms are common in quiescent IBD. IBS-like symptoms of recurrent abdominal pain and altered bowel habits can also be attributed to a wide range of overlapping etiologies and systemic disorders with GI manifestations that often do not respond to conventional IBS therapies. Figure 15.2 shows a colonoscopic image of scarring and associated colonic pseudo-diverticulae resulting from chronic, clinically inactive ulcerative colitis. Under such circumstances, neuromodulators, instead of anti-inflammatory agents or biologics, are advised.

Delay in diagnosis of these conditions can lead to ongoing patient suffering, reduced quality of life, repetition of invasive testing, increased healthcare utilization, and potentially unnecessary empirical escalation of IBD-related treatments [12].

Intestinal motility and secretion are locally controlled by enteric neural networks within the wall of the gut. The integrity of these functions depends on the precision of intercellular signaling among enteric neurons, epithelial cells, immune cells, and glia, all of which are vulnerable to inflammation-induced neuroplasticity. In response to inflammation, changes include increased epithelial serotonin availability, hyperexcitability of intrinsic primary afferent neurons, facilitation of synaptic activity among enteric neurons, and attenuated neuromuscular transmission. Other cells implicated in inflammation-induced neuroplasticity include muscularis macrophages and enteric glia. Targeted treatments include 5-hydroxytryptamine receptor 4 agonists, cyclooxygenase inhibitors, antioxidants, B cell depletion therapy, intravenous immunoglobulin, and activation of anti-inflammatory pathways [13].

Crohn's Disease The risk of colorectal cancer in long-standing Crohn's disease (CD) involving the colon is uncertain, although increased incidence of squamous cell carcinoma of the anus and skin, adenocarcinoma of the small bowel, duodenal and testicular cancer, and hematologic malignancies have all been reported [14]. Crohn's disease, proctocolectomy, total colectomy, ileostomy, and age younger than 60 years are all risk factors for adhesion formation. In such cases, outside of a bowel obstruction where a clear transition point can be identified, diagnosis using imaging is challenging.

***Clostridium difficile* Infection** *Clostridioides difficile* is a spore-forming, toxin-producing, gram-positive anaerobic bacterium that may colonize the human intestinal tract, typically after disruption of the normal gut microbiota by the use of antibiotics. *C. difficile* infection (CDI) is a significant cause of morbidity and mortality, especially among older hospitalized patients and those with cancer and underlying dysmotility. CDI manifestations range from asymptomatic carriage to fulminant disease with toxic megacolon [15]. Infrequently, CDI presents acutely as ileus, with no diarrhea, due to pooling of secretions in a dilated, atonic colon. Such patients are usually severely ill, with colonic (and possibly small bowel) dilation, often with colonic thickening, fever, and leukocytosis [16]. The *C. difficile* toxins have variable and profound effects on intestinal smooth muscle, frequently leading to colonic wall thickening (Fig. 15.3) [17, 18].

Neutropenic Enterocolitis (NEC) Neutropenic enterocolitis is a life-threatening condition occurring in severely neutropenic patients, following intensive chemotherapy for leukemia. Its pathogenesis is multifactorial, including mucosal injury from cytotoxic drugs, profound neutropenia, impaired host defenses, and possibly alterations in the microbiome. Symptoms usually occur within 1 month of initiation of chemotherapy or within 2 weeks following its completion, and they coincide with the neutropenia nadir. Key features of NEC include profound neutropenia, high fever, right lower quadrant abdominal pain, rebound tenderness, diarrhea, abdominal distension, nausea, vomiting, and bloody diarrhea. Conservative supportive management is preferred over surgery [19].

Chronic Colonic Pseudo-Obstruction (CCPO) Clinically, this is part of the spectrum of CIPO. There are four networks of the interstitial cells of Cajal (ICC) in the human colon associated with its musculature: (1) ICC-MP (ICC associated with the myenteric plexus), hypothesized to be stimulus-dependent pacemaker cells

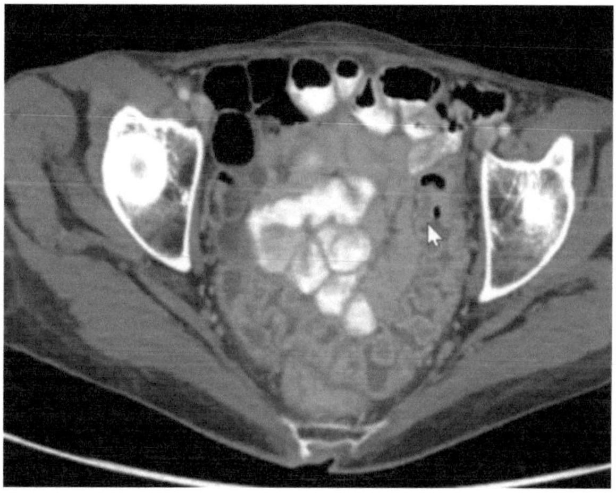

Fig. 15.3 Abdominal CT imaging in a patient with diarrhea revealing profound colonic wall thickening in the context of *C. difficile* infection. The diagnosis needs to be always entertained in cancer patients

orchestrating high-amplitude propagating pressure waves (HAPWs); (2) ICC-SMP (ICC associated with the submuscular plexus), the dominant pacemaker cells generating rhythmic depolarization at ~3 cycles/min; (3) ICC-IM (intramuscular ICC), present in both the longitudinal and circular muscle, transmitting pacemaker activity throughout the musculature and mediating neural stimuli; and (4) ICC-SS (ICC associated with the subserosa) that may perform pacemaker functions to the longitudinal muscle layer [20]. In studies on colonic motor dysfunction requiring surgery, ICC are almost always abnormal or significantly reduced. However, there are still gaps in our knowledge about the role of ICC in the control of colonic motility and the mechanistic link(s) between ICC abnormalities and colonic motor dysfunction, manifesting as severe chronic constipation and colonic distention. Using high-resolution manometry, our understanding of human colonic motility, and autonomic reflexes that generate motor patterns, is poised to increase markedly.

Opioid-Induced Constipation (OIC) Daily use of opioid analgesics has significantly increased in recent years due to an increasing prevalence of conditions associated with chronic pain, particularly cancer. Yet, opioid-induced constipation (OIC) is commonly under-recognized and under-treated. OIC significantly reduces the quality of life by causing psychological distress, lowering work productivity, and imposing significant economic and social burden to patients. First-line therapy typically involves the use of osmotic (preferably polyethylene glycol) and stimulant laxatives. Peripherally acting μ-opioid receptor antagonists, such as methylnaltrexone and naloxegol, should be used in non-responders. Gastrointestinal motility depends on a fine balance between excitatory and inhibitory pathways, mostly mediated by submucosal and myenteric neurons. Exogenous opioids disrupt intestinal motility by increasing gut wall musculature tone, slowing propulsion, and triggering tonic spasms in the colon and small intestine. Opioid receptors also affect the secretion and absorption of water in the gut. Further reduction in the intestinal fluid content is

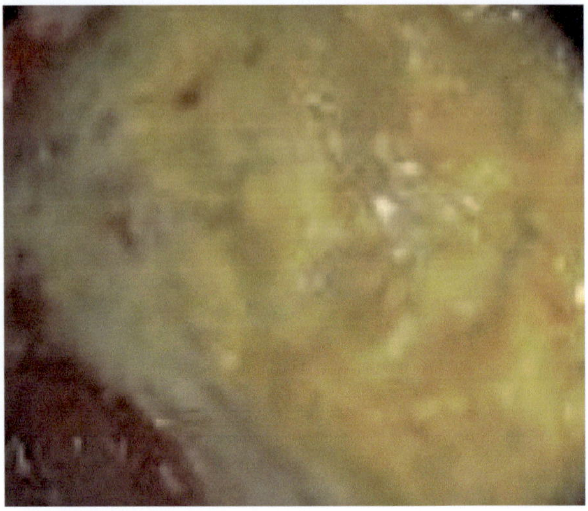

Fig. 15.4 Large, malignant ulcer due to endometrial cancer invading the rectal wall

facilitated by prolonged fecal stasis due to altered intestinal motility and activation of mechanoreceptors. This is why patients on opioids frequently complain of dry and hard stools. Opioids may also inhibit saliva production, causing dry mouth, and reduce biliary and pancreatic secretions, impairing digestion. Finally, stimulation of opioid receptors increases the resting tone of all sphincters in the digestive tract. The increased tone of the internal anal sphincter (anismus) produces straining, functional anal obstruction, hemorrhoids, or even colon perforation [21].

Structural Anorectal Disorders Clinically, these diverse conditions may present with constipation, bloating, obstructive defecation and incomplete evacuation, straining, rectal urgency, and fecal soiling. Various degrees of rectal prolapse, intussusception, rectocele and enterocele, descending perineum, anal or anastomotic stricture, or bowel/pouch kink while bearing down need to be considered, mainly using endoscopic visualization and MR defecography. Hemorrhoids and anal fissures may co-exist, adding to the complexity of the management of symptoms. Fig. 15.4 shows a large semi-circumferential rectal ulcer originating from locally advanced endometrial carcinoma causing obstructive defecation due to scarring and fecal urgency due to poor rectal compliance due to rectal wall encasement by the tumor.

Pelvic Floor Prolapse The female pelvic floor anatomy is complex, and pelvic floor integrity, provided by the interaction between muscles, ligaments, and associated connective tissue, may be altered after oncologic urogynecologic surgery. Clinically, such surgery may result in adverse events not only affecting the anterior and midpelvic compartments but also rectal integrity, thereby requiring careful and well-orchestrated multidisciplinary evaluation and management [22].

Table 15.1 Common abnormalities in HRAM, RST, and BET in patients with LARS

Variable	Value
HPZ length (*n* = 4.1–4.5 cm)	Normal or short
Resting pressure (*n* = 83–96 mmHg)	Normal
Squeeze pressure (*n* = 245–287 mmHg)	Low
Squeeze duration (*n* = 28–30 s)	Short
Residual anal pressure (*n* = 28–52)	High
RAIR (*n* = present)	Absent
First rectal sensation (*n* = 20–25 ml)	Low
Urge to defecate (*n* = 140–167 ml)	Low
Discomfort (*n* = 192–222 ml)	Low
Balloon expulsion (50 cc expulsion in <60 s)	Normal

LAR Syndrome (LARS) Low anterior resection syndrome (LARS) refers to a functional defecatory problem that occurs after sphincter-saving surgery for rectal cancer and is associated with fecal urgency, frequency, and incontinence that may significantly affect quality of life. Although many risk factors have been identified, LARS is mostly related to the reduction of storage capacity of the rectum. Key risk factors for LARS are anal sphincter muscle or nerve damage during recto-anal resection or anastomosis construction and intersphincteric resection for low-lying tumors or hand-sewing anastomosis. Preoperative radiotherapy and postoperative complications, such as anastomosis leakage or longer duration of stoma, may also have an impact. The severity of LARS can be confirmed using the LARS score questionnaire. Various empirical treatments, such as loperamide, fiber, probiotics, or enemas, have been tried, but their efficacy remains uncertain. Ramosetron, a 5-hydroxytryptamine (5-HT) receptor antagonist used in IBS, is a potential drug symptom relief [23]. High-resolution anorectal manometry (HRAM) may be useful in guiding the clinician managing patients with LARS by highlighting areas in need for improvement, such as rectal hypersensitivity, dyssynergia, or anal pressure abnormalities, using pelvic floor physical therapy. Table 15.1 shows typical HRAM, RST, and BET findings in LARS.

In a multicenter randomized, double-blinded, placebo-controlled, crossover study, ondansetron 4 mg orally daily was a safe and simple treatment that improves both symptoms and QoL in LARS patients [24].

Dyssynergic Defecation Dyssynergic defecation (DD) is defined as a lack of coordination among the recto-anal, abdominal, and pelvic floor muscles that leads to excessive straining, incomplete evacuation, hard stools, infrequent bowel movements, and need for use of digital maneuvers to assist with evacuation. DD is characterized by paradoxical anal contraction (an increase in anal sphincter pressure), inadequate relaxation of the resting anal sphincter pressure (<20%), or insufficient effort of abdominal or rectal muscles (Table 15.2) [25]. The severity and duration of DD and its associated symptoms cause psychological distress and significantly

Table 15.2 Common findings in HRAM, RST, and BET in patients with dyssynergic defecation (DD)

Variable	Value
HPZ length (*n* = 4.1–4.5 cm)	Normal
Resting pressure (*n* = 83–96 mmHg)	High
Squeeze pressure (*n* = 245–287 mmHg)	Normal or high
Squeeze duration (*n* = 28–30 s)	Normal or high
Residual anal pressure (*n* = 28–52)	High
RAIR (*n* = present)	Present or absent
First rectal sensation (*n* = 20–25 ml)	Low or high
Urge to defecate (*n* = 140–167 ml)	Low or high
Discomfort (*n* = 192–222 ml)	Low or high
Balloon expulsion (50 cc expulsion in <60 s)	Prolonged or absent

impair patients' quality of life (QoL). Both secretagogues and biofeedback therapy have been shown to improve constipation and QoL [26].

Radiation Proctopathy (RP) In the rectum and distal colon, acute radiation injury usually occurs within 6 weeks of beginning therapy and is characterized by nausea, diarrhea, urgency, tenesmus, mucus discharge, and, occasionally, minor rectal bleeding. These symptoms usually resolve within 6 months without the need for therapy, and they are typically associated with visible changes on colonoscopic examination. Radiation proctitis (RP), or radiation proctopathy, is characterized by damage to the rectal mucosa secondary to ionizing radiation therapy, adjuvantly or neoadjuvantly delivered either by external beam radiation or brachytherapy to the pelvis. Based on the onset of signs and symptoms, RP can be classified as acute or chronic. Chronic radiation proctitis has a delayed onset, occurring approximately a year or later after exposure to radiation. This type of chronic injury is caused by obliterative endarteritis and chronic mucosal ischemia, resulting in epithelial atrophy and fibrosis. The result of this process is stricture formation and bleeding within the colon and rectum. Patients with radiation proctitis can present with diarrhea, bleeding, tenesmus, urgency, difficulties with defecation, and, less commonly, fecal incontinence. The diagnosis of radiation proctitis is made by colonoscopy revealing mucosal edema, erythema, friability, and the presence of telangiectasias. In severe cases, mucosal ulcerations and strictures may be seen. Treatment for radiation proctitis should focus on the pattern of symptoms. Some patients will present mostly with pain, diarrhea, and tenesmus and others exclusively with bleeding. Sucralfate, administered orally or topically, may improve symptoms without significant adverse events; other treatments that have shown some benefit in small clinical trials include hyperbaric oxygen, short-chain fatty acid enemas, and rectal instillation of formaldehyde. External beam or interstitial radiation therapy in men with localized prostate cancer may lead to urinary, gastrointestinal, and sexual complications. Improvements in surgical and radiation techniques have reduced the incidence of many of these complications [27]. In a similar fashion, patients who receive pelvic radiation for gynecologic malignancies may experience toxicity because of the anatomic locations, combination with concurrent chemotherapy, and/or surgery. Late radiation toxicity can significantly increase the risk of morbidity [28]. Chronic radiation injury may manifest as radiation proctopathy, defined as epithelial damage to the rectum due to radiation that is associated with minimal or no inflammation. Chronic radiation injury may occur as a continuation of acute radiation proctitis or have a delayed onset (9–14 months following radiation exposure to 30 years after exposure). The reported incidence of chronic radiation injury ranges from 2% to 5% [29]. External beam radiotherapy (EBRT) reduces anal resting pressure, decreases rectal distensibility, and frequently induces telangiectasias of rectal mucosa. Such changes may be associated with fecal incontinence, urgency, frequent bowel movements, and rectal bleeding [30]. In one study, EBRT reduced maximal rectal capacity and rectal compliance, but sensory pressure thresholds did not significantly change. Patients with urgency had a more reduced anal squeeze and maximum pressure compared with patients without complaints, suggesting a deteriorated external anal sphincter function [31]. In another study, fecal incontinence and rectal urgency were the symptoms with the largest influence on QoL, as measured by the Fecal Incontinence Quality of Life Scale (FIQL) and the Expanded Prostate Cancer Index Composite Bowel domain (EPICB)-bother subscale. Impaired anal resting pressure was the objective function parameter with the largest influence [32]. At 6 weeks and 6 months after treatment, respectively, the proctitis symptom scores and the incontinence symptom scores increased. Urgency, frequency of defecation, anorectal pain, incontinence to liquid stool and to flatus, and alteration in lifestyle were significant symptoms after treatment. The following measurements decreased: anal canal resting pressure, the squeeze increment, and the maximum tolerated rectal volume [33]. A study using univariate logistical regression analysis showed that the frequency of defecation at 4–6 weeks and the rectal volumes at baseline both for perception and desire to defecate predicted significantly the patients who had symptoms and signs of anorectal dysfunction at 1 year. Individual patient tumor and treatment-related variables tested, in contrast, had no predictive significance [34].

Using perfusion anorectal manometry in men with chronic radiation proctitis and symptoms of urgency, frequency, and occasional incontinence of feces, dysfunction of the internal anal sphincter was seen, contributing to anorectal symptoms. Histological evidence suggests that damage to the myenteric plexus is mainly responsible. The manometric function of the external sphincter remains relatively unaffected [35]. All the above studies were performed using outdated, water perfusion, not high-resolution anorectal manometry (HR-ARM) systems, and up-to-date objective classifications, such as the London classification [36], and without objective assessments of rectal sensation and balloon expulsion.

A new method, impedance planimetry (IP; EndoFLIP), may obtain simultaneous measurements of pressure and rectal cross-sectional area (CSA) during balloon inflations. Rectal distensions are done with an intraluminal balloon using specified pressures up to 40 cmH2O above baseline rectal pressure. Typically, balloon inflation elicits a phase of rapid increase in rectal CSA followed by a phase of slow increase until a steady state is reached. Impedance planimetry offers new possibilities for investigation of anorectal physiology through the study of segmental biomechanical wall properties of the human rectum in patients with chronic radiation proctopathy [37]. Patients with chronic RP may have additional symptoms secondary to full-thickness bowel ischemia and fibrotic changes, such as severe bleeding, stricture formation, perforation, or fistulas. Involvement of the anal sphincter may lead to fecal incontinence [38].

Chemotherapy-Associated Constipation Constipation causing abdominal pain and distention may occur in 30–50% of cancer patients receiving chemotherapy; it is usually of moderate severity, but it impacts significantly the patients' quality of life [39]. Although mostly multifactorial, reflecting drug use (antiemetics, opioid analgesics, antidepressants, etc.), physical inactivity, fluid consumption, performance status, or diet, constipation could be an adverse effect of chemotherapy agents on the enteric nervous system (ENS), mitigating the normal peristaltic effect of proximal contraction occurring in conjunction with distal colonic relaxation, thereby delaying transit, and enhancing fluid reabsorption. Common agents associated with constipation include vincristine, vinblastine, oxaliplatin, cisplatin, and thalidomide [40, 41]. Early diagnosis and treatment of constipation using various therapeutic approaches are crucial in improving symptoms and quality of life, and it may prevent interruption or discontinuation of chemotherapy, avoid surgical complications, and shorten the duration of hospital stay.

Postoperative Bile Acid Malabsorption (BAM) Although typically a result of postoperative loss of the ileocecal valve, postoperative bile acid malabsorption presents with watery diarrhea and at times steatorrhea, rectal urgency, and abdominal cramping, and it requires a high index of suspicion. A trial of bile acid sequestrants, such as cholestyramine, has both diagnostic and therapeutic value. Increasingly recognized is the role of the gut microbiome and its interplay with altered bile acid profiles in such patients. BAM is a potential cause of loose stools after right-sided colon surgery, and it can be classified as type 1 (secondary to bowel dysfunction due to ileal resection or inflammation), type 2 (primary or idiopathic BAM), and type 3 (secondary to other disorders, such as pancreatic dysfunction, cholecystectomy, or small intestinal bacterial overgrowth) [42]. While type 1 represents true malabsorption, types 2 and 3 are characterized by an excessive amount of bile acids in the bowel, potentially stimulating the colonic epithelial cells to secrete fluid and electrolytes [43].

Resection of the ileocecal valve may lead to retrograde passage of colonic bacteria resulting in small intestinal bacterial overgrowth (SIBO). The bacteria may induce brush border injury in the small intestine, leading to malabsorption of carbohydrates, which results in loose stools. Furthermore, excess of bacteria in the small bowel may also deconjugate bile acids and thereby induce BAM type 3 [44]. Hepatic overproduction of bile acids may be another cause of BAM following ileal resection [45]. A recent study investigated the frequency of BAM and SIBO in patients having undergone right-sided hemicolectomy for cancer and found that both BAM and SIBO are common [46].

The spatiotemporal structures of the human microbiome, proteome, and metabolome reflect and determine regional intestinal physiology and may have implications for disease [47, 48]. Yet, little is known about the distribution of microorganisms, their environment, and their biochemical activity in the gut because of reliance on stool samples and limited access to only some regions of the gut using endoscopy in fasting or sedated individuals. To address these deficiencies, an ingestible device that collects samples from multiple regions of the human intestinal tract during normal digestion has been introduced [49]. Collection of intestinal samples from healthy individuals using the device and subsequent multi-omics analyses identified significant differences between bacteria, phages, host proteins, and metabolites in the intestines vs. stool. Certain microbial taxa were differentially enriched in the intestines than in stool. The host proteome and bile acid profiles varied along the intestines and were highly distinct from those of stool. Correlations between gradients in bile acid concentrations and microbial abundance predicted species that altered the bile acid pool through deconjugation.

Diverticulosis Coexistent diverticulosis and adenomas are frequently found at routine diagnostic and screening colonoscopy. Colonic diverticulosis is very prevalent in Caucasians, particularly the old, although 5–10% of subjects with diverticula are under age 40, with a shifting incidence to a younger age [50]. Similarly, colorectal cancer remains among the most incident tumors in the West, and most of them arise from adenomas [51]. Moreover, an increased incidence of this cancer in subjects aged below 50 years was recently reported in a large US study [52]. Diverticulosis and colonic neoplasia may share some risk factors, since a diet low in fiber and rich in saturated fats, the so-called Western diet, largely consumed in developed countries, may favor their development. A diet rich in fiber reduces hypercontractility in the sigmoid tract that triggers diverticula formation, while a fat-rich diet and obesity increase the risk of adenomas [53]. Nevertheless, data from systematic reviews are conflicting [54]. Indeed, an increased risk of colon neoplastic lesions in diverticulosis subjects was found to be increased in some studies, but not in others.

The presence of diverticulosis may distort the structure of the colon and alter motor and sensory function [55]. Structural changes may include shortened teniae, thickened segments of circular muscle, and luminal narrowing impeding the safe passage of the colonoscope (Fig. 15.5). These may be due to abnormal elastin deposition, collagen crosslinking and an increased ratio of type 3 collagen, and high levels of tissue-degrading metalloproteinases [56, 57].

Abnormal motor activity could increase luminal pressure, causing pain and predisposing to mucosal herniation [58]. Colonic manometry studies in patients with diverticulosis have demonstrated greater intraluminal pressure and higher amplitude contractions following meals [59].

Segmental Colitis Associated with Diverticulosis (SCAD) Segmental colitis associated with diverticulosis (SCAD) is characterized by a chronic inflammatory response involving the inter-diverticular colonic mucosa, sparing the rectum and the

Fig. 15.5 CT colonography showing scattered diverticulosis with a moderate degree of sigmoid colon wall hypertrophy. The mid-sigmoid colon is tortuous and rigid with wall hypertrophy that impaired the passage of the small-caliber colonoscope

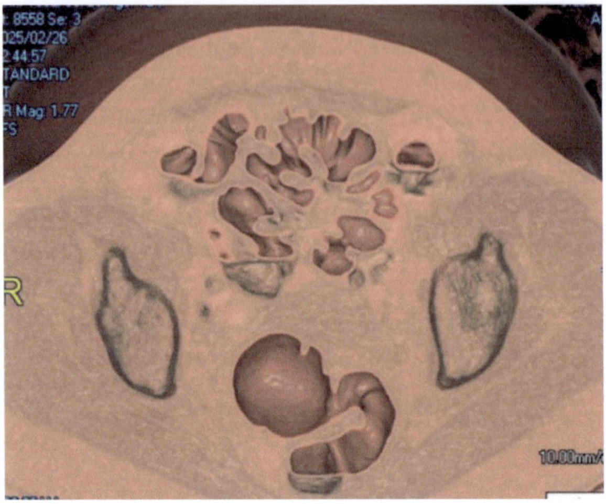

right colon. SCAD can be diagnosed in about 5% of population undergoing screening colonoscopy and in 12% of those with diverticulosis. SCAD seems to be associated with a reduced rate of adenomas or CRC, as compared with diverticulosis [60].

Pelvic Floor Neuropathy A sequel of pelvic or anorectal surgery, pelvic floor neuropathy is characterized by inability to evacuate stool from the rectum caused by both functional and structural disorders that cause paradoxical contraction or inadequate relaxation of pelvic floor muscles (i.e., dyssynergic defecation) and/or inadequate propulsive force during attempted defecation [61]. It may also be associated with urinary dysfunction (i.e., urinary retention or incontinence), bladder or uterine prolapse, as well as various posterior compartment issues, such as rectocele or rectal prolapse. Dyssynergic defecation can present with obstructive constipation, alternating bowel habits, fecal incontinence, diarrhea, and rectal discomfort. Examples of structural rectal evacuation disorders include enterocele, rectocele, rectal prolapse, pelvic organ prolapse, intussusception, and benign or malignant strictures. These issues can be identified by MR defecography, which provides a dynamic assessment of defecatory structure and function. Depending on the severity of these abnormalities, the patient may benefit from biofeedback or need evaluation by colorectal surgeon and/or urogynecologist. Pelvic floor biofeedback is the first-line therapy and involves interactive retraining of the pelvic floor muscles and anal sphincters to restore normal defecation. Good response rates to biofeedback can be accomplished in both ileal pouch anal anastomosis (IPAA) or J-pouch IPAA and non-IPAA patients. Defecography is a useful diagnostic test for evaluating functional defecatory disorders of the pouch and can provide valuable information regarding pouch emptying dynamics and assess for underlying structural abnormalities [62].

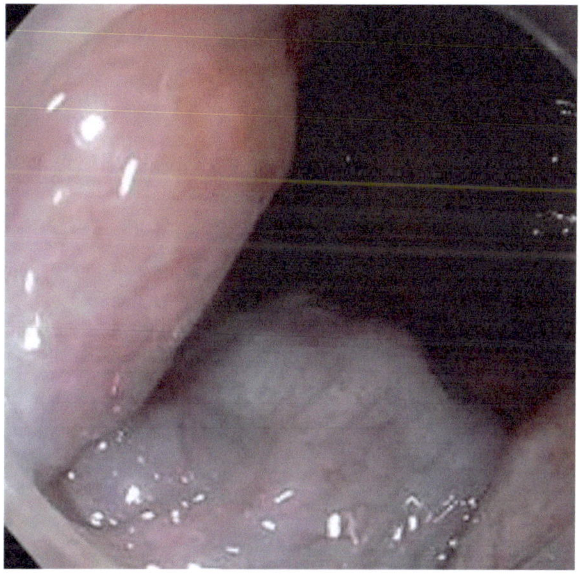

Fig. 15.6 Internal hemorrhoids seen on antegrade view of the anorectum at colonoscopy

Hemorrhoids Evaluation of hemorrhoids should always include a careful perianal and digital rectal examination and, if possible, an office-based anoscopy. Hemorrhoids are generally classified as internal, if they originate proximal to the dentate line; external if distal to the dentate line; or mixed if they are crossing the dentate line. Risk factors for symptomatic hemorrhoids include long-standing ascites, excessive sitting or squatting, low dietary fiber intake, obesity, and sedentary lifestyle or inanition, often seen in the cancer population. Recurrent straining at defecation and alternating constipation or diarrhea may lead to engorgement of the hemorrhoidal plexuses, causing bleeding, prolapse, and swelling. Age-related or post-treatment pelvic floor changes and sarcopenia may cause the hemorrhoids to slide back and forth during defecation, resulting in mucoid anal discharge, perianal wetness, soiling, and anal irritation and itching. If pain is present, it should raise suspicion for hemorrhoidal thrombosis, ischemia, incarceration from prolapse, or the possibility of anal fissure, infection, or perianal abscess.

Symptomatic hemorrhoids should be differentiated from rectal mucosal or full-thickness prolapse or a prolapsing rectal polyp. Colonoscopy under anesthesia should be considered if alarm features are present or rectal bleeding persists after empiric hemorrhoid treatment or for guideline-based colorectal cancer screening (Fig. 15.6). First-line therapy for hemorrhoids includes increased fiber and liquid intake and avoidance of straining at defecation. Various topical agents, used once or twice daily for a minimum of several weeks, may reduce hemorrhoid symptoms. Patients with significant rectal bleeding from internal hemorrhoids that are unresponsive to medical therapy should be considered for banding, usually performed endoscopically. Hemorrhoidal sclerotherapy and infrared coagulation are less effective. Thrombosed external hemorrhoids, typically associated with very painful anal swelling, are best treated with surgical excision. Surgical hemorrhoidectomy should be reserved for refractory hemorrhoids, large external hemorrhoids, or combined internal and external hemorrhoids with rectal prolapse [63].

Anal Fissure A classic combination of altered motility (high anal canal pressure; anismus) and altered sensation (anal pain), an anal fissure is a longitudinal mucosal tear of the anal canal, which usually results from trauma due to passage of hard stool (dyschezia), and it is characterized by anorectal pain that is worsened by defecation and sitting. Rectal bleeding with bowel movements or wiping is common. Acute anal fissures generally resolve within a few weeks with the use of sitz baths, psyllium, bulking agents, and topical anesthetics and anti-inflammatory agents. Anal fissures lasting more than 8–12 weeks are considered chronic, with edema, fibrosis, and anal spasticity. Chronic anal fissures may be treated preferably with topical calcium channel blockers or nitrates. Those who are unresponsive to these therapies should be referred for endoscopic anal sphincter botulinum toxin injection (100 IU in four quadrants) or, less frequently, surgical internal lateral sphincterotomy [64].

References

1. Fan R, Zhang J, Shen J, Mao C, Li S, Zhuang Z. Causal relationships of chronic constipation and irritable bowel syndrome with digestive tract cancers: a Mendelian randomization study. Recent Pat Anticancer Drug Discov. 2024;20:432.
2. Andreyev HJ, Davidson SE, Gillespie C, Allum WH, Swarbrick E, British Society of Gastroenterology, Association of Colo-Proctology of Great Britain and Ireland; Association of Upper Gastrointestinal Surgeons; Faculty of Clinical Oncology Section of the Royal College of Radiologists. Practice guidance on the management of acute and chronic gastrointestinal problems arising as a result of treatment for cancer. Gut. 2012;61(2):179–92.
3. Yi JC, Syrjala KL. Anxiety and depression in cancer survivors. Med Clin North Am. 2017;101(6):1099–113.
4. Lee C, Doo E, Choi JM, Jang SH, Ryu HS, Lee JY, Oh JH, Park JH, Kim YS, Brain-Gut Axis Research Group of Korean Society of Neurogastroenterology and Motility. The increased level of depression and anxiety in irritable bowel syndrome patients compared with healthy controls: systematic review and meta-analysis. J Neurogastroenterol Motil. 2017;23(3):349–62.
5. Bajic JE, Johnston IN, Howarth GS, Hutchinson MR. From the bottom-up: chemotherapy and gut-brain Axis dysregulation. Front Behav Neurosci. 2018;12:104.
6. Camilleri M, Yang DY. Algorithms or biomarkers in patients with lower DGBI? Neurogastroenterol Motil. 2024;36(11):e14856.
7. Mellacheruvu SP, Lekkala SP, Chauhan S, Mohammed AS, Mundla SR, Shenoy A, Mohammed BK, Bawa J, Nallapothula S, Gurram P, Jain A, Desai R, Nayeem MM. Link between irritable bowel syndrome, depression, and colorectal cancer risk in young patients: age-matched nationwide population-based study. World J Gastrointest Pathophysiol. 2024;15(3):93408.
8. Hanna-Jairala I, Drossman DA. Central neuromodulators in irritable bowel syndrome: why, how, and when. Am J Gastroenterol. 2024;119(7):1272–84. https://doi.org/10.14309/ajg.0000000000002800. Epub 2024 Apr 9. PMID: 38595149; PMCID: PMC11208063.

9. Fernández-Bañares F. Carbohydrate Maldigestion and intolerance. Nutrients. 2022;14(9):1923.
10. Omer A, Quigley EMM. Carbohydrate Maldigestion and malabsorption. Clin Gastroenterol Hepatol. 2018;16(8):1197–9.
11. Yadav A, Jena A, Arpitha K, Shah J, Vaiphei K, Dutta U, Singh AK. Colon cancer in ulcerative colitis: a mimicker of a flare of disease. Inflamm Bowel Dis. 2022;28(8):e116–7. https://doi.org/10.1093/ibd/izac033.
12. Lim J, Rezaie A. Irritable bowel syndrome-like symptoms in quiescent inflammatory bowel disease: a practical approach to diagnosis and treatment of organic causes. Dig Dis Sci. 2023;68(11):4081–97.
13. Spear ET, Mawe GM. Enteric neuroplasticity and dysmotility in inflammatory disease: key players and possible therapeutic targets. Am J Physiol Gastrointest Liver Physiol. 2019;317(6):G853–61. https://doi.org/10.1152/ajpgi.00206.2019. Epub 2019 Oct 11. PMID: 31604034; PMCID: PMC6962496.
14. Kiran RP, Khoury W, Church JM, Lavery IC, Fazio VW, Remzi FH. Colorectal cancer complicating inflammatory bowel disease: similarities and differences between Crohn's and ulcerative colitis based on three decades of experience. Ann Surg. 2010;252(2):330–5. https://doi.org/10.1097/SLA.0b013e3181e61e69.
15. Kelly CR, Fischer M, Allegretti JR, LaPlante K, Stewart DB, Limketkai BN, Stollman NH. ACG clinical guidelines: prevention, diagnosis, and treatment of clostridioides difficile Infections. Am J Gastroenterol. 2021;116(6):1124–47. https://doi.org/10.14309/ajg.0000000000001278. Erratum in: Am J Gastroenterol. 2022 Feb 1;117(2):358. 10.14309/ajg.0000000000001529. PMID: 34003176.
16. Triadafilopoulos G, Hallstone AE. Acute abdomen as the first presentation of pseudomembranous colitis. Gastroenterology. 1991;101(3):685–91. https://doi.org/10.1016/0016-5085(91)90526-q.
17. Gilbert RJ, Pothoulakis C, LaMont JT. Effect of purified *Clostridium difficile* toxins on intestinal smooth muscle. II. Toxin B. Am J Physiol. 1989;256(4 Pt 1):G767–72. https://doi.org/10.1152/ajpgi.1989.256.4.G767. PMID: 2495734.
18. Gilbert RJ, Triadafilopoulos G, Pothoulakis C, Giampaolo C, LaMont JT. Effect of purified *Clostridium difficile* toxins on intestinal smooth muscle. I. Toxin A. Am J Physiol. 1989;256(4 Pt 1):G759–66. https://doi.org/10.1152/ajpgi.1989.256.4.G759. PMID: 2495733.
19. Babakhanlou R, Ravandi-Kashani F, Kontoyiannis DP. Neutropenic Enterocolitis: an uncommon, but fearsome complication of leukemia. J Hematol. 2023;12(2):59–65. 10.14740/jh1105. Epub 2023 Apr 30. PMID: 37187499; PMCID: PMC10181327
20. Huizinga JD, Hussain A, Chen JH. Interstitial cells of Cajal and human colon motility in health and disease. Am J Physiol Gastrointest Liver Physiol. 2021;321(5):G552–75.
21. Squeo F, Celiberto F, Ierardi E, Russo F, Riezzo G, D'Attoma B, Di Leo A, Losurdo G. Opioid-induced constipation: old and new concepts in diagnosis and treatment. J Neurogastroenterol Motil. 2024;30(2):131–42. https://doi.org/10.5056/jnm23144. PMID: 38576366; PMCID: PMC10999847.
22. Daykan Y, Rotem R, O'Reilly BA. Robot-assisted laparoscopic pelvic floor surgery: review. Best Pract Res Clin Obstet Gynaecol. 2023;91:102418. https://doi.org/10.1016/j.bpobgyn.2023.102418.
23. Ryoo SB. Low anterior resection syndrome. Ann Gastroenterol Surg. 2023;7(5):719–24. https://doi.org/10.1002/ags3.12695. PMID: 37663958; PMCID: PMC10472409.
24. Popeskou SG, Roesel R, Faes S, Vanoni A, Galafassi J, di Tor Vajana AF, Piotet LM, Christoforidis D. Ondansetron for low anterior resection syndrome (LARS): a double-blind, placebo-controlled, cross-over, randomized study. Ann Surg. 2024;279(2):196–202.
25. Shahsavari D, Rao SSC. Review article: advances in the diagnosis and management of anorectal motility disorders. Aliment Pharmacol Ther. 2024;60(6):701–14. https://doi.org/10.1111/apt.18170. Epub 2024 Jul 25. PMID: 39051556.
26. Rao SSC, Go JT, Valestin J, Schneider J. Home biofeedback for the treatment of dyssynergic defecation: does it improve quality of life and is it cost-effective? Am J Gastroenterol. 2019;114:938–44.

27. Michaelson MD, Cotter SE, Gargollo PC, Zietman AL, Dahl DM, Smith MR. Management of complications of prostate cancer treatment. CA Cancer J Clin. 2008;58(4):196–213. https://doi.org/10.3322/CA.2008.0002. Epub 2008 May 23
28. Viswanathan AN, Lee LJ, Eswara JR, Horowitz NS, Konstantinopoulos PA, Mirabeau-Beale KL, Rose BS, von Keudell AG, Wo JY. Complications of pelvic radiation in patients treated for gynecologic malignancies. Cancer. 2014;120(24):3870–83.
29. Kennedy GD, Heise CP. Radiation colitis and proctitis. Clin Colon Rectal Surg. 2007;20:64–72.
30. Krol R, Smeenk RJ, van Lin EN, Yeoh EE, Hopman WP. Systematic review: anal and rectal changes after radiotherapy for prostate cancer. Int J Color Dis. 2014;29(3):273–83.
31. Krol R, Hopman WP, Smeenk RJ, Van Lin EN. Increased rectal wall stiffness after prostate radiotherapy: relation with fecal urgency. Neurogastroenterol Motil. 2012;24(4):339–e166.
32. Krol R, Smeenk RJ, van Lin EN, Hopman WP. Impact of late anorectal dysfunction on quality of life after pelvic radiotherapy. Int J Color Dis. 2013;28(4):519–26.
33. Kushwaha RS, Hayne D, Vaizey CJ, Wrightham E, Payne H, Boulos PB. Physiologic changes of the anorectum after pelvic radiotherapy for the treatment of prostate and bladder cancer. Dis Colon Rectum. 2003;46(9):1182–8.
34. Yeoh EE, Botten R, Russo A, McGowan R, Fraser R, Roos D, Penniment M, Borg M, Sun W. Chronic effects of therapeutic irradiation for localized prostatic carcinoma on anorectal function. Int J Radiat Oncol Biol Phys. 2000;47(4):915–24.
35. Varma JS, Smith AN, Busuttil A. Function of the anal sphincters after chronic radiation injury. Gut. 1986;27(5):528–33.
36. Carrington EV, Heinrich H, Knowles CH, Fox M, Rao S, Altomare DF, Bharucha AE, Burgell R, Chey WD, Chiarioni G, Dinning P, Emmanuel A, Farouk R, Felt-Bersma RJF, Jung KW, Lembo A, Malcolm A, Mittal RK, Mion F, Myung SJ, O'Connell PR, Pehl C, Remes-Troche JM, Reveille RM, Vaizey CJ, Vitton V, Whitehead WE, Wong RK, Scott SM. All members of the International Anorectal Physiology Working Group. The international anorectal physiology working group (IAPWG) recommendations: standardized testing protocol and the London classification for disorders of anorectal function. Neurogastroenterol Motil. 2020;32(1):e13679.
37. Dall FH, Jørgensen CS, Houe D, Gregersen H, Djurhuus JC. Biomechanical wall properties of the human rectum. A study with impedance planimetry. Gut. 1993;34(11):1581–6.
38. Dahiya DS, Kichloo A, Tuma F, Albosta M, Wani F. Radiation Proctitis and management strategies. Clin Endosc. 2022;55(1):22–32. https://doi.org/10.5946/ce.2020.288. Epub 2021 Nov 18. PMID: 34788934; PMCID: PMC8831406.
39. Pehlivan Z, Nural N. Prevalence of constipation in patients undergoing chemotherapy and the effect of constipation on quality of life. Support Care Cancer. 2022;30(10):8019–28. https://doi.org/10.1007/s00520-022-07244-7. Epub 2022 Jun 28. PMID: 35761103.
40. Escalante J, McQuade RM, Stojanovska V, Nurgali K. Impact of chemotherapy on gastrointestinal functions and the enteric nervous system. Maturitas. 2017;105:23–9. https://doi.org/10.1016/j.maturitas.2017.04.021.
41. Wong ML, Paul SM, Cooper BA, Dunn LB, Hammer MJ, Conley YP, Miaskowski C. Predictors of the multidimensional symptom experience of lung cancer patients receiving chemotherapy. Support Care Cancer. 2017;25(6):1931–9. https://doi.org/10.1007/s00520-017-3593-z.
42. Camilleri M. Bile acid diarrhea: prevalence, pathogenesis, and therapy. Gut Liver. 2015;9(3):332–9.
43. BouSaba, et al. Bile acid diarrhea - as bad as it gets? Curr Opin Gastroenterol. 2023;39(3):184–91. https://doi.org/10.1097/MOG.0000000000000916. Epub 2023 Mar 2
44. Mathias JR, et al. Review: pathophysiology of diarrhea caused by bacterial overgrowth of the small intestine. Am J Med Sci. 1985;289(6):243–8.
45. Walters JR, et al. A new mechanism for bile acid diarrhea: defective feedback inhibition of bile acid biosynthesis. Clin Gastroenterol Hepatol. 2009;7(11):1189–94.
46. Larsen HM, et al. Chronic loose stools following right-sided hemicolectomy for colon cancer and the association with bile acid malabsorption and small intestinal bacterial overgrowth. Color Dis. 2023;25(4):600–7.

47. Hillman ET, et al. Microbial ecology along the gastrointestinal tract. Microbes environ. 2017;32(4):300-313. 10.1264/jsme2.ME17017. Epub 2017 Nov 10. PMID: 29129876; PMCID: PMC5745014.Lichtman J et al. The effect of microbial colonization on the host proteome varies by gastrointestinal location. ISME J. 2016;10(5):1170–81. https://doi.org/10.1038/ismej.2015.187. Epub 2015 Nov 17
48. Zhou H, et al. Bile acids are nutrient signaling hormones. Steroids. 2014; 86:62-8. 10.1016/j.steroids.2014.04.016. Epub 2014 may 10. Lynch SV et al. The human intestinal microbiome in health and disease. N Engl J Med. 2016;375(24):2369–79.
49. Shalon D, et al. Profiling the human intestinal environment under physiological conditions. Nature. 2023;617(7961):581–91.
50. Wlodarczyk JR, Yoon D, Owens J, et al. Prevalence of and risk factors for incidental colonic diverticulosis. J Surg Res. 2022;280:348–34.
51. Pinheiro M, Moreira DN, Ghidini M. Colon and rectal cancer: an emergent public health problem. World J Gastroenterol. 2024;30:644–51.
52. Wang L, Xu R, Kaelber DC, et al. Time trend and association of early-onset colorectal cancer with diverticular disease in the United States: 2010-2021. Cancers (Basel). 2022;14:4948. https://doi.org/10.3390/cancers14194948.
53. Morini S, Zullo A, Hassan C, et al. Diverticulosis and colorectal cancer: between lights and shadows. J Clin Gastroenterol. 2008;42:763–70.
54. Lee HJ, Park SJ, Cheon JH, et al. The relationship between diverticulosis and colorectal neoplasia: a meta-analysis. PLoS One. 2019;14:e0216380. eCollection 2019
55. Williams S, Bjarnason I, Hayee B, Haji A. Diverticular disease: update on pathophysiology, classification and management. Frontline Gastroenterol. 2023;15(1):50–8. https://doi.org/10.1136/flgastro-2022-102361. PMID: 38487561; PMCID: PMC10935533.
56. Bode MK, Karttunen TJ, Mäkelä J, Risteli L, Risteli J. Type I and III collagens in human colon cancer and diverticulosis. Scand J Gastroenterol. 2000;35(7):747–52. https://doi.org/10.1080/003655200750023435. PMID: 10972180.
57. Rosemar A, Ivarsson M-L, Börjesson L, et al. Increased concentration of tissue-degrading matrix metalloproteinases and their inhibitor in complicated diverticular disease. Scand J Gastroenterol. 2007;42:215–20. https://doi.org/10.1080/00365520600960104.
58. Hodgson J. Effect of methylcellulose on rectal and colonic pressures in treatment of diverticular disease. Br Med J. 1972;3:729–31. https://doi.org/10.1136/bmj.3.5829.729.
59. Bassotti G, Battaglia E, De Roberto G, et al. Alterations in colonic motility and relationship to pain in colonic diverticulosis. Clin Gastroenterol Hepatol. 2005;3:248–53. https://doi.org/10.1016/s1542-3565(04)00614-7.
60. Imperatore N, Cordone G, Martorelli L, Rispo A, Familiari V, Musto D, Avellino M, Franzese MD, Ricciolino S, Lamanda R. Segmental colitis associated with diverticulosis (SCAD) in a colorectal cancer screening population: prevalence, endoscopic features and oncological outcomes. Dig Liver Dis. 2024;S1590-8658(24):00871–5.
61. Rao SS, Bharucha AE, Chiarioni G, Felt-Bersma R, Knowles C, Malcolm A, Wald A. Functional anorectal disorders. Gastroenterology. 2016;150:1430. https://doi.org/10.1053/j.gastro.2016.02.009.
62. Stellingwerf ME, Maeda Y, Patel U, Vaizey CJ, Warusavitarne J, Bemelman WA, et al. The role of the defaecating pouchogram in the assessment of evacuation difficulty after restorative proctocolectomy and pouch-anal anastomosis. Color Dis. 2016;18:O292–300.
63. Akinmoladun O, Oh W. Management of hemorrhoids and anal fissures. Surg Clin North Am. 2024;104(3):473–90. https://doi.org/10.1016/j.suc.2023.11.001. Epub 2023 Dec 9. PMID: 38677814.
64. Thippeswamy KM, Gruber M, Abdelaziz H, Abdel-Dayem M. Efficacy and safety of botulinum toxin injection in the management of chronic symptomatic anal fissure: a systematic review and meta-analysis of randomized controlled trials. Tech Coloproctol. 2025;29(1):44. https://doi.org/10.1007/s10151-024-03087-y.

16 Multi-regional Disorders

George Triadafilopoulos

16.1 Multi-regional Disorders

Disorders of Gut-Brain Interaction (DGBI) These disorders manifest as gastrointestinal symptoms resulting from visceral hypersensitivity, altered motility, microbiota composition, or mucosal and immune dysfunction and associated with disordered central nervous system processing. DGBI may be focal or diffuse and may chronically or intermittently involve the esophagus, stomach, and small bowel and/or the colon, causing abnormalities of esophageal motility, gastric emptying and accommodation, small bowel and colonic motility and transit, as well as altered colonic volume and rectal evacuation that can be measured objectively with special noninvasive tests in patients who are not responding to behavioral, empirical dietary, or pharmacological treatments [1]. IBS represents one of the most common disorders of the gut-brain interaction (DGBI). The clinical presentation of IBS is complex and varies widely among individuals. Currently, IBS is present when all of the following criteria are met: [1] there are chronic symptoms, i.e., lasting longer than 3 months (e.g., abdominal pain, flatulence) and accompanied by altered bowel movements; [2] the complaints should justify the patient seeking help and/or worrying about them and be so severe resulting in impaired quality of life; and [3] there are no other clinical features responsible for these symptoms [2]. Compared with the general population, IBS does not increase the overall risk of cancer. Conversely, IBS is associated with lower risk of incident colorectal cancer and cancer-specific mortality [3]. Nevertheless, there are studies suggestive that IBS might be associated with cancer of the digestive organs as well as with non-digestive cancer entities, but without proof of causality [4].

G. Triadafilopoulos (✉)
Department of Gastroenterology, Hepatology and Nutrition, UT MD Anderson Cancer Center, Houston, TX, USA
e-mail: GTriadafilopoulo@mdanderson.org

G. Triadafilopoulos (ed.), *Onco-Neurogastroenterology*,
https://doi.org/10.1007/978-3-031-98848-6_16

Radiation Injury The small intestine is the organ at most risk during abdominal-pelvic irradiation, and this risk is increased when the intestinal loops occupy the place of removed organ(s) after abdominal-pelvic organ resection, such as after total hysterectomy for cancer, or after proctectomy for rectal cancer, where the small intestinal loops fall into the pelvis. The position of the small intestine can be technically challenging, especially in case of postoperative enterocele, and omentopexy to fill the pelvic space or fixation of the greater omentum to the pelvic brim posteriorly and to the bladder anteriorly or the use of absorbable mesh may be considered [5]. Acute toxicity reflects mucosal injury. The normal villous epithelium of the intestine is renewed by non-functional cells, causing loss of the barrier effect and, consequently, abdominal pain and accelerated intestinal transit. Conversely, late effects reflect a combination of submucosal fibrosis and vascular degeneration. This chronic involvement, typically of the muscular and serosal layers, can have uni- or multi-segmental involvement. The main late effect of RT is chronic diarrhea due to malabsorption, microbial overgrowth, or protein-losing enteropathy. Mucosal ulcers, or strictures with perforation, abscess, and/or fistula formation, may possibly cause chronic obstruction and microbial overgrowth [6].

Abdomino-pelvic radiation results in acute toxicity in nearly 80% of patients and late toxicity in 20%. Acute toxicity occurs within 3 months following irradiation, and it reaches a maximum between the 4th and 5th week, causing diarrhea, abdominal pain, and weight loss. If there is associated radiation proctitis, hematochezia, rectal pain, or fecal incontinence may be seen. Symptoms usually resolve after therapy discontinuation. Late toxicity occurs between 18 and 60 months after irradiation, but cases have been reported as early as 3 months or as late as 30 years. Chronic radiation enteropathy most frequently presents with chronic diarrhea, which is more severe if there is associated loss of sigmoid-rectal compliance. If obstructive symptoms are prominent, they are typically related to ileal stricture. Because of the delay in diagnosis and long-standing symptoms, malabsorption is frequently observed, potentially requiring total parenteral nutrition (TPN). Rarely, radiation enteropathy can be diagnosed based on findings at emergency operation for complications (i.e., obstruction, abscess, perforations, fistulas) [7].

Imaging is necessary to confirm the diagnosis, to identify the single or multi-segmental site of involvement, and to search for a potential complication and/or associated pelvic involvement (i.e., colorectal stricture, ureteral dilation). Imaging is also essential to rule out cancer recurrence. Colonoscopy is necessary to rule out colonic or terminal ileal involvement. MR enterography, followed possibly by video capsule enteroscopy, should also be considered to provide precise mapping of intestinal involvement (short or long segment, single or multiple strictures, distance between the most distal stricture and the ileocecal valve) and determine its upstream impact or even detect complications, such as fistulas or abscesses. The use of intravenous enhancement is important since it highlights any inflammatory signs within the mesentery. Video capsule endoscopy must be preceded by MR enterography or a patency-type test to ensure that the capsule will pass without causing intestinal obstruction.

Therapy is symptomatic, particularly using anti-diarrheal medication bile acid binders, antibiotics for microbial overgrowth, and local treatment of associated radiation proctitis. Nutritional management with supplements, or TPN, for episodes of obstruction or to manage short bowel syndrome due to surgical resections, may be needed. Intravenous steroid therapy and parenteral nutrition decrease the risk of recurrence. Hyperbaric oxygen therapy has been associated with mixed results. Glutamine, as an intestinal trophic factor, has no significant effect on the prevention and treatment of severe radiation injury. Surgical management is indicated in 30% of patients when faced with complicated or severe radiation enteritis, refractory to medical treatment [8]. There is no consensus concerning intestinal resection or enteric bypass, in the absence of perforation or fistula. The disadvantage of internal bypass, which is simpler and quicker to perform, is that the diseased bowel remains in place with the risk of bleeding, abscess, perforation, and bacterial translocation. The natural history of radiation enteritis, is characterized by multiple lesions, frequent recurrences, and repeated resections, which can lead to short gut syndrome and intestinal insufficiency, Management requires an individualized approach for optimal decision making.

Intra-abdominal Adhesions Abdominal adhesions are bands of scar tissue that can form after surgery or due to inflammation or neoplasia, extrinsically affecting the small intestine or the colon or both. Adhesions can cause bowel problems, including classic intestinal obstruction, chronic nonspecific abdominal pain, cramps, and changes in bowel habits. In contrast to other etiologies, patients report transient, short-lived episodes of pain (hours to few days) associated with constipation. Bloating and abdominal distention are common. The diagnosis of adhesive bowel disease, particularly when it is not acute, is challenging, and it is based on history, clinical evaluation, biological tests, and, importantly, CT imaging. In the acute setting, ultrasonography also represents a user-friendly and inexpensive diagnostic tool that could be performed at bedside since it has a high sensitivity (92%) and specificity (97%) for small bowel obstruction [9]. Acute adhesive small bowel obstruction (ASBO) resolves with NPO, IV fluids, NG decompression, and analgesics in up to 80% of cases, unless strangulation or ischemia is present. Unfortunately, if surgery is required, it may leave adhesions, potentially inducing future episodes of bowel obstruction. When an extensive resection is required, it may lead to short bowel syndrome [10].

Notably, in patients without prior abdomino-pelvic surgery (virgin abdomen), there is a high prevalence of malignant etiologies (7.7–13.4% in one study), most of which not suspected before surgery. In almost half of these patients, a trial of non-operative management fails, and patients require operative interventions [11]. The risk of ASBO is the highest following colorectal and oncologic gynecological surgery [12]. Laparoscopy is associated with a significant reduction in the rate of adhesions across multiple abdominal procedures compared to open surgery. There is a general reluctance for the use of laparoscopy for ASBO possibly due to the fact that laparoscopic adhesiolysis can be technically demanding, associated with a higher risk of iatrogenic bowel injury [13]. The onco-neurogastroenterologist should work closely with the surgeon to risk stratify patients for operability and jointly consider further clinical assessment, longitudinal monitoring, and therapy. High-resolution small bowel manometry is not generally available, but it could be useful in elucidating the patients' symptoms by demonstrating evidence of partial small obstruction by detecting the minute rhythm (MRP) or prolonged simultaneous contractions (PSC) postprandially in only a small percentage of cases [14]. Anecdotally, the use of high dose (17 g bid) of polyethylene glycol may improve abdominal symptoms by maintaining intestinal fluidity and improving colonic cleansing.

Endometriosis Endometriosis is defined by the presence of endometrial-like tissue outside the uterine cavity, including the gut. It affects 11.4% of reproductive-aged females and commonly causes chronic pelvic pain and infertility. Laparoscopy remains the gold standard for diagnosis of small-volume disease, with pelvic imaging recognized as being diagnostic in severe or invasive disease [15]. Endometriosis can be challenging for the onco-neurogastroenterologist since it gives rise to various abdomino-pelvic symptoms and adhesion formation. Endometriosis has also been associated with an increased risk of ovarian cancer [16]. Since it is a chronic condition, a multidisciplinary approach among gynecologists, laparoscopists, and gastroenterologists is fruitful for diagnosis and management. Endometriosis has long been treated with hormonal therapies that impact estrogen. First-line therapies include the combined oral contraceptive pill (COCP), progestogens, and nonsteroidal anti-inflammatory drugs. Second-line suppressive treatments, such as gonadotropin-releasing hormone agonists (GnRHa) and antagonists (GnRHant), can be offered to those whose symptoms fail to be controlled by first-line agents. Nonhormonal complementary and alternative medicines are increasingly investigated as possible treatments for endometriosis.

Postural Orthostatic Tachycardia Syndrome (POTS) Patients with cancer may often suffer from orthostatic intolerance, with symptoms that develop in response to upright posture and, classically, resolve upon recumbency. Such orthostatic intolerance is due to generalized autonomic failure (e.g., from diabetes mellitus and amyloidosis) or most commonly due to postural orthostatic tachycardia syndrome (POTS). Non-orthostatic symptoms commonly seen in POTS include dry eyes or mouth and a variety of urinary and gastrointestinal (GI) complaints [17].

The dysautonomia seen in POTS may cause symptoms of abnormal gut motility, such as nausea (86%), irregular bowel movements (71%), abdominal pain (70%), constipation (70%), heartburn (64%), and bloating (59%). Most patients report multiple symptoms occurring more than once weekly and not improving with supine positioning and fluctuating along with autonomic symptoms. GI symptoms may lead to a reduction in nutrient and fluid intake resulting in volume shifts and dehydration, further aggravating the autonomic symptoms. Abnormalities in both gastric emptying (mostly rapid gastric emptying) and in the gastric electrical activity may be noted. In one study using small intestinal manometry, 93% (11/12) demonstrated signs of intestinal neuropathy, such as bursts of uncoordinated phasic activity in both fasting (58%) and postprandial (42%) states, low contractility in the fed state

(67%), and lack of development of the fed state (42%). Colon transit was slow in 80% of cases. Esophageal manometry and anorectal manometry studies showed abnormalities in 67% and 86% of cases, respectively. Abdominal imaging may show signs of pseudo-obstruction in 58%, such as dilated bowel loops and/or air-fluid levels. These data suggest that the perturbations in POTS involve multiple segments of the gut [18]. The management is symptom-driven and palliative, mostly aiming at improving quality of life. The most common pharmacologic treatment options for POTS include midodrine, bisoprolol, fludrocortisone, desmopressin, and propranolol.

Cancer Therapy-Induced Gastrointestinal Dysfunction Intra-abdominal adhesions resulting from prior abdominal and/or pelvic surgery and radiation therapy may present with chronic abdominal bloating, crampy abdominal pain, altered bowel habits, and nausea and may contribute to partial or complete bowel obstruction and small intestinal bacterial overgrowth. Peritoneal carcinomatosis causing CIPO needs to be excluded. Diagnostic tests, such as barium small bowel follow-through or MR enterography, and antro-duodenal manometry to assess for repeated phase 3 migrating motor complexes in fasting state, and ultimately diagnostic laparoscopy to intraoperatively identify of abdominal adhesions may be required to make a definitive diagnosis. Treatment options include abdominal visceral massage, smooth muscle relaxants (i.e., dicyclomine, hyoscyamine, or peppermint oil), low-residue diet, and minimization of fiber supplements and stimulant laxatives. Obviously, elective lysis of adhesions—when found at laparoscopy—is the preferred approach, but it is not always feasible and carries the risk for recurrences [19].

Opioid-Induced Bowel Dysfunction (OIBD) Since constipation is not the only opioid side effect on the gut, we prefer the term "opioid-induced bowel dysfunction" (OIBD), which includes dry mouth, dysphagia, heartburn, gastroesophageal reflux, early satiety, and postprandial epigastric discomfort, nausea and vomiting, bloating, and distention, consistent with the role of mu, delta, and kappa opioid receptors (MOR, DOR, and KOR, respectively) in modulating gastrointestinal motility and secretion, in turn leading to decreased peristalsis, delayed intestinal transit time, increased sphincter constriction, decreased small bowel water and electrolyte secretion, and water resorption with development of hard stools [20, 21].

Paraneoplastic Neurological syndromes (PNS) Paraneoplastic neurological syndromes are rare, affecting fewer than 1% of all patients with cancer. Paraneoplastic chronic intestinal pseudo-obstruction (CIPO) is mainly associated with small cell lung carcinoma (SCLC), but it may be seen with prostate cancer, extraskeletal myxoid chondrosarcoma, and thymoma. Typically, such patients have detectable onconeural (mostly anti-Hu) autoantibodies. Paraneoplastic CIPO is attributed to humoral mediators secreted by tumor cells or an immune response targeting tumor antigens [22].

Multiple Endocrine Neoplasias (MEN) Multiple endocrine neoplasias are rare but potentially malignant hereditary syndromes. Multiple endocrine neoplasia type 2 (MEN 2) is an autosomal dominant hereditary cancer syndrome with two distinct clinical subtypes: (1) MEN 2A is associated with medullary thyroid carcinoma (MTC), pheochromocytoma, primary hyperparathyroidism, cutaneous lichen amyloidosis, and Hirschsprung's disease, and (2) MEN 2B is associated with MTC, pheochromocytoma, ganglioneuromatosis of the aerodigestive tract, and musculoskeletal and ophthalmologic abnormalities. The definitive diagnosis of MEN 2 is made by *RET* sequencing (which is positive in 98% of cases). Genetic counseling and genetic testing for *RET* germline variants should be offered to first-degree relatives of patients with a proven pathogenic *RET* germline variant, followed by examinations for MEN 2-related tumors in affected members [23].

Neurofibromatosis Neurofibromatosis type 1 (NF1) is a rare autosomal dominant genetic disorder characterized by multiple café au lait macules and neurofibromas. An increased risk of constipation and irritable bowel syndrome may be seen with NF1 and predisposes to gastrointestinal stromal tumors (GISTs) [24].

Cannabinoid Gut For various reasons, the percentage of cannabis users in the USA increased significantly from 11% (or 25.8 million people) in 2002 to 17.5% (or 48.2 million people) in 2019. Among adult cancer survivors, approximately 50% used cannabis for medical reasons during coronavirus pandemic [25]. Overall, cannabinoid hyperemesis or withdrawal and cyclic vomiting syndrome are increasingly recognized. The metabolism of endocannabinoids, the location of cannabinoid (CB) receptors, and their impact on immune/inflammatory, neuromuscular, sensory, and motility functions in the gut and disorders of gut-brain interaction have been extensively studied [26]. In general, cannabinoids inhibit gastrointestinal motor function; yet they relieve symptoms of gastroparesis, nausea, and abdominal pain. In particular, agents that affect CB_2 mechanisms have therapeutic potential in gut inflammatory conditions, gastroparesis, pain, and disorders of gut-brain interaction.

Amyloidosis Amyloidosis is characterized by the extracellular deposition of autologous, insoluble, fibrillar misfolded proteins that deposit in tissues aggregated in ß-pleated sheets and causing distortion to the tissue architecture and function [27]. In cancer patients, amyloidosis is associated with plasma cell dyscrasias, chronic inflammatory conditions, or hemodialysis. Gastrointestinal amyloidosis may be systemic or localized. Systemic amyloidosis is more common than localized amyloidosis; secondary systemic amyloidosis (AA) represents only a small fraction of all cases. Infiltration of extracellular misfolded proteins can be seen in the different layers of the GI tract. AA amyloid deposition is seen mainly in the mucosa, potentially leading to friability, erosions, diarrhea, or malabsorption. Neuromuscular infiltration is characterized by the deposition of the amyloid proteins in the neuromuscular layer of the GI tract, affecting the myenteric or submucosal nerve plexuses and longitudinal and circular muscles, and leading to abnormal peristalsis, abnormal GI transit times, or bowel obstruction [28]. The clinical manifestations of GI amyloidosis depend on the amount and location of the amyloid deposits, irrespective of whether it is in the context of primary or secondary systemic amyloidosis. Patients with localized amyloidosis may have similar clinical features as those with systemic disease. All patients share common presenting symptoms, such as fatigue, lightheadedness, anorexia, and weight loss.

Gastrointestinal bleeding may occur in up to 57% of patients with amyloidosis and is due to mucosal lesions (amyloidoma ulcers, erosions, polypoid lesions, hematomas, or submucosal hemorrhages), vascular friability, or bowel ischemia. Malabsorption may present with diarrhea, weight loss, steatorrhea, anorexia, or dizziness, and it is usually secondary to mucosal infiltration, pancreatic insufficiency, protein-losing gastroenteropathy, or small intestinal bacterial overgrowth (SIBO). Chronic gastrointestinal dysmotility may present with nausea, vomiting, dysphagia, gastroparesis, gastroesophageal reflux, loss of appetite, constipation or diarrhea, abdominal pain, bloating, or clinical features of chronic intestinal pseudo-obstruction. Dysmotility can be secondary to myopathic and neuropathic dysfunction [29].

The gold standard test for establishing a diagnosis of amyloidosis is tissue biopsy followed by Congo red staining and apple-green birefringence of the Congo red-stained deposits under polarized light. However, not all patients may have a positive tissue confirmation of the disease. Along with symptomatic management, the treatment for GI amyloidosis consists of observation or localized surgical excision in patients with localized disease and treatment of the underlying pathology, in cases of systemic amyloidosis (i.e., treatment of multiple myeloma).

Adrenal Insufficiency Adrenal insufficiency in patients with cancer may result from a primary adrenal disorder (tumor infiltration, bilateral adrenalectomy, hemorrhage), secondary to adrenocorticotropic hormone deficiency (hypophyseal tumor infiltration, surgery, radiation), or by suppression of adrenocorticotropic hormone by exogenous glucocorticoids or opioid medications [30]. Key clinical features are unintentional weight loss, anorexia, postural hypotension, profound fatigue, muscle and abdominal pain, and hyponatremia. Chronic gastrointestinal symptoms are common. Additionally, patients with primary adrenal insufficiency usually develop skin hyperpigmentation and crave salt. The diagnosis of adrenal insufficiency is usually delayed because the initial presentation is often nonspecific; physician awareness must be improved to avoid adrenal crisis, which may still occur in about 50% of patients after diagnosis. Gastrointestinal symptoms are frequent in both acute and chronic adrenal insufficiency. Abdominal pain with features of irritable bowel syndrome and affecting the patient's quality of life has been described in 30–50% of patients [31]. Such digestive symptoms may also be related to impairment of the hypothalamic-pituitary-adrenal axis or other coexistent hormone deficiencies (i.e., thyroid or gonadotropic). Loss of physiological secretion of cortisol or an inappropriate replacement therapy may also impact intestinal permeability, even in treated patients, and therefore might induce digestive symptoms. Hence, assessment and management of digestive symptoms should be considered, preferably by an onco-neurogastroenterologist in conjunction with an endocrinologist.

Thyroid Disorders Thyroid disorders are a frequent reason for altered motility in patients with cancer and will need consideration on every patient with suggestive symptoms. Hyperthyroidism is a condition where the thyroid gland produces and inappropriately secretes high amounts of thyroid hormone, which can lead to thyrotoxicosis. The diagnosis can be made clinically and confirmed with biochemical tests and imaging, such as ultrasound and radioactive iodine uptake scans. Causes of hyperthyroidism include TSH-producing pituitary tumors, trophoblastic and germ cell tumors, struma ovarii, thyroid adenoma, and cancer [32].

The clinical manifestations of hyperthyroidism can be diverse, as thyroid hormones can have an impact on a variety of systemic and gastrointestinal symptoms, such as intermittent dysphagia (from extrinsic compression of the esophagus), hyperdefecation (frequently described as diarrhea), and hunger with hyperphagia without weight gain [33]. Such symptoms are intensified during a thyroid storm and will need to be managed by an endocrinologist. TSH is the most sensitive and specific first-line biochemical test to examine thyroid function, at times confirmed with free T4 and total serum T3. In cancer patients, surgery may involve a total thyroidectomy for toxic multinodular goiters and a thyroid lobectomy for toxic adenomas and cancer. Advantages of surgery for hyperthyroidism allow for nearly 100% cure rates, identification of incidental cancers, and rapid achievement of euthyroid or hypothyroid states.

Hypothyroidism is a common condition of thyroid hormone deficiency, which can be defined as elevated thyroid-stimulating hormone (TSH) levels, associated with low free thyroxine concentrations. Hypothyroidism can be classified as primary (due to thyroid hormone deficiency) or secondary (due to TSH deficiency). In cancer patients, hypothyroidism most frequently reflects prior total thyroidectomy for thyroid cancer. The clinical manifestations of hypothyroidism range from asymptomatic to life-threatening (myxedema coma). The most common symptoms of hypothyroidism are fatigue, lethargy, cold intolerance, weight gain, constipation, change (hoarseness) in voice, and dry skin [34]. The onco-neurogastroenterologist should always consider hypothyroidism as a cause of delayed gastric emptying (gastroparesis) and refractory, slow-transit constipation and treat it aggressively by optimally regulated thyroid hormone supplementation, prokinetics, and laxatives.

Autoimmune Gastrointestinal Dysmotility (AGID) Autoimmune gastrointestinal dysmotility is an idiopathic or paraneoplastic phenomenon, reflecting limited autoimmune dysautonomia. The use of WMC identifies the key areas of involvement, such as the stomach, small intestine, and colon involved in the process (Fig. 16.1).

Anti-neuronal autoantibodies are often detected in patients with AGID. Although autoantibodies play a key role in GI dysmotility, whether they cause neuronal destruction is unknown. Immunomodulatory therapies are used as the first-line therapy. A comprehensive autoimmune evaluation and cancer screening are essential for clinical diagnosis. Well-accepted diagnostic criteria, treatment protocols, and

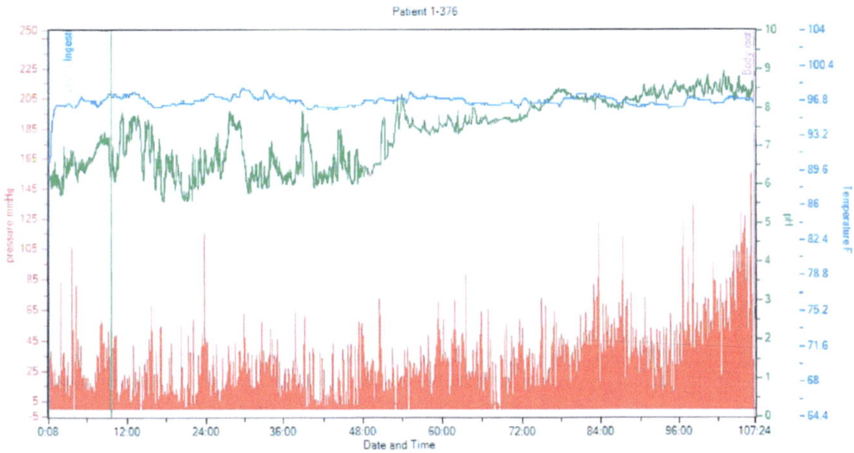

Fig. 16.1 Wireless motility capsule (WMC) testing in a patient with long-standing AGID who presented with postprandial bloating, constipation, and recurrent SIBO. The combination of the pressure profiles (in red), temperature (in blue), and pH (in green) allows the assessment of gastric, small intestinal, and colonic transit times in such patients. In this tracing from a patient with paraneoplastic autoimmune intestinal dysmotility, there is a lack of gastric acidity, while the capsule was in the stomach since the patient had associated achlorhydria and the T ½ gastric emptying time was only assessed scintigraphically at 4 h and 42 min (not shown). Nevertheless, WMC (shown) assessed the small intestinal transit to be 6 h and 37 min and the colonic transit to be 97 h and 40 min

outcome definitions for AGID are required for prompt diagnosis and treatment and appropriate management of immunotherapy, which will circumvent the need for surgeries and improve patient outcomes [35].

References

1. Camilleri M. Abnormal gastrointestinal motility is a major factor in explaining symptoms and a potential therapeutic target in patients with disorders of gut-brain interaction. Gut. 2023;72(12):2372–80.
2. Palsson OS, Whitehead WE, van Tilburg MA, Chang L, Chey W, Crowell MD, Keefer L, Lembo AJ, Parkman HP, Rao SS, Sperber A, Spiegel B, Tack J, Vanner S, Walker LS, Whorwell P, Yang Y. Rome IV diagnostic questionnaires and tables for investigators and clinicians. Gastroenterology. 2016:S0016-5085(16)00180-3.
3. Wu S, Yuan C, Liu S, Zhang Q, Yang Z, Sun F, Zhan S, Zhu S, Zhang S. Irritable bowel syndrome and long-term risk of cancer: a prospective cohort study among 0.5 million adults in UK biobank. Am J Gastroenterol. 2022;117(5):785–93.
4. Loosen SH, Jördens MS, Luedde M, Modest DP, Labuhn S, Luedde T, Kostev K, Roderburg C. Incidence of cancer in patients with irritable bowel syndrome. J Clin Med. 2021;10(24):5911.
5. Loge L, Florescu C, Alves A, Menahem B. Radiation enteritis: diagnostic and therapeutic issues. J Visc Surg. 2020;157(6):475–85.
6. Hauer-Jensen M, Denham JW, Andreyev HJ. Radiation enteropathy–pathogenesis, treatment and prevention. Nat Rev Gastroenterol Hepatol. 2014;11:470–9.
7. Fuccio L, Guido A, Andreyev HJ. Management of intestinal complications in patients with pelvic radiation disease. Clin Gastroenterol Hepatol. 2012;10:1326–34.

8. Theis VS, Sripadam R, Ramani V, Lal S. Chronic radiation enteritis. Clin Oncol (R Coll Radiol). 2010;22:70–83.
9. Gottlieb M, Peksa GD, Pandurangadu AV, Nakitende D, Takhar S, Seethala RR. Utilization of ultrasound for the evaluation of small bowel obstruction: a systematic review and meta-analysis. Am J Emerg Med. 2018;36(2):234–42. https://doi.org/10.1016/j.ajem.2017.07.085. Epub 2017 Jul 29. PMID: 28797559.
10. Podda M, Khan M, Di Saverio S. Adhesive small bowel obstruction and the six w's: who, how, why, when, what, and where to diagnose and operate? Scand J Surg. 2021;110(2):159–69. https://doi.org/10.1177/1457496920982763.
11. Choi J, Fisher AT, Mulaney B, Anand A, Carlos G, Stave CD, Spain DA, Weiser TG. Safety of foregoing operation for small bowel obstruction in the virgin abdomen: systematic review and meta-analysis. J Am Coll Surg. 2020;231(3):368–375.e1. https://doi.org/10.1016/j.jamcollsurg.2020.06.010. Epub 2020 Jun 20. PMID: 32574687.
12. ten Broek RP, Issa Y, van Santbrink EJ, Bouvy ND, Kruitwagen RF, Jeekel J, Bakkum EA, Rovers MM, van Goor H. Burden of adhesions in abdominal and pelvic surgery: systematic review and meta-analysis. BMJ. 2013;347:f5588. https://doi.org/10.1136/bmj.f5588. PMID: 24092941; PMCID: PMC3789584.
13. Di Saverio S, Birindelli A, Broek RT, Davies JR, Mandrioli M, Sallinen V. Laparoscopic adhesiolysis: not for all patients, not for all surgeons, not in all centres. Updates Surg. 2018;70(4):557–61. https://doi.org/10.1007/s13304-018-0534-4. Epub 2018 May 16. PMID: 29767333; PMCID: PMC6244716.
14. Alcalá-González LG, Malagelada C, Monrroy H, Mego M, Accarino A, Malagelada JR, Azpiroz F. Clinical significance of small bowel manometry patterns suggestive of intestinal obstruction. Neurogastroenterol Motil. 2023;35(1):e14462. https://doi.org/10.1111/nmo.14462. Epub 2022 Sep 14. PMID: 36102622; PMCID: PMC10078417.
15. Alonso A, Gunther K, Maheux-Lacroix S, Abbott J. Medical management of endometriosis. Curr Opin Obstet Gynecol. 2024;36(5):353–61. https://doi.org/10.1097/GCO.0000000000000983. Epub 2024 Aug 17. PMID: 39159261; PMCID: PMC11356688.
16. Barnard ME, Farland LV, Yan B, Wang J, Trabert B, Doherty JA, Meeks HD, Madsen M, Guinto E, Collin LJ, Maurer KA, Page JM, Kiser AC, Varner MW, Allen-Brady K, Pollack AZ, Peterson KR, Peterson CM, Schliep KC. Endometriosis typology and ovarian cancer risk. JAMA. 2024;332(6):482–9. https://doi.org/10.1001/jama.2024.9210. PMID: 39018030; PMCID: PMC11255975.
17. DiBaise JK, Harris LA, Goodman B. Postural tachycardia syndrome (POTS) and the GI tract: a primer for the gastroenterologist. Am J Gastroenterol. 2018;113(10):1458–67. https://doi.org/10.1038/s41395-018-0215-4. Epub 2018 Aug 3. PMID: 30072778.
18. Huang RJ, Chun CL, Friday K, Triadafilopoulos G. Manometric abnormalities in the postural orthostatic tachycardia syndrome: a case series. Dig Dis Sci. 2013;58(11):3207–11. https://doi.org/10.1007/s10620-013-2865-9. Epub 2013 Sep 26. PMID: 24068608.
19. Lim J, Rezaie A. Irritable bowel syndrome-like symptoms in quiescent inflammatory bowel disease: a practical approach to diagnosis and treatment of organic causes. Dig Dis Sci. 2023;68(11):4081–97.
20. Farmer AD, Drewes AM, Chiarioni G, De Giorgio R, O'Brien T, Morlion B, Tack J. Pathophysiology and management of opioid-induced constipation: European expert consensus statement. United Eur Gastroenterol J. 2019;7(1):7–20.
21. van Malderen K, Halawi H, Camilleri M. Insights on efficacious doses of PAMORAs for patients on chronic opioid therapy or opioid-naïve patients. Neurogastroenterol Motil. 2018;30(5):e13250. https://doi.org/10.1111/nmo.13250. Epub 2017 Nov 9. PMID: 29119706.
22. Ren XJ, Shi ZH, Cheng YX, Luo Y. Paraneoplastic syndrome with intestinal pseudo-obstruction in a patient with small cell lung carcinoma: a case report and literature review. J Int Med Res. 2025;53(1):3000605241245868. https://doi.org/10.1177/03000605241245868. PMID: 39819129; PMCID: PMC11748382.

23. Mathiesen JS, Effraimidis G, Rossing M, Rasmussen ÅK, Hoejberg L, Bastholt L, Godballe C, Oturai P, Feldt-Rasmussen U. Multiple endocrine neoplasia type 2: a review. Semin Cancer Biol. 2022;79:163–79. https://doi.org/10.1016/j.semcancer.2021.03.035. Epub 2021 Apr 1. PMID: 33812987.
24. Landry JP, Schertz KL, Chiang YJ, Bhalla AD, Yi M, Keung EZ, Scally CP, Feig BW, Hunt KK, Roland CL, Guadagnolo A, Bishop AJ, Lazar AJ, Slopis JM, McCutcheon IE, Torres KE. Comparison of cancer prevalence in patients with Neurofibromatosis type 1 at an academic cancer center vs in the general population from 1985 to 2020. JAMA Netw Open. 2021;4(3):e210945.
25. Camilleri M, Zheng T. Cannabinoids and the gastrointestinal tract. Clin Gastroenterol Hepatol. 2023;21(13):3217–29.
26. Maselli DB, Camilleri M. Pharmacology, clinical effects, and therapeutic potential of cannabinoids for gastrointestinal and liver diseases. Clin Gastroenterol Hepatol. 2021;19(9):1748–58.
27. Dahiya DS, Kichloo A, Singh J, Albosta M, Wani F. Gastrointestinal amyloidosis: a focused review. World J Gastrointest Endosc. 2021;13(1):1–12. https://doi.org/10.4253/wjge.v13.i1.1. PMID: 33520102; PMCID: PMC7809597.
28. Petre S, Shah IA, Gilani N. Review article: gastrointestinal amyloidosis - clinical features, diagnosis and therapy. Aliment Pharmacol Ther. 2008;27(11):1006–16. https://doi.org/10.1111/j.1365-2036.2008.03682.x. Epub 2008 Mar 17. PMID: 18363891.
29. Guirl MJ, Högenauer C, Santa Ana CA, Porter JL, Little KH, Stone MJ, Fordtran JS. Rapid intestinal transit as a primary cause of severe chronic diarrhea in patients with amyloidosis. Am J Gastroenterol. 2003;98(10):2219–25. https://doi.org/10.1111/j.1572-0241.2003.07695.x.
30. Husebye ES, Pearce SH, Krone NP, Kämpe O. Adrenal insufficiency. Lancet. 2021;397(10274):613–29. https://doi.org/10.1016/S0140-6736(21)00136-7. Epub 2021 Jan 20. PMID: 33484633.
31. Quénéhervé L, Drui D, Blin J, Péré M, Coron E, Barbara G, Barbaro MR, Cariou B, Neunlist M, Masson D, Bach-Ngohou K. Digestive symptoms in daily life of chronic adrenal insufficiency patients are similar to irritable bowel syndrome symptoms. Sci Rep. 2021;11(1):8077. https://doi.org/10.1038/s41598-021-87158-2. PMID: 33850177; PMCID: PMC8044180.
32. Doubleday AR, Sippel RS. Hyperthyroidism. Gland Surg. 2020;9(1):124–35. https://doi.org/10.21037/gs.2019.11.01. PMID: 32206604; PMCID: PMC7082267.
33. Sippel RS, Chen H. The handbook of endocrine surgery hyperthyroidism Hackensack. New York: World Scientific Publishing Co. Pte. Ltd; 2010.
34. Chaker L, Bianco AC, Jonklaas J, Peeters RP. Hypothyroidism. Lancet. 2017;390(10101):1550–62. https://doi.org/10.1016/S0140-6736(17)30703-1. Epub 2017 Mar 20. PMID: 28336049; PMCID: PMC6619426.
35. Nakane S, Mukaino A, Ihara E, Ogawa Y. Autoimmune gastrointestinal dysmotility: the interface between clinical immunology and neurogastroenterology. Immunol Med. 2021;44(2):74–85. https://doi.org/10.1080/25785826.2020.1797319. Epub 2020 Jul 27. PMID: 32715927.

Pharmacotherapy of Gastrointestinal Sensory-Motor Disorders

17

George Triadafilopoulos, David M. Richards, Mehnaz A. Shafi, and Lavanya Viswanathan

There is a wide range of options to manage gastrointestinal sensory-motor function in cancer patients. Table 17.1 highlights the various agents used in the pharmacologic management of gastrointestinal sensory-motor disorders. Although these agents are used extensively in cancer patients, they have not been selectively tested for safety, tolerability, and efficacy, and their impact on cancer-related outcomes is uncertain.

Analgesics Abdominal pain may be very difficult to manage because many pain medications slow intestinal transit. In patients with cancer, management by a physician specialized in pain management is often necessary. Analgesics typically prescribed for neuropathy, such as tricyclic antidepressants (amitriptyline, nortriptyline, and imipramine), and antiepileptic medications, such as gabapentin and pregabalin, can be used with caution. Opioids should be avoided, because their side effects (e.g., sphincter of Oddi dysfunction, constipation) may worsen symptoms. Transdermal buprenorphine has a high receptor affinity combined with a high potency and a low risk for euphorigenic effects and may be used in selected patients. Percutaneous/endoscopic placement of a decompressive tube gastrostomy and/or jejunostomy or tube cecostomy may relieve symptoms (including pain) associated with intestinal distension or malignant obstruction [1].

Coating agents/sucralfate In a prospective study, patients with radiation-induced proctosigmoiditis were randomized to receive a course of either 3.0 g oral sulfasalazine plus 20 mg twice daily rectal prednisolone enemas or 2.0 g twice daily rectal sucralfate enemas plus oral placebo. The two groups were comparable with respect to demographic features, duration of symptoms, and clinical and endoscopic staging

G. Triadafilopoulos (✉) · D. M. Richards · M. A. Shafi · L. Viswanathan
Department of Gastroenterology, Hepatology and Nutrition, UT MD Anderson Cancer Center, Houston, TX, USA
e-mail: gtriadafilopoulo@mdanderson.org

G. Triadafilopoulos (ed.), *Onco-Neurogastroenterology*,
https://doi.org/10.1007/978-3-031-98848-6_17

Table 17.1 Agents used in the pharmacologic management of gastrointestinal sensory-motor disorders

Class	Agents and dosage ranges
Analgesics	Acetaminophen Non-steroidal anti-inflammatory drugs (NSAIDs) Gabapentin/pregabalin Opioids
Coating agents	Sucralfate
Prokinetics	Dopamine receptor antagonists (metoclopramide, domperidone) Motilin agonists (erythromycin, clarithromycin) Ghrelin receptor agonists (relamorelin) 5-HT4 receptor agonists (prucalopride)
Antiemetics	Phenothiazines (promethazine, prochlorperazine) 5-HT3 receptor antagonists (ondansetron, granisetron) Neurokinin-1 receptor antagonists (aprepitant)
Laxatives	Osmotics (PEG, lactulose) Stimulants (senna) Magnesium Chloride channel activators (lubiprostone) Guanylate cyclase receptor activators (linaclotide, plecanatide) Sodium/hydrogen exchange-3 inhibitors (tenapanor) Misoprostol Peripherally acting mu-opioid receptor antagonists (PAMORA) (methylnaltrexone, naloxegol, alvimopan)
Antidiarrheals	Loperamide Diphenoxylate with atropine Octreotide 5-HT3 antagonists (alosetron) Mixed opioid receptor antagonists (eluxadoline)
Opium	Tincture of opium
Antispasmodics	Dicyclomine Hyoscyamine Peppermint oil
Antibiotics	Rifaximin Neomycin
Acid blockers	Antacids H2 receptor antagonists Proton pump inhibitors Potassium-competitive acid blockers
Bile acid sequestrants	Cholestyramine, colestipol, colesevelam, obeticholic acid
Topical anti-inflammatory	Budesonide, suppositories, enemas
Neuromodulators	TCAs (tricyclic antidepressants) SSRIs (selective serotonin reuptake inhibitors) SNRIs (serotonin and noradrenaline reuptake inhibitors) TNAS (tetracyclics or noradrenergic and specific serotonergic antidepressants) AAP (atypical antipsychotics)
Somatostatin analogs (SSAs)	Octreotide, lanreotide
Others	Pyridostigmine, midodrine
Steroids	Prednisone, fludrocortisone

of the disease. At 4 weeks, both groups showed significant clinical improvement and endoscopic healing. When the two groups were compared, sucralfate enemas showed a significantly better response as assessed clinically, although endoscopically the response was not statistically different. Sucralfate enemas give a better clinical response, are tolerated better, and because of their lower cost should be the preferred mode of short-term treatment [2].

Prokinetics Prokinetics are drugs that enhance gastrointestinal motility by increasing the frequency or strength of gastrointestinal contractions without disrupting their rhythm. These drugs are frequently used in the management of patients with heartburn, abdominal bloating, nausea, vomiting, early satiety, and constipation. Examples of these agents include the dopamine receptor antagonists, such as metoclopramide and domperidone; motilin agonists, such as erythromycin and clarithromycin; ghrelin receptor agonists, such as relamorelin; or 5-HT4 receptor agonists, such as prucalopride.

Antiemetics These drugs are used mostly for the control of nausea and vomiting, either acutely or chronically. Several classes of antiemetics may antagonize the neurotransmitter receptors involved in the induction of nausea and vomiting, and they are classified according to their primary action (M1, muscarinic; D2, dopamine; H1, histamine; 5-hydroxytryptamine (HT)-3, serotonin; and neurokinin-1 (NK1) receptor, substance P); some agents affect multiple receptors.

Laxatives Generally, any substance that stimulates bowel movements is called a "laxative." Many of these agents are available over the counter, safe, and inexpensive. There is no evidence that any one laxative is superior to any other. The treatment of constipation should be individualized, dependent on patient preferences or comorbidities, and considering the presence or not of fecal impaction. Glycerol or bisacodyl suppositories may be effective in patients with stool in the rectum, but they will not affect the whole colon. Rectal interventions should be reserved as a last resort since they are burdensome for the patient and caretakers. Polyethylene glycol (PEG) 3550, also available over the counter, promotes a dose-dependent bowel cleansing by pulling water into the gut lumen and promoting soft stools without increasing gut motility. To be effective, an optimal dose needs to be found and used daily, not as needed. The effective dose can be titrated, with fecal incontinence being the dose-limiting factor. If that is reached, slow reduction in the daily dose usually suffices. In a randomized, double-blind crossover study of 72 cancer patients with OIC, patients taking PEG were more likely to optimize bowel evacuation before taking senna as a rescue [3].

Polyethylene glycol (PEG), an osmotic laxative, is soluble in water and is minimally absorbed in the gastrointestinal tract. Since it forms hydrogen bonds with water molecules, PEG causes water retention in the gut lumen, which softens the stool, and bowel movements occur more frequently [4, 5]. Overall, polyethylene glycol is preferred over lactulose [6].

Poorly absorbed or nonabsorbable sugars and saline laxatives cause intestinal water secretion and thereby increase stool frequency. Excessive use of these agents may result in electrolyte and volume shifts in patients with renal and cardiac dysfunction [7]. Magnesium and sulfate both individually exert a laxative action, mainly mediated by an osmotic effect due to their incomplete absorption in the gastrointestinal tract [8]. Daily consumption of 1 L magnesium sulfate-rich natural mineral water reduced constipation and hard or lumpy stools in women with constipation [9].

Lubiprostone is a locally acting chloride channel activator that enhances chloride-rich intestinal fluid secretion [10].

Linaclotide is a polypeptide that binds to guanylate cyclase-C receptors located on the luminal surface of the gastrointestinal tract, causing a cyclic GMP-mediated increase in chloride and bicarbonate secretion while inhibiting absorption of sodium ions, thereby increasing the net secretion of fluid in the gut lumen [11].

Plecanatide is also a minimally absorbed peptide agonist of the guanylate cyclase-C receptor that stimulates intestinal fluid secretion and transit [12, 13].

Prucalopride stimulates contractions in colonic longitudinal smooth muscles by promoting acetylcholine release via activation of 5-HT4 receptors on presynaptic, cholinergic enteric neurons. They all increase spontaneous bowel movements and improve bloating, discomfort, stool frequency, and straining [14].

Misoprostol is a prostaglandin analog, which may also treat some patients with severe constipation. Colchicine may be effective for the treatment of chronic constipation [15].

Tenapanor is a potent small-molecule inhibitor of the sodium/hydrogen exchanger isoform 3 (NHE3) localized in the apical membrane of intestinal epithelial cells, which is minimally absorbed and acts locally to inhibit sodium absorption. It also modulates tight junctions in the small intestine and increases transepithelial electrical resistance (TEER) reducing phosphate ion permeability and paracellular phosphate absorption in the presence of NHE3. The resulting increase of sodium in the gut leads to increased fluid secretion [16].

The peripherally acting mu-opioid receptor antagonists (PAMORA) methylnaltrexone, naloxegol, and naldemedine are derivatives of naloxone or naltrexone that do not cross the blood-brain barrier, and they are a new treatment option for OIC. Importantly, PAMORA do not reverse the analgesic effect of opioids, but by preferentially binding to opioid receptors in the gut and by significantly increasing the frequency of spontaneous bowel movement, they effectively relieve constipation and improve quality of life [17]. PAMORA affect all peripheral tissues that may help the management of gastroparesis, opioid-induced dysphagia, and xerostomia [18]. The American Gastroenterological Association strongly recommended traditional laxatives as first-line agents and PAMORA as superior to no treatment, particularly using naldemedine and naloxegol and, less so, methylnaltrexone [19, 20].

Methylnaltrexone does not permeate the blood-brain barrier (BBB) and is poorly absorbed. When given subcutaneously with weight-based dosing of 8 mg or 12 mg every other day, it is an effective and well-tolerated treatment, with 50–60% of patients experiencing laxation within 4–24 h after dosing, twice as much than placebo [21]. In cancer patients, subcutaneous administration is preferable, given that opioid-induced gastroparesis (OIG) impedes absorption [22].

Naloxegol is an orally administered naloxone derivative, with proven effectiveness in opioid-induced constipation (OIC) [23]. In the form of 25 mg and 12.5 mg tablets, it is used for the treatment of OIC in adults with chronic cancer pain [24]. Adverse effects are infrequent (<10%), primarily mild to moderate, mainly abdominal pain, diarrhea, flatulence, and nausea.

Naldemedine is a potent antagonist of mu-, delta-, and kappa-opioid receptors that is not crossing the brain barrier. It is administered in 0.2 mg tablets once daily, regardless of meals. In a meta-analysis of 6 randomized controlled trials with 2991 cancer and non-cancer patients, the odds ratio (OR) for spontaneous bowel movement response was 3, in favor of naldemedine [25]. An efficacy and safety trial of naldemedine 0.2 mg daily, specifically in cancer patients with OIC, showed a spontaneous bowel movement response rate of 71%, significantly higher than placebo 34% [26]. Naldemedine does not affect opioid-mediated analgesia and is not associated with symptoms of opioid withdrawal syndrome.

Axelopran is a highly potent peripheral mu-opioid receptor antagonist with limited ability to cross the brain barrier. In non-cancer pain, axelopran is better than placebo, with a durable increase in bowel movement frequency and return toward normal bowel function [27].

The classical mu-opioid receptor antagonists naloxone and naltrexone revert all the peripheral and central opioid effects, including analgesia, since they cross the brain barrier. Naloxone has antagonistic effect on opioid receptors in the gut, with minimal impact on analgesia. There are several oral combinations of naloxone with oxycodone and pentazocine for pain treatment. There is also a naloxone/buprenorphine sublingual tablet to treat opioid addiction and a hydromorphone/naloxone, prolonged-release tablet formulation. Naloxone 5, 10, and 20 mg slow-release tablets administered once daily for OIC in non-cancer patients show significant increase in laxation, twice as much as placebo [28]. Naltrexone is available in combination with morphine or oxycodone tablets for severe pain treatment. Oxycodone/naloxone in fixed-ratio 2:1 dose extended-release tablets are widely used to treat severe pain, with the premise that naloxone counteracts OIC by blocking the action of oxycodone at opioid receptors locally in the gut.

Alvimopan is indicated only for the treatment of post-abdominal surgery ileus and is available only to hospitals for short-term inpatient use because of an increased risk of ischemic cardiovascular events associated with long-term therapy. It is administered in 12 mg capsules once prior to surgery and up to 7 days postoperatively in hospitalized patients [18].

Colchicine Colchicine is used mostly as an anti-inflammatory drug in gout, but it induces diarrhea as a dose-dependent side effect, probably through an increase in prostaglandin synthesis, intestinal secretion, and GI motility [29]. The drug also reduces water and electrolyte intestinal absorption and increases secretion through a cyclic AMP-mediated activity, ultimately leading to an increased net intestinal secretion [30]. Colchicine (1 mg daily) is mostly used in patients with refractory slow-transit constipation [31].

Misoprostol Misoprostol, a PGE1 analog, through a dose-dependent inhibition of both gastric acid and pepsin release, is effective in preventing gastric and duodenal ulcers in patients using long-term NSAIDs usually given as 200–400 mcg orally daily. It protects against gut irradiation injury, enteropathy, and constipation. Misoprostol rectal suppositories may also be useful in the prevention of acute and chronic symptoms of radiation proctopathy. The drug cannot be used in fertile women because of its abortigenic potential [32].

Antidiarrheal agents In general, the use of antidiarrheal agents is best avoided in patients with unclear etiology of diarrhea, particularly if infectious or inflammatory causes have not been fully evaluated. Loperamide is a synthetic opioid that reduces peristalsis by inhibiting the release of acetylcholine through activation of the mu-opioid receptors, slowing GI transit time, allowing more time for absorption of water in the intestine, in turn leading to a reduction in stool frequency [33, 34]. Inhibition of acetylcholine release also leads to antisecretory activity because muscarinic acetylcholine receptors exist on secretory intestinal epithelial cells [35]. Loperamide treatment delays both small bowel and whole gut transit. Loperamide also has a relaxing effect on localized and segmental colonic contractions, improving stool consistency and reducing pain intensity [36].

Diphenoxylate is a synthetic opioid that, by acting on the presynaptic opioid receptors (predominantly mu receptors) in the enteric nervous system, inhibits motility and decreases segmental contractions, thereby prolonging gastrointestinal transit time. It also reduces the epithelial secretion of fluid and electrolytes and enhances active absorption by mild action on delta receptors. Commercial preparations contain a subtherapeutic amount of atropine to discourage abuse. High doses of diphenoxylate-atropine can result in symptoms of excess cholinergic and central narcotic effects, such as drowsiness, flushing, dry mouth, tachycardia, dilated pupils, rash, and nausea [37].

5-HT3 antagonists Alosetron slows down fecal transit through the colon and provides more time for water absorption, resulting in a decrease in total moisture and volume of fecal contents. Alosetron is a selective 5-HT3 antagonist acting both centrally and peripherally. The FDA has restricted its use to the treatment of severe IBS-D in women under a risk management program. The initial recommended starting dosage is 0.5 mg twice per day [38]. Contraindications to the drug include history of chronic or severe constipation, strictures of the GI tract, history of perforation or adhesions, ischemic colitis, inflammatory bowel disease, diverticulitis, and severe hepatic impairment.

Mixed opioid receptor antagonists Eluxadoline is a μ- and κ-opioid receptor agonist and δ-opioid receptor antagonist that acts locally on the gut mucosa and enteric nervous system. Local μ receptor agonism reduces colonic secretion and slows gut transit, while δ-opioid receptor antagonism counteracts any excessive μ receptor inhibition and prevents excessive constipation from unopposed μ receptor stimulation. In addition, concomitant μ agonism and δ antagonism have synergistic analgesic effects, relieving associated abdominal discomfort in patients with IBS. Kappa-opioid receptor agonism reduces visceral hypersensitivity [39].

Octreotide Octreotide is a synthetic somatostatin analog that when given intravenously, subcutaneously, or as a depot injection diminishes diarrhea by acting directly on epithelial cells to reduce the secretion of a number of pancreatic and GI hormones, such as VIP, serotonin, gastrin, secretin, and pancreatic polypeptide, and is particularly useful in patients with neuroendocrine tumors. It prolongs intestinal transit time, promotes intestinal absorption, and decreases secretion of fluids and electrolytes [40, 41].

Opium tincture By interacting with opioid receptors, the opioids increase smooth muscle tone of the gastrointestinal tract, inhibit motility and propulsion, and reduce digestive secretions. As normal bowel movements are inhibited, the transit of intestinal contents is delayed, which permits increased water absorption, thereby desiccating the feces, and subsequent constipation. Relatively small doses, which do not produce significant analgesia, are effective in controlling diarrhea. Importantly, tolerance does not develop, unlike antinociceptive tolerance that requires increasing doses of opioids to provide the same level of analgesia over time.

In a randomized, double-blinded, placebo-controlled, crossover trial in subjects with refractory chronic diarrhea, the number of daily bowel movements was reduced during opium tincture treatment. Opium tincture prolonged the colonic transit time compared to placebo (17 h vs. 12 h, $p < 0.001$). There were no CNS effects or addiction [42].

Opium tincture has been reprofiled as Dropizol, a liquid formulation, that enables rapid absorption with adequate binding and drug effect through intestinal opioid μ receptors. In the CLARIFY study, Dropizol was given on day 1 at a dose of 5.6 ± 2.8 (mean ± SD) mg/day and after 2 months at a dose of 11.6 ± 8.7 mg per day. A similar opioid solution Elixir Paregorico was given at a daily dose of 12 mL, corresponding to 12 mg opioid drops per day [43].

Using a detailed pan-alimentary MRI framework in healthy volunteers, opium tincture, compared to placebo, increased postprandial gastric accommodation and delayed gastric emptying, delayed GI transit, increased the volume of the colon, and decreased colonic water content [44].

Antispasmodics Dicyclomine, 10–20 mg up to 4 times daily, is an anticholinergic agent used for control of abdominal pain in patients with irritable bowel syndrome and painful diverticular disease. Dicyclomine causes anticholinergic side effects, such as blurred vision, dizziness, dry mouth, and impaired cognitive function. These side effects may require dose reductions or drug discontinuation; resolution typically occurs within 12–24 h after discontinuation.

Hyoscyamine, 0.125 mg sublingually or orally up to 4 times daily, has anticholinergic properties inhibiting gastrointestinal smooth muscle and reducing stimulated colonic motor activity, and it may be beneficial in patients with postprandial abdominal pain, gas, bloating, and fecal urgency. Anticholinergic side effects, such as blurred vision, dizziness, dry mouth, and impaired cognitive function, may limit its use.

Peppermint oil is a widely used therapy for crampy abdominal pain and bloating. Although predominantly an antispasmodic, it has antinociceptive, anti-inflammatory, and carminative effects [45].

Antibiotics Small intestinal bacterial overgrowth (SIBO) is almost universally present in CIPO, causing abdominal distension and promoting intestinal bacterial translocation. Although not approved for this indication, rifaximin, a nonabsorbable antibiotic, can be used to treat microbial overgrowth. Alternative or sequential treatments with other antibiotics may be offered. For SIBO due to methane-producing bacteria, oral neomycin is preferred, usually in combination with rifaximin [46].

Acid blockers It is estimated that more than 25% of cancer patients undergoing anticancer treatment use PPIs [47]. PPI use among cancer patients has been associated with a higher risk of all-cause mortality compared to non-users or H2RA users (HRs, 2.34–2.72). Compared with H2RA users, PPI users demonstrated a higher rate of all-cause mortality (HR, 1.51; 95% CI, 1.41–1.69), emphasizing the need for cautious use of PPIs in cancer patients and suggesting that alternative treatments should be considered when clinically feasible [48]. Clinicians should weigh the risks and benefits of prolonged PPI use in cancer patients, considering alternative management strategies for acid-related symptoms when feasible. This is particularly relevant during chemotherapy, where PPI use might negatively impact treatment efficacy.

Table 17.2 outlines common oral acid blockers and their dosage ranges. Although the exact prevalence of PPI use in cancer patients is unknown, their use is widespread. PPIs are generally well-tolerated and carry an excellent safety profile [49]. However, increasing and longer-term PPI use has raised concerns about the risk of pneumonia, bone fractures, and enteric infections and a possible interaction with clopidogrel that could increase the risk of cardiovascular events. PPI-induced acid suppression may increase the risk of *Clostridium difficile* or other enteric infections, nutritional deficiencies, and community-acquired pneumonia, all particularly important in cancer patients. Further, PPIs are associated with hypergastrinemia, which can lead to gastric mucosal changes. The indications for PPI use in cancer patients should be carefully reviewed prior to use. The newer potassium-competitive acid blockers (P-CABs), such as vonoprazan, are more potent than proton pump inhibitors but carry no increased risk of malignant epithelial cell alterations and gastric NETs [50].

Figure 17.1 depicts the outcomes encountered during PPI use. Accomplishing complete symptomatic response obviously restores the QoL of such patients, but in

Table 17.2 Common oral acid blockers and their dosage ranges

Class	Common oral acid blockers and dosage ranges
Antacids	Tums PRN (OTC) Pepcid AC (combination) (OTC) PRN and qhs
Histamine receptor 2 blockers (H2RA)	Famotidine 10–40 mg daily to twice a day
Proton pump inhibitors (PPIs)	Omeprazole 20–40 mg daily to twice a day Lansoprazole 30 mg daily to twice a day Pantoprazole 40 mg daily to twice a day Rabeprazole 20 mg daily to twice a day Esomeprazole 20–40 mg daily to twice a day
Potassium-competitive acid blockers (PCAB)	Vonoprazan 20–40 mg qd

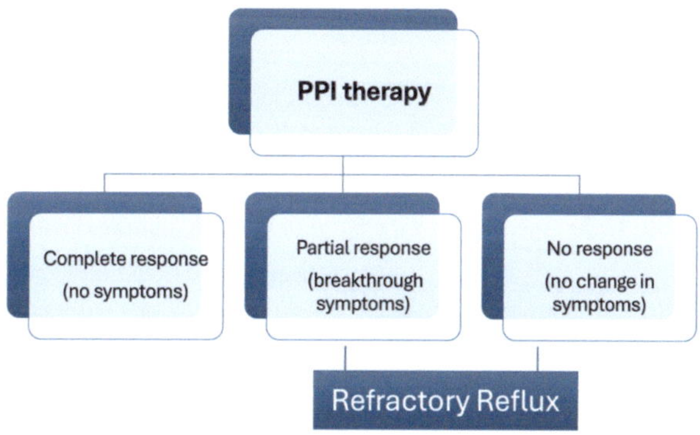

Fig. 17.1 Potential outcomes encountered during PPI use. The management of refractory GERD will require multidimensional and multidisciplinary approach to optimize care

some cases where esophageal pH control is important (i.e., patients with BE), pH monitoring, performed with patient on PPI, may reveal inadequacy of such therapy in pH normalization. In cases where patients may present with breakthrough GERD symptoms despite PPI therapy, ambulatory esophageal pH monitoring can be very useful in guiding the clinician in pharmacologic treatment optimization or other (endoscopic or surgical) considerations. When there is no response to properly prescribed (and adhered to) PPI therapy, the likelihood of underlying GERD is low, and other differential diagnoses (i.e., achalasia) need to be considered. In the latter two scenarios of "refractory GERD," the combined utilization of structural and functional tests (particularly esophageal pH monitoring) is paramount.

The long-term use of PPI may also be associated with efficacy drawbacks (Fig. 17.2).

Bile acid sequestrants (BASs) Bile acid diarrhea (BAD) typically after ileal resection, right hemicolectomy, or pelvic radiation increases intestinal motility and may contribute to impaired quality of life. Various agents show promise in the symptomatic management of BAD (Table 17.3). Bile acid sequestrants (BASs), such as cholestyramine, colestipol, and colesevelam, lead to significant improvement in liquid stools to normal fecal consistency and cessation of diarrhea, but they have been associated with low patient adherence and a high incidence of side effects, such as abdominal cramps and nausea. There are no significant differences in the frequency

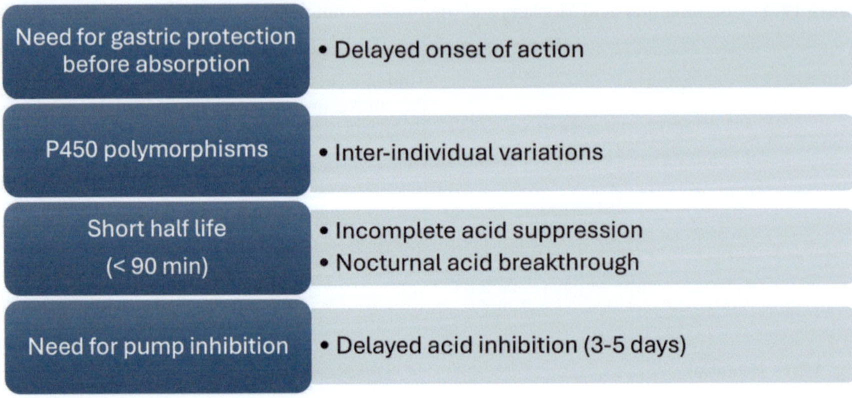

Fig. 17.2 Important issues to be considered when using PPI agents. Fine-tuning of the timing and dosage of administration of these agents is important

Table 17.3 Agents used for control of bile acid diarrhea (BAD)

Class	Common agents and dosage ranges
Bile acid sequestrants (BASs)	Cholestyramine (4 g daily or twice daily) Colestipol (15–30 mg orally per day in 2–4 doses) Colesevelam (three 625 mg capsules twice daily)
Farnesoid X receptor (FXR) agonists	Obeticholic acid (5 mg orally daily)
Glucagon-like peptide 1 receptor agonists	Liraglutide (daily subcutaneous injection uptitrated from 0.6 mg to 1.8 mg over 3 weeks)

of diarrhea, incidence of nausea, and other side effects among various BASs, but availability and costs may play a role [51]. In certain patients, idiopathic bile acid malabsorption may be the cause of diarrhea, and treatment with a bile acid binder cholestyramine may be effective [52].

The glucagon-like peptide 1 receptor agonist liraglutide is a potential new treatment modality for bile acid diarrhea, since it is superior to colesevelam in reducing daily stool frequency [53]. Drugs that are agonists of the FXR pathway, such as obeticholic acid, are attractive candidates for the treatment of BAD but have not been adequately studied [54]. Rather than just controlling symptoms with BASs, dietary effects and changes in the intestinal microbiome, which are key to bile acid metabolism and feedback, may be potentially curative [55].

Topical anti-inflammatory agents Several topical agents are available to control rectal inflammation and symptoms. Mesalamine (5-ASA) suppositories, 1 g once to twice daily, are first-line therapy for patients with mild to moderate rectal inflammation (proctitis) due to ulcerative colitis or Crohn's disease causing diarrhea, bleeding, and tenesmus. If the disease is limited to the rectum (≤18 cm from the anal verge), hydrocortisone suppositories once daily for 2 weeks for induction of remission may be used. If the disease extends beyond 18 cm, hydrocortisone enema once daily is preferred and may be advanced to twice daily, if needed. Budesonide rectal foam is well-tolerated and efficacious in inducing remission in patients with mild to moderate ulcerative proctitis and ulcerative proctosigmoiditis. For patients with persistent rectal pain, tenesmus, or bleeding due to XRT proctopathy, sucralfate enemas (20 mL of a 10% sucralfate twice daily) may improve symptoms. Sodium butyrate enemas are also effective in the treatment of acute radiation-induced proctitis.

Neuromodulators Neuromodulators work by enhancing the synaptic transmission of 5-hydroxytryptamine, noradrenalin, and dopamine, leading to desensitization of their postsynaptic receptors along the brain-gut axis. These agents, in doses lower than those used in psychiatry, not only are useful in treating psychiatric comorbidities but also, importantly, in modifying gut motility, improving central downregulation of visceral signals in irritable bowel syndrome (IBS) (Table 17.4) [56]. Typically, the first-line treatment for pain management in IBS is using tricyclic antidepressants or the serotonin and noradrenaline reuptake inhibitors. When selecting a neuromodulator to treat IBS, clarifying the predominant bowel symptom is important; selective serotonin reuptake inhibitors help constipation, not pain, but may cause diarrhea, while tricyclic antidepressants help diarrhea but may cause constipation. A clinical response may occur in 6–8 weeks, but long-term treatment is often needed to prevent relapse. Augmentation therapy may also be needed.

Somatostatin analogs (SSAs) The SSAs, such as octreotide and lanreotide, are key therapeutic agents in the management of NETs because they are more potent

Table 17.4 Various options and dose ranges of neuromodulators for patients with IBS and DBGI

Class	Neuromodulating agents and dosage ranges
TCA (tricyclic antidepressants)	Amitriptyline 25–150 mg qd Imipramine 25–150 mg qd Desipramine 25–150 mg qd Nortriptyline 25–150 mg qd
SSRIs (selective serotonin reuptake inhibitors)	Citalopram 10–40 mg qd Escitalopram 5–20 mg qd Fluoxetine 10–40 mg qd Paroxetine 10–40 mg qd Sertraline 50–150 mg qd Fluvoxamine 50–150 mg qd
SNRIs (serotonin and noradrenaline reuptake inhibitors)	Venlafaxine 75–225 mg qd Duloxetine 30–90 mg qd Milnacipran 50–100 mg bid
TNAS (tetracyclics or noradrenergic and specific serotonergic antidepressants)	Mirtazapine 7.5–45 mg qhs
AAP (atypical antipsychotics)	Quetiapine 25–200 mg qd Olanzapine 2.5–10 mg qd Brexpiprazole 1–1.5 mg qd Aripiprazole 2.5–5 mg qd

Modified from: Hanna-Jairala and Drossman [56]

and have a longer duration of action than somatostatin. Octreotide is available in two forms: a short-acting one for subcutaneous or intravenous use and a long-acting release (LAR) form, given as 30 mg intramuscularly every 4 weeks. Lanreotide Autogel® is a depot formulation available in doses of 60, 90, and 120 mg. Given 120 mg subcutaneously every 4 weeks, it achieves a steady-state concentration on the first day. Both drugs inhibit the secretion of various hormones and peptides produced by neuroendocrine cells, providing significant symptom relief. SSAs also exhibit antiproliferative actions on certain well-differentiated, slow-growing NETs potentially reducing tumor growth and possibly mitigating tumor progression and metastasis. Similarly, lanreotide improves progression-free survival in patients with metastatic enteropancreatic NETs [57]. One-third of patients treated with SSAs may develop abdominal bloating, nausea, weight loss, loose stools, and/or steatorrhea since these agents reversibly inhibit secretion of pancreatic enzymes and bile acids. These symptoms typically occur during the first few weeks of therapy, eventually spontaneously subsiding. Symptoms of pancreatic insufficiency that persist or worsen may be treated with pancreatic enzyme supplementation [40]. SSAs reduce postprandial gallbladder contractility and delay gallbladder emptying, potentially leading to sludge or gallstone formation in up to 25% of patients during the first 18 months of therapy (Fig. 17.3) [58].

Steroids Budesonide, an orally administered steroid with minimal systemic absorption, is an effective induction and maintenance treatment for microscopic colitis and diarrhea. The long-term use of budesonide at the lowest effective dose appears to be safe, with limited adverse effects. Unfortunately, after drug discontinuation, there is a high risk of recurrence [59].

Pyridostigmine Although primarily used for myasthenia gravis, the cholinomimetic agent pyridostigmine, at doses of 30–60 mg orally every 4 h, may be used in refractory patients with CIPO after true mechanical intestinal obstruction has been excluded, since it increases colonic motility with a low side effect profile [60].

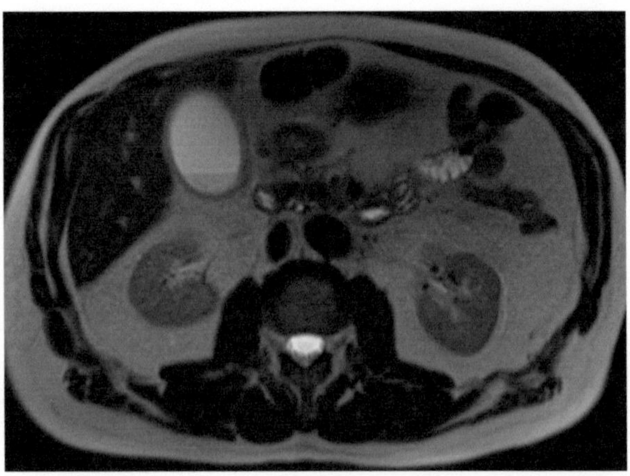

Fig. 17.3 Abdominal MR image of a patient treated with octreotide for NET who presented with symptoms of biliary dyskinesia. There is evidence of fluid layering in the gallbladder, suggestive of sludge and gallstone formation. Symptoms resolved after elective cholecystectomy

Midodrine Midodrine, a selective α-adrenergic agonist, at a dose of 10 mg orally tid, is beneficial in POTS management since it reduces venous capacitance and improves venous return at low doses that do not increase blood pressure. Its peripheral action, owing to the inability to cross the blood-brain barrier, ensures minimal central nervous system side effects [61].

Intravenous immunoglobulin (IVIG) Autoimmune gastrointestinal dysmotility (AGID), an organ manifestation of autoimmune dysautonomia, can be idiopathic or a paraneoplastic phenomenon. Immunotherapy using intravenous methylprednisolone and high-dose immune globulin (IVIG) are considered safe and appropriate therapies, since they may improve symptoms, such as constipation, nausea or vomiting, weight loss, bloating, and early satiety, as well as autonomic testing, scintigraphy, and manometry [62].

References

1. Prapaitrakool S, Hollmann MW, Wartenberg HC, Preckel B, Brugger S. Use of buprenorphine in children with chronic pseudo-obstruction syndrome: case series and review of literature. Clin J Pain. 2012;28(8):722–5. https://doi.org/10.1097/AJP.0b013e318243f609.
2. Kochhar R, Patel F, Dhar A, Sharma SC, Ayyagari S, Aggarwal R, Goenka MK, Gupta BD, Mehta SK. Radiation-induced proctosigmoiditis. Prospective, randomized, double-blind controlled trial of oral sulfasalazine plus rectal steroids versus rectal sucralfate. Dig Dis Sci. 1991;36(1):103–7. https://doi.org/10.1007/BF01300096.
3. Hawley P, MacKenzie H, Gobbo M. PEG vs. sennosides for opioid-induced constipation in cancer care. Support Care Cancer. 2020;28(4):1775–82.
4. Dipalma JA, Cleveland MV, McGowan J, Herrera JL. A randomized, multicenter, placebo-controlled trial of polyethylene glycol laxative for chronic treatment of chronic constipation. Am J Gastroenterol. 2007;102(7):1436–41. https://doi.org/10.1111/j.1572-0241.2007.01199.x. Epub 2007 Mar 31.
5. Corazziari E, Badiali D, Bazzocchi G, Bassotti G, Roselli P, Mastropaolo G, Lucà MG, Galeazzi R, Peruzzi E. Long term efficacy, safety, and tolerability of low daily doses of isosmotic polyethylene glycol electrolyte balanced solution (PMF-100) in the treatment of functional chronic constipation. Gut. 2000;46(4):522–6. https://doi.org/10.1136/gut.46.4.522. PMID: 10716682; PMCID: PMC1727881.
6. Lee-Robichaud H, Thomas K, Morgan J, Nelson RL. Lactulose versus polyethylene glycol for chronic constipation. Cochrane Database Syst Rev. 2010;7:CD007570. https://doi.org/10.1002/14651858.CD007570.pub2.
7. Lembo A, Camilleri M. Chronic constipation. N Engl J Med. 2003;349(14):1360–8. https://doi.org/10.1056/NEJMra020995.
8. Dupont C, Hébert G. Magnesium sulfate-rich natural mineral waters in the treatment of functional constipation-a review. Nutrients. 2020;12(7):2052. https://doi.org/10.3390/nu12072052. PMID: 32664341; PMCID: PMC7400933.
9. Dupont C, Campagne A, Constant F. Efficacy and safety of a magnesium sulfate-rich natural mineral water for patients with functional constipation. Clin Gastroenterol Hepatol. 2014;12(8):1280–7. https://doi.org/10.1016/j.cgh.2013.12.005. Epub 2013 Dec 14.
10. Sada H, Kajizono M, Ushio S, Esumi S, Kitamura Y, Sendo T. The efficacy and safety of lubiprostone for constipation in cancer patients compared with non-cancer patients: a retrospective cohort study. Biol Pharm Bull. 2020;43(11):1699–706. https://doi.org/10.1248/bpb.b20-00398.

11. Layer P, Stanghellini V. Review article: linaclotide for the management of irritable bowel syndrome with constipation. Aliment Pharmacol Ther. 2014;39(4):371–84. Bassotti G, Usai-Satta P, Bellini M. Linaclotide for the treatment of chronic constipation. Expert Opin Pharmacother 2018;19(11):1261–1266. https://doi.org/10.1080/14656566.2018.1494728. Epub 2018 Jul 9.
12. Brenner DM, Fogel R, Dorn SD, Krause R, Eng P, Kirshoff R, et al. Efficacy, safety, and tolerability of plecanatide in patients with irritable bowel syndrome with constipation: results of two phase 3 randomized clinical trials. Am J Gastroenterol. 2018;113(5):735–45.
13. Menees SB, Franklin H, Chey WD. Evaluation of plecanatide for the treatment of chronic idiopathic constipation and irritable bowel syndrome with constipation in patients 65 years or older. Clin Ther. 2020;42(7):1406–1414.e4. https://doi.org/10.1016/j.clinthera.2020.05.012. Epub 2020 Jul 10.
14. Bassotti G, Usai Satta P, Bellini M. Prucalopride for the treatment of constipation: a view from 2015 and beyond. Expert Rev Gastroenterol Hepatol. 2019;13(3):257–62. https://doi.org/10.1080/17474124.2019.1568238. Epub 2019 Jan 23.
15. Soffer EE, Metcalf A, Launspach J. Misoprostol is effective treatment for patients with severe chronic constipation. Dig Dis Sci. 1994;39(5):929–33. https://doi.org/10.1007/BF02087539.
16. King AJ, Siegel M, He Y, Nie B, Wang J, Koo-McCoy S, et al. Inhibition of sodium/hydrogen exchanger 3 in the gastrointestinal tract by tenapanor reduces paracellular phosphate permeability. Sci Transl Med. 2018;10(456):eaam6474.
17. Argoff CE. Opioid-induced constipation. Clin J Pain. 2020;36(9):716–22.
18. Farmer AD, Drewes AM, Chiarioni G, De Giorgio R, O'Brien T, Morlion B, Tack J. Pathophysiology and management of opioid-induced constipation: European expert consensus statement. United Eur Gastroenterol J. 2019;7(1):7–20.
19. Hanson B, Siddique SM, Scarlett Y, Sultan S. American Gastroenterological Association Institute technical review on the medical management of opioid-induced constipation. Gastroenterology. 2019;156(1):229.
20. Crockett SD, Greer KB, Heidelbaugh JJ, Falck-Ytter Y, Hanson BJ, Sultan S. American Gastroenterological Association Institute guideline on the medical management of opioid-induced constipation. Gastroenterology. 2019;156(1):218–26.
21. Bull J, Wellman CV, Israel RJ, Barrett AC, Paterson C, Forbes WP. Fixed-dose subcutaneous methylnaltrexone in patients with advanced illness and opioid-induced constipation: results of a randomized, placebo-controlled study and open-label extension. J Palliat Med. 2015;18(7):593–600.
22. Murphy DB, Sutton JA, Prescott LF, Murphy MB. Opioid-induced delay in gastric emptying. Anesthesiology. 1997;87(4):765–70.
23. Daniali M, Nikfar S, Abdollahi M. Evaluating naloxegol for the treatment of opioid-induced constipation. Expert Opin Pharmacother. 2020;21(8):883–91.
24. Cobo Dols M, Beato Zambrano C, Cabezón Gutiérrez L, et al. Efficacy of naloxegol on symptoms and quality of life related to opioid-induced constipation in patients with cancer: a 3-month follow-up analysis. BMJ Support Palliat Care. 2021;11(1):25–31.
25. Esmadi M, Ahmad D, Hewlett A. Efficacy of naldemedine for the treatment of opioid-induced constipation: a meta-analysis. J Gastrointest Liver Dis. 2019;28(1):41–6.
26. Katakami N, Harada T, Murata T, Shinozaki K, Tsutsumi M, Yokota T, Arai M, Tada Y, Narabayashi M, Boku N. Randomized phase III and extension studies of naldemedine in patients with opioid-induced constipation and cancer. J Clin Oncol. 2017;35(34):3859–66.
27. Vickery R, Li Y, Schwertschlag U, Singla N, Webster L, Canafax D. With a durable increase in bowel movement frequency and return toward normal bowel function in a 5-week Ph2b Opioid-Induced Constipation (OIC) study. J Pain. 2013;14(4):S78. https://doi.org/10.1016/j.jpain.2013.01.651.
28. Sanders M, Jones S, Löwenstein O, Jansen J-P, Miles H, Simpson K. New formulation of sustained release naloxone can reverse opioid induced constipation without compromising the desired opioid effects. Pain Med. 2015;16(8):1540–50.
29. Sninsky CA, Lynch DF. Why should microtubular inhibitors induce frequent activity fronts (AF) of the migrating myoelectric complex (MMC)? Gastroenterology. 1986;90:1641.

30. Rachmilewitz D, Karmeli F. Effect of colchicine on jejunal adenylate cyclase activity, PGE2 and cAMP contents. Eur J Pharmacol. 1980;67(2–3):235–9. https://doi.org/10.1016/0014-2999(80)90503-8.
31. Taghavi SA, Shabani S, Mehramiri A, Eshraghian A, Kazemi SM, Moeini M, Hosseini-Asl SM, Saberifiroozi M, Alizade-Naeeni M, Mostaghni AA. Colchicine iş effective for short-term treatment of slow transit constipation: a double-blind placebo-controlled clinical trial. Int J Color Dis. 2010;25(3):389–94. https://doi.org/10.1007/s00384-009-0794-z. Epub 2009 Aug 25.
32. Davies NM, Longstreth J, Jamali F. Misoprostol therapeutics revisited. Pharmacotherapy. 2001;21(1):60–73. https://doi.org/10.1592/phco.21.1.60.34442.
33. Regnard C, Twycross R, Mihalyo M, Wilcock A. Loperamide. J Pain Symptom Manag. 2011;42(2):319–23. https://doi.org/10.1016/j.jpainsymman.2011.06.001. Epub 2011 Jun 23.
34. Cann PA, Read NW, Holdsworth CD, Barends D. Role of loperamide and placebo in management of irritable bowel syndrome (IBS). Dig Dis Sci. 1984;29(3):239–47. https://doi.org/10.1007/BF01296258. PMID: 6365490.
35. Ooms LA, Degryse AD, Janssen PA. Mechanisms of action of loperamide. Scand J Gastroenterol Suppl. 1984;96:145–55.
36. Efskind PS, Bernklev T, Vatn MH. A double-blind placebo-controlled trial with loperamide in irritable bowel syndrome. Scand J Gastroenterol. 1996;31(5):463–8. https://doi.org/10.3109/00365529609006766.
37. Penfold D, Volans GN. Overdose from lomotil. Br Med J. 1977;2(6099):1401–2. https://doi.org/10.1136/bmj.2.6099.1401. PMID: 589232; PMCID: PMC1632364.
38. Lembo A, Sultan S, Chang L, Heidelbaugh JJ, Smalley W, Verne GN. AGA clinical practice guideline on the pharmacological management of Irritable Bowel Syndrome with diarrhea. Gastroenterology. 2022;163(1):137–51.
39. Lacy BE. Emerging treatments in neurogastroenterology: eluxadoline - a new therapeutic option for diarrhea-predominant IBS. Neurogastroenterol Motil. 2016;28(1):26–35.
40. Lamberts SW, van der Lely AJ, de Herder WW, Hofland LJ. Octreotide. N Engl J Med. 1996;334(4):246–54. https://doi.org/10.1056/NEJM199601253340408.
41. Dueno MI, Bai JC, Santangelo WC, Krejs GJ. Effect of somatostatin analog on water and electrolyte transport and transit time in human small bowel. Dig Dis Sci. 1987;32(10):1092–6. https://doi.org/10.1007/BF01300194.
42. Okdahl T, Høyer KL, Knoph CS, Davidsen L, Larsen IM, Mark EB, Hvas CL, Krogh K, Drewes AM. Opium tincture has anti-propulsive effects in patients with chronic diarrhea: a randomized, placebo-controlled, and cross-over trial. Scand J Gastroenterol. 2024;59(9):1023–34.
43. Dahlgren D, Hellström PM. Medicinal grade opium tincture for severe diarrhea: effect revisited in observational study. Curr Opin Gastroenterol. 2024;40(3):196–202.
44. Mark EB, Okdahl T, Kahlke DG, Hansen LEM, Krogh K, Frøkjær JB, Drewes AM. Effects of opium tincture on gastrointestinal function and motility in healthy volunteers: a magnetic resonance imaging study. Neurogastroenterol Motil. 2024;36(12):e14941.
45. Hills JM, Aaronson PI. The mechanism of action of peppermint oil on gastrointestinal smooth muscle. An analysis using patch clamp electrophysiology and isolated tissue pharmacology in rabbit and Guinea pig. Gastroenterology. 1991;101(1):55–65.
46. Pimentel M, Chang C, Chua KS, Mirocha J, DiBaise J, Rao S, Amichai M. Antibiotic treatment of constipation-predominant irritable bowel syndrome. Dig Dis Sci. 2014;59(6):1278–85. https://doi.org/10.1007/s10620-014-3157-8. Epub 2014 May 1.
47. Raoul JL, Guérin-Charbonnel C, Edeline J, Simmet V, Gilabert M, Frenel JS. Prevalence of proton pump inhibitor use among patients with cancer. JAMA Netw Open. 2021;4(6):e2113739. https://doi.org/10.1001/jamanetworkopen.2021.13739. PMID: 34132796; PMCID: PMC8209575.
48. Krishnan A, Schneider CV, Walsh D. Proton pump inhibitors and all-cause mortality risk among cancer patients. World J Clin Oncol. 2025;16(1):99240. https://doi.org/10.5306/wjco.v16.i1.99240. PMID: 39867734; PMCID: PMC11528898.

49. Triadafilopoulos G, Roorda AK, Akiyama J. Indications and safety of proton pump inhibitor drug use in patients with cancer. Expert Opin Drug Saf. 2013;12(5):659–72. https://doi.org/10.1517/14740338.2013.797961. Epub 2013 May 7.
50. Uemura N, Kinoshita Y, Haruma K, Kushima R, Yao T, Akiyama J, Aoyama N, Baba Y, Suzuki C, Ishiguro K. Vonoprazan as a long-term maintenance treatment for erosive esophagitis: VISION, a 5-year, randomized, open-label study. Clin Gastroenterol Hepatol. 2024;S1542-3565(24):00770–5. https://doi.org/10.1016/j.cgh.2024.08.004. Epub ahead of print.
51. Soares GAR, Godoi A, Marcolin P, Piredda G, Laia E, Rodrigues AZ. Efficacy of bile acid sequestrants in the treatment of bile acid diarrhea: a meta-analysis of randomized controlled trials. J Clin Pharmacol. 2024;65:478. https://doi.org/10.1002/jcph.6154. Epub ahead of print.
52. Wedlake L, A'Hern R, Russell D, Thomas K, Walters JR, Andreyev HJ. Systematic review: the prevalence of idiopathic bile acid malabsorption as diagnosed by SeHCAT scanning in patients with diarrhoea-predominant irritable bowel syndrome. Aliment Pharmacol Ther. 2009;30(7):707–17. https://doi.org/10.1111/j.1365-2036.2009.04081.x. Epub 2009 Jun 30.
53. Kårhus ML, Brønden A, Forman JL, Haaber A, Knudsen E, Langholz E, Dragsted LO, Hansen SH, Krakauer M, Vilsbøll T, Sonne DP, Knop FK. Safety and efficacy of liraglutide versus colesevelam for the treatment of bile acid diarrhoea: a randomised, double-blind, active-comparator, non-inferiority clinical trial. Lancet Gastroenterol Hepatol. 2022;7(10):922–31. https://doi.org/10.1016/S2468-1253(22)00198-4. Epub 2022 Jul 20.
54. Walters JR, Johnston IM, Nolan JD, Vassie C, Pruzanski ME, Shapiro DA. The response of patients with bile acid diarrhoea to the farnesoid X receptor agonist obeticholic acid. Aliment Pharmacol Ther. 2015;41(1):54–64. https://doi.org/10.1111/apt.12999. Epub 2014 Oct 20.
55. Walters JRF, Sikafi R. Managing bile acid diarrhea: aspects of contention. Expert Rev Gastroenterol Hepatol. 2024;18(9):521–8. https://doi.org/10.1080/17474124.2024.2402353. Epub 2024 Sep 16.
56. Hanna-Jairala I, Drossman DA. Central neuromodulators in irritable bowel syndrome: why, how, and when. Am J Gastroenterol. 2024;119(7):1272–84. https://doi.org/10.14309/ajg.0000000000002800. Epub 2024 Apr 9. PMID: 38595149; PMCID: PMC11208063.
57. Marasco M, Dell'Unto E, Laviano A, Campana D, Panzuto F. Gastrointestinal side effects of somatostatin analogs in neuroendocrine tumors: a focused review. J Gastroenterol Hepatol. 2024;39(9):1737–44. https://doi.org/10.1111/jgh.16638. Epub 2024 May 23.
58. Newman CB, Melmed S, Snyder PJ, Young WF, Boyajy LD, Levy R, Stewart WN, Klibanski A, Molitch ME, Gagel RF. Safety and efficacy of long-term octreotide therapy of acromegaly: results of a multicenter trial in 103 patients--a clinical research center study. J Clin Endocrinol Metab. 1995;80(9):2768–75. https://doi.org/10.1210/jcem.80.9.7673422. Erratum in: J Clin Endocrinol Metab 1995 Nov;80(11):3238.
59. Tome J, Tariq R, Hassett LC, Khanna S, Pardi DS. Effectiveness and safety profile of budesonide maintenance in microscopic colitis: a systematic review and meta-analysis. Inflamm Bowel Dis. 2024;30(7):1178–88. https://doi.org/10.1093/ibd/izad178.
60. Wilkie BD, Noori J, Johnston M, Woods R, Keck JO, Behrenbruch C. Pyridostigmine in chronic intestinal pseudo-obstruction - a systematic review. ANZ J Surg. 2023;93(9):2086–91. https://doi.org/10.1111/ans.18478. Epub 2023 May 2.
61. Ghazal M, Akkawi AR, Fancher A, Oundo E, Tanzeem H, Sajjad L, Briasoulis A. Pathophysiology and management of postural orthostatic tachycardia syndrome (POTS): a literature review. Curr Probl Cardiol. 2025;50(3):102977. https://doi.org/10.1016/j.cpcardiol.2024.102977. Epub 2024 Dec 18.
62. Flanagan EP, Saito YA, Lennon VA, McKeon A, Fealey RD, Szarka LA, Murray JA, Foxx-Orenstein AE, Fox JC, Pittock SJ. Immunotherapy trial as diagnostic test in evaluating patients with presumed autoimmune gastrointestinal dysmotility. Neurogastroenterol Motil. 2014;26(9):1285–97. https://doi.org/10.1111/nmo.12391. Epub 2014 Jul 20. PMID: 25039328; PMCID: PMC4149849.

Common Therapies in Onco-neurogastroenterology

18

George Triadafilopoulos

18.1 Constipation in the Cancer Patient

Constipation is a common problem in patients undergoing cancer treatment. In this setting, constipation is usually caused by a combination of poor oral intake, decreased physical activity, and the action of drugs, such as opioid analgesics or antiemetic agents, which slow intestinal transit time, and it has a multifaceted impact (Figs. 18.1 and 18.2).

Constipation has also been reported in patients taking vinca alkaloids, in particular vincristine and thalidomide [1]. Impaction, bowel obstruction, and colonic pseudo-obstruction must be ruled out before initiating therapy for constipation by obtaining an abdominal radiograph. HRAM, RST, and BET may also be useful in the evaluation of patients with slow-transit constipation (Table 18.1).

Electrolyte abnormalities and other reversible causes should be corrected first. Drugs that cause constipation should be discontinued if possible. Laxatives, with or without stool softeners, can also be used in the initial treatment of constipation. Stimulant laxatives such as bisacodyl and senna alter electrolyte transport by the intestinal mucosa and increase intestinal motor activity. If these agents are not effective, osmotic agents such as lactulose or sorbitol can be effective at improving stool frequency and consistency [2]. Polyethylene glycol solutions (without electrolytes) are available in powder form and have been found to be effective at improving chronic constipation.

Chronic GVHD can occur in up to 50% of patients who survive long term after receiving a transplant from an HLA-identical sibling. The esophagus is the most common site of involvement in patients with chronic GVHD, and these patients can

G. Triadafilopoulos (✉)
Department of Gastroenterology, Hepatology and Nutrition, UT MD Anderson Cancer Center, Houston, TX, USA
e-mail: gtriadafilopoulo@mdanderson.org

G. Triadafilopoulos (ed.), *Onco-Neurogastroenterology*,
https://doi.org/10.1007/978-3-031-98848-6_18

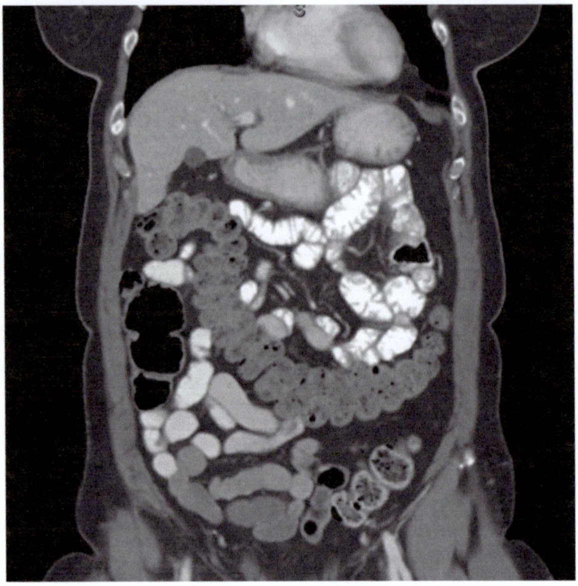

Fig. 18.1 CT of the abdomen and pelvis in a woman with long-standing bloating and constipation, revealing moderate to severe stool burden, particularly along the transverse colon

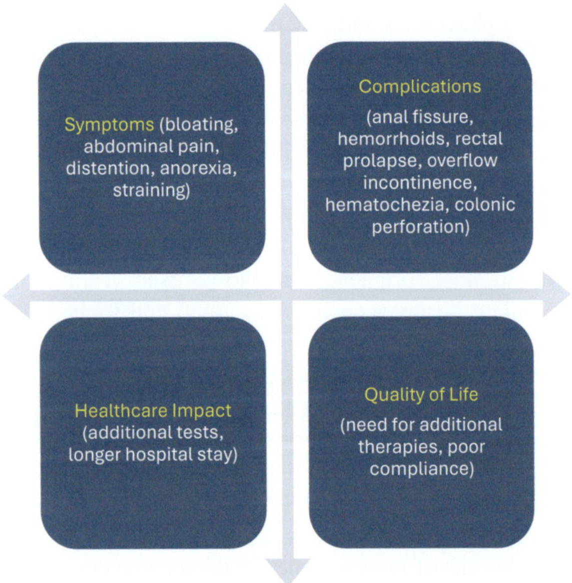

Fig. 18.2 Impact of constipation in patients with cancer

develop painful esophageal ulcerations, webs, rings, and strictures [3]. The oral mucosa can be dry, resulting in ulceration and pain. The small bowel and colon are not as frequently involved as in acute GVHD, but when they are involved, patients can present with diarrhea, malabsorption, fibrosis of the submucosa, and sclerosis of the intestine [4]. Constipation is one of the most frequent problems in cancer

Table 18.1 Common findings in HRAM, RST, and BET in patients with slow-transit constipation

Variable	Value
HPZ length (n = 4.1–4.5 cm)	Normal or short
Resting pressure (n = 83–96 mmHg)	Normal
Squeeze pressure (n = 245–287 mmHg)	Low
Squeeze duration (n = 28–30 s)	Short
Residual anal pressure (n = 28–52)	High
RAIR (n = present)	Absent
First rectal sensation (n = 20–25 ml)	Low
Urge to defecate (n = 140–167 ml)	Low
Discomfort (n = 192–222 ml)	Low
Balloon expulsion (50 cc expulsion in ˂60 s)	Normal

patients, with prevalence ranging from 30% to 90%, significantly affecting the quality of life, mostly of the elderly and those with advanced cancer [5]. Constipation may also be associated with nausea, vomiting, anal pain, and hematochezia due to anal fissure or hemorrhoids, and it may contribute to bowel obstruction and urinary retention. Further it causes significant psychological distress, indirectly affecting patients' compliance to opioid use for pain, thereby impeding treatment. Because of its chronicity and severity, it frequently requires additional therapies, thereby increasing direct and indirect healthcare costs. Contributing factors to constipation are a poor general performance status, low food and fluid intake, use of drugs that slow down gut motility and secretion, caregiver dependency, and limited mobility due to cancer pain and fatigue [6].

Despite its high prevalence, constipation remains underdiagnosed and undertreated in advanced cancer, due to lack of a widely accepted definition and diagnostic criteria in palliative care or end-stage cancer patients [7]. According to the clinical practice guidelines of the European Society for Medical Oncology (ESMO), all cancer patients should be regularly assessed for constipation using validated scales, preferably in conjunction with patient-reported outcome measures, when feasible. Since opioids are pivotal for treating moderate and severe pain, they are often the main culprit, depending on the frequency, type, and route of administration [8]. Opioid-induced constipation (OIC) affects opioid therapy, with patients seeking a balance between pain relief and the occurrence of constipation, modifying or discontinuing their opioid use [9]. The Rome IV criteria for opioid-induced constipation (OIC) are moderately sensitive (85%) and specific (77%) [10, 11]. There are no significant differences between transdermal therapeutic systems and orally administered opioids [12]. A pyramidal schematic of options available for the management of chronic constipation is presented in Fig. 18.3.

Dietary and behavioral interventions Chemotherapy, as well as opioid and antiemetic drugs, can contribute to constipation in patients with cancer. The effectiveness of non-pharmacological measures for constipation in cancer patients is unclear. There is potential of specific rehabilitation strategies and alternative strategies for improving constipation and minimizing the use of laxatives [13]. Most

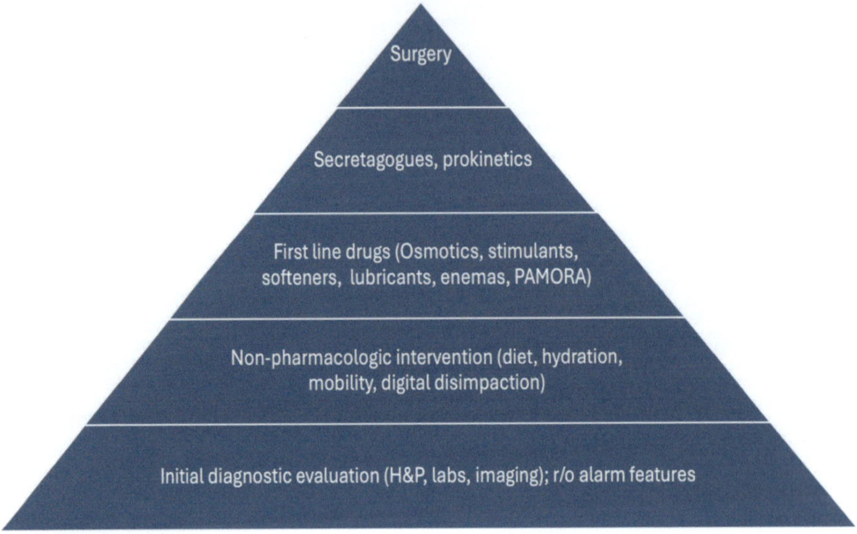

Fig. 18.3 Pyramidal scheme outlining the diagnosis and stepwise management of chronic constipation

studies show that physical exercise, abdominal massage, acupuncture, and education on the correct defecation position have a positive symptomatic impact and improvement of quality of life. Physiotherapy involving massages as well as aerobic and resistance training improves constipation in women, regardless of age, sex, and frailty. The outcomes regarding TENS are inconsistent. Adequate hydration and nutrition, proper access and positioning for defecation using a commode or footstool placing the knees above the wait and caregiver help can aid in successful defecation. However, fiber-rich diet or aggressive hydration is generally contraindicated [14]. In terms of non-pharmacologic interventions, acupuncture and acupressure have not been well studied for OIC [15]. Abdominal massage may reduce symptoms and improve bowel evacuation. An automated intermittent colonic exoperistalsis (ICE) treatment device increased the number of complete bowel movements and reduced symptoms of chronic constipation and laxative use, with infrequent mild to moderate side effects [16]. The best type, timing, and duration of treatment and the impact of the cause, stage, and location of cancer remain unclear.

Pharmacological options Linaclotide, 70-290 ug μg tablets, is a guanylate cyclase C receptor agonist that upregulates cyclic guanosine monophosphate (cGMP) within enterocytes, resulting in intraluminal secretions and accelerated intestinal transit, which promotes laxation. It also has analgesic properties by reducing visceral hypersensitivity [17]. Lubiprostone, 24 μg tablets taken twice daily, activates chloride type 2 channels (CIC-2) located on the apical membrane of epithelial cells in the intestine resulting in an intraluminal efflux. Prucalopride 2 mg and 4 mg daily is a selective serotonin (5-HT4) receptor agonist, which induces a prokinetic effect with an increase of ≥1 spontaneous complete bowel movement (SCBM) per week, significantly higher in patients treated with prucalopride than placebo [18]. There is no evidence for the efficacy of these substances in cancer patients.

Vibrating capsule The vibrating capsule is a non-pharmacologic, orally ingested, programmable capsule that vibrates intraluminally to induce bowel movements. In a double-blind, placebo-controlled trial of 312 patients with chronic constipation, who were randomized to receive either a vibrating or placebo capsule, once daily, 5 days a week for 8 weeks, a greater percentage of patients receiving the vibrating capsule achieved both primary efficacy end points compared with placebo (39.3% vs 22.1%, $P=0.001$ for CSBM; 22.7% vs 11.4%, $P=0.008$ for CSBM). Significantly greater improvements were also seen with the vibrating capsule for stool consistency and quality-of-life measures compared with placebo. A mild vibrating sensation was reported by 11% of patients in the vibrating capsule group [19].

Footstool The use of a in front of footstool may improve rectal balloon expulsion in patients with defecatory disorders, particularly in younger women with defecatory dyssynergia with optimal stool consistency (Bristol stool 3 or 4), who have lower anal resting pressures and higher recto-anal pressure gradients and fail balloon expulsion test (BET) [20].

18.2 Diarrhea in Cancer Patient

Diarrhea is a common complication of cytotoxic therapy and occurs most commonly in cancer patients treated with fluoropyrimidines (particularly 5-fluorouracil [5-FU]), irinotecan hydrochloride, methotrexate, or cisplatin. The diarrhea can be debilitating, has a multidimensional impact (Fig. 18.4), and in severe cases can even be life-threatening. The onset of diarrhea can lead to cancer treatment delays, reduced quality of life, and diminished drug compliance. In fact, diarrhea is the dose-limiting factor and the major toxic adverse effect of regimens containing a fluoropyrimidine and/or irinotecan. Other causes of diarrhea in patients undergoing cancer treatment include radiation therapy, small-molecule therapy, monoclonal antibody therapy, neutropenic enterocolitis, and *Clostridium difficile* colitis. Neutropenic enterocolitis (typhlitis) causes diarrhea in the unique setting of intense cytotoxic chemotherapy for leukemia. GVHD in patients who have received an allogeneic hematopoietic stem cell transplant is also associated with severe diarrhea.

Chemotherapy-induced diarrhea The severity of chemotherapy-induced diarrhea is often described, based on the number of stools passed per day, the passing of nocturnal stools, and the need for parenteral support or intensive care, using the National Cancer Institute Common Toxicity Criteria (NCI-CTC) [21]. The severity and prevalence of diarrhea caused by 5-FU treatment is increased by the addition of leucovorin (also known as folinic acid) to the treatment regimen. Diarrhea is reported in up to 50% of patients receiving weekly 5-FU/leucovorin combined

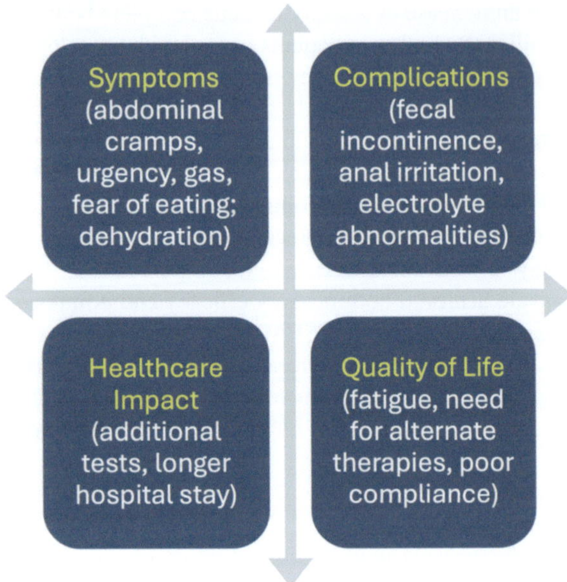

Fig. 18.4 Impact of chronic diarrhea in patients with cancer

treatment. Moreover, the severity of the diarrhea can worsen when 5-FU is administered by bolus injection, as opposed to intravenous infusion. Other factors that can raise the risk of 5-FU-induced diarrhea include female sex, the presence of an unresected primary tumor, previous episodes of chemotherapy-induced diarrhea, and treatment during the summer season [22].

Irinotecan can cause an early-onset diarrhea accompanied by abdominal cramping, lacrimation, and salivation, mediated by cholinergic receptors. These symptoms can be effectively treated with loperamide and anticholinergic agents [23]. The late-onset diarrhea associated with irinotecan is dose-unrelated and unpredictable, but it occurs less frequently when irinotecan is given every 3 weeks [24]. Diarrhea caused by the combined treatment regimen of irinotecan, 5-FU, and leucovorin tends to be more severe, compared with diarrhea caused by 5-FU and leucovorin [25]. Diarrhea is a dose-limiting toxicity of capecitabine, an oral fluoropyrimidine that is converted to 5-FU [26]. Diarrhea also occurs frequently in patients with cancer treated with combination of 5-FU, leucovorin, and oxaliplatin, particularly when 5-FU is administered as a weekly or daily bolus [27].

Diarrhea induced by small molecules and monoclonal antibodies Diarrhea is also common in patients with cancer receiving small-molecule epidermal growth factor receptor (EGFR) tyrosine kinase inhibitors. For example, grade 1–2 diarrhea as defined by the NCI-CTC has been reported in up to 56% of patients receiving erlotinib [28]. Another small-molecule inhibitor of tyrosine kinases in the vascular endothelial growth factor (VEGF) pathway, sorafenib, has been associated with diarrhea in approximately 34% of patients [29]. Unlike the small-molecule EGFR inhibitors, cetuximab, which is a chimeric monoclonal antibody that binds EGFR, may cause diarrhea of any grade in only 12.7% of patients and grade 3 diarrhea in only 1.2% of patients [30].

Radiation-induced diarrhea Radiation therapy can injure the gastrointestinal mucosa. The extent of injury and associated diarrhea usually peaks 1–2 weeks after initiation of irradiation. Worsening diarrhea occurs when radiation is given in combination with chemotherapy, for example, with 5-FU for the treatment of rectal cancer [31].

Treatment of chemotherapy-induced and radiation-induced diarrhea The treatment of chemotherapy- or radiation-induced diarrhea involves aggressive oral rehydration and electrolyte replacement and the use of drugs to reduce fluid loss and decrease intestinal motility. Loperamide and diphenoxylate are the most commonly used agents in varying doses, based on severity. An initial dose of 4 mg loperamide should be given, followed by a further 2 mg every 2–4 h [32]. Octreotide, a synthetic long-acting somatostatin analog, at a dose of 100–150 μg subcutaneously three times daily, is used in patients who do not respond to opioids. Octreotide may also be used as 25–50 μg every hour intravenously, and it can be titrated to higher doses (500–2500 μg three times daily) for the treatment of those individuals who do not respond to lower doses [33]. Other agents have been used as adjunctive therapy in the treatment of mild to moderate chemotherapy-induced and radiation-induced diarrhea, including absorbents, such as kaolin and charcoal, deodorized tincture of opium, paregoric, and codeine phosphate.

Stem cell transplantation-associated diarrhea Patients undergoing stem cell transplantation can suffer from diarrhea caused by the conditioning regimen, GVHD, or an infection related to immunosuppressive therapy. Pretransplant conditioning regimens (including total body irradiation and/or a combination of chemotherapeutic agents) can injure the intestinal mucosa, causing a secretory diarrhea that resolves after mucosal restitution. Recipients of allogeneic stem cell transplants can also develop GVHD, which usually starts 3 weeks or longer after transplantation.

Carcinoid syndrome-induced diarrhea Carcinoid syndrome (CS) occurs in about 20% of patients with neuroendocrine tumors [34]. CD is characterized by diarrhea, flushing, and bronchoconstriction, which result from tumor production of biogenic amines, such as serotonin, which regulates intestinal motility, secretion, and visceral sensitivity. Telotristat ethyl (Xermelo) is a tryptophan hydroxylase inhibitor, which is used in combination with a somatostatin analog (SSA) for the treatment of inadequately controlled carcinoid syndrome diarrhea. The parenteral SSAs octreotide (Sandostatin and others) and lanreotide (Somatuline Depot) have been used for years to treat carcinoid syndrome-associated diarrhea because they bind to somatostatin receptors on tumor cells and inhibit the release of serotonin and other peptides [35, 36].

A clinical response (≥30% reduction from baseline in the number of bowel movements for ≥50% of the time) was achieved in 44% of patients taking telotristat ethyl 250 mg [37]. Common side effects of telotristat are nausea, anorexia, and constipation. The recommended dosage is 250 mg taken three times daily with food. Telotristat ethyl should only be used in combination with an SSA.

References

1. Singhal S, et al. Antitumor activity of thalidomide in refractory multiple myeloma. N Engl J Med. 1999;341:1565–71.
2. Brandt LJ, Prather CM, Quigley EM, Schiller LR, Schoenfeld P, Talley NJ. Systematic review on the management of chronic constipation in North America. Am J Gastroenterol. 2005;100(Suppl 1):S5–S21.
3. Atkinson K. Chronic graft-versus-host disease. Bone Marrow Transplant. 1990;5(2):69–82.
4. Akpek G, Chinratanalab W, Lee LA, Torbenson M, Hallick JP, Anders V, Vogelsang GB. Gastrointestinal involvement in chronic graft-versus-host disease: a clinicopathologic study. Biol Blood Marrow Transplant. 2003 Jan;9(1):46–51.
5. Dzierżanowski T, Mercadante S. Constipation in cancer patients – an update of clinical evidence. Curr Treat Options in Oncol. 2022;23(7):936–50. https://doi.org/10.1007/s11864-022-00976-y. Epub 2022 Apr 20. PMID: 35441979.
6. Hess B, Bernardi M, Klotz HP. Attitude of Swiss physicians towards opioid-induced constipation: a national survey. Eur J Intern Med. 2011;22(5):527–31. https://doi.org/10.1016/j.ejim.2011.02.014. Epub 2011 Mar 21. PMID: 21925066.
7. Larkin PJ, Cherny NI, La Carpia D, Guglielmo M, Ostgathe C, Scotté F, Ripamonti CI. Diagnosis, assessment and management of constipation in advanced cancer: ESMO clinical practice guidelines. Ann Oncol. 2018;29(Supplement_4):iv111–25.
8. Davis MP. Cancer constipation: are opioids really the culprit? Support Care Cancer. 2008;16(5):427–9.
9. Argoff CE. Opioid-induced constipation. Clin J Pain. 2020;36(9):716–22.
10. Lacy BE, Mearin F, Chang L, Chey WD, Lembo AJ, Simren M, Spiller R. Bowel disorders. Gastroenterology. 2016;150(6):1393–140.
11. Davies A, Leach C, Butler C, Gregory A, Henshaw S, Minton O, Shorthose K, Batsari KM. Opioid-induced constipation in patients with cancer: a "real-world," multi-centre, observational study of diagnostic criteria and clinical features. Pain. 2021;162(1):309–18.
12. Ueberall MA, Mueller-Schwefe G. Opioid-induced constipation – a frequent and distressing side effect in daily practice affecting oral and transdermal opioid applications. Eur J Pain. 2006;10(S1):S172.
13. Chiaramonte R, Bonfiglio M, Caramma S, Condorelli R. The role of rehabilitation in the treatment of constipation in oncological patients. J Clin Med. 2023;12(15):5083.
14. Crawford GB, Dzierżanowski T, Hauser K, Larkin P, Luque-Blanco AI, Murphy I, Puchalski CM, Ripamonti CI. Care of the adult cancer patient at the end of life: ESMO clinical practice guidelines. ESMO Open. 2021;6(4):100225. https://doi.org/10.1016/j.esmoop.2021.100225.
15. Yang P, Wang Y, Xiao Y, Ma Q, Ma R, Mi J, Hui J. Acupuncture for opioid-induced constipation. Medicine (Baltimore). 2020;99(49):e23352. https://doi.org/10.1097/MD.0000000000023352.
16. McClurg D, Booth L, Herrero-Fresneda I. Safety and efficacy of intermittent colonic exoperistalsis device to treat chronic constipation: a prospective multicentric clinical trial. Clin Transl Gastroenterol. 2020;11(12):e00267. https://doi.org/10.14309/ctg.0000000000000267.
17. Davis M, Gamier P. New options in constipation management. Curr Oncol Rep. 2015;17(12):55. https://doi.org/10.1007/s11912-015-0481-x. There are no trials in cancer patients.
18. Sloots CEJ, Rykx A, Cools M, Kerstens R, De Pauw M. Efficacy and safety of prucalopride in patients with chronic noncancer pain suffering from opioid-induced constipation. Dig Dis Sci. 2010;55(10):2912–21.

19. Rao SSC, Quigley EMM, Chey WD, Sharma A, Lembo AJ. Randomized placebo-controlled phase 3 trial of vibrating capsule for chronic constipation. Gastroenterology. 2023;164(7):1202–1210.e6. https://doi.org/10.1053/j.gastro.2023.02.013. Epub 2023 Feb 21. PMID: 36822371.
20. Ulsh L, Halawi H, Triadafilopoulos G, Gurland B, Nguyen L, Garcia P, Sonu I, Fernandez-Becker N, Becker L, Sheth V, Neshatian L. Use of a footstool improves rectal balloon expulsion in some patients with defecatory disorders. Neurogastroenterol Motil. 2024;36(7):e14781.
21. National Cancer Institute Common Toxicity Criteria. http://www.ctep.cancer.gov/forms/CTCAEv3.pdf/
22. Sloan JA, Goldberg RM, Sargent DJ, Vargas-Chanes D, Nair S, Cha SS, Novotny PJ, Poon MA, O'Connell MJ, Loprinzi CL. Women experience greater toxicity with fluorouracil-based chemotherapy for colorectal cancer. J Clin Oncol. 2002;20(6):1491–8.
23. Abigerges D, Chabot GG, Armand JP, Hérait P, Gouyette A, Gandia D. Phase I and pharmacologic studies of the camptothecin analog irinotecan administered every 3 weeks in cancer patients. J Clin Oncol. 1995;13(1):210–21.
24. Fuchs CS, Moore MR, Harker G, Villa L, Rinaldi D, Hecht JR. Phase III comparison of two irinotecan dosing regimens in second-line therapy of metastatic colorectal cancer. J Clin Oncol. 2003;21(5):807–14.
25. Rothenberg ML, Meropol NJ, Poplin EA, Van Cutsem E, Wadler S. Mortality associated with irinotecan plus bolus fluorouracil/leucovorin: summary findings of an independent panel. J Clin Oncol. 2001;19(18):3801–7.
26. Haller DG, Cassidy J, Clarke SJ, Cunningham D, Van Cutsem E, Hoff PM, Rothenberg ML, Saltz LB, Schmoll HJ, Allegra C, Bertino JR, Douillard JY, Gustavsson BG, Milano G, O'Connell M, Rustum Y, Tabernero J, Gilberg F, Sirzén F, Twelves C. Potential regional differences for the tolerability profiles of fluoropyrimidines. J Clin Oncol. 2008;26(13):2118–23.
27. Delaunoit T, Goldberg RM, Sargent DJ, Morton RF, Fuchs CS, Findlay BP, Thomas SP, Salim M, Schaefer PL, Stella PJ, Green E, Mailliard JA. Mortality associated with daily bolus 5-fluorouracil/leucovorin administered in combination with either irinotecan or oxaliplatin: results from intergroup trial N9741. Cancer. 2004;101(10):2170–6.
28. Pérez-Soler R, Chachoua A, Hammond LA, Rowinsky EK, Huberman M, Karp D, Rigas J, Clark GM, Santabárbara P, Bonomi P. Determinants of tumor response and survival with erlotinib in patients with non-small-cell lung cancer. J Clin Oncol. 2004;22(16):3238–47.
29. Strumberg D, et al. Safety, pharmacokinetics, and preliminary antitumor activity of sorafenib: a review of four phase I trials in patients with advanced refractory solid tumors. Oncologist. 2007;12:426–37.
30. Lenz HJ, et al. Multicenter phase II and translational study of cetuximab in metastatic colorectal carcinoma refractory to irinotecan, oxaliplatin, and fluoropyrimidines. J Clin Oncol. 2006;24:4914–21.
31. O'Connell MJ, et al. Improving adjuvant therapy for rectal cancer by combining protracted infusion-fluorouracil with radiation therapy after curative surgery. N Engl J Med. 1994;331:502–7.
32. Benson AB, et al. Recommended guidelines for the treatment of cancer treatment-induced diarrhea. J Clin Oncol. 2004;22:2918–26.
33. Barbounis V, Koumakis G, Vassilomanolakis M, Demiri M, Efremidis AP. Control of irinotecan-induced diarrhea by octreotide after loperamide failure. Support Care Cancer. 2001;9(4):258–60.
34. Halperin DM, Shen C, Dasari A, Xu Y, Chu Y, Zhou S, Shih YT, Yao JC. Frequency of carcinoid syndrome at neuroendocrine tumour diagnosis: a population-based study. Lancet Oncol. 2017;18(4):525–34. https://doi.org/10.1016/S1470-2045(17)30110-9. Epub 2017 Feb 24. PMID: 28238592; PMCID: PMC6066284.
35. Wolin EM. The expanding role of somatostatin analogs in the management of neuroendocrine tumors. Gastrointest Cancer Res. 2012;5(5):161–8. PMID: 23112884; PMCID: PMC3481148. Although initially effective recurrent symptoms may occur.

36. Cives M, Strosberg J. Treatment strategies for metastatic neuroendocrine tumors of the gastrointestinal tract. Curr Treat Options in Oncol. 2017;18(3):14. https://doi.org/10.1007/s11864-017-0461-5. PMID: 28286921.
37. Kulke MH, Hörsch D, Caplin ME, Anthony LB, Bergsland E, Öberg K, Welin S, Warner RR, Lombard-Bohas C, Kunz PL, Grande E, Valle JW, Fleming D, Lapuerta P, Banks P, Jackson S, Zambrowicz B, Sands AT, Pavel M. Telotristat ethyl, a tryptophan hydroxylase inhibitor for the treatment of carcinoid syndrome. J Clin Oncol. 2017;35(1):14–23. https://doi.org/10.1200/JCO.2016.69.2780. Epub 2016 Oct 28. PMID: 27918724.

Minimally Invasive Therapies for Gastrointestinal Sensory-Motor Disorders

19

George Triadafilopoulos

Although the onco-neurogastroenterologist is mostly engaged in the diagnosis and pharmacologic treatment of disordered motility and sensation, they have a panoply of minimally invasive therapies that they may choose to utilize, either as a single or adjunctive—even temporary—measure, aiming at symptom relief and QoL improvement. Table 19.1 shows various minimally invasive therapies for gastrointestinal sensory-motor disorders that are available if other measures have been inadequate or have failed.

Table 19.1 Minimally invasive therapies for gastrointestinal sensory-motor disorders

Route	Minimally invasive intervention
Endoscopic	Endoscopic stricture dilation Botulinum toxin injection Pneumatic balloon dilation of EGJ Peroral endoscopic myotomy (POEM), gastric POEM (G-POEM) Endoscopic therapies for GERD (Stretta, transoral fundoplication) Endoscopic food disimpaction Foreign body extraction Celiac plexus block Colonoscopic decompression EUS-guided gastro- and jejuno-jejunostomy
Radiologic	Venting G-tube Feeding G and J tube
Nutritional	Enteral feeding Total parenteral nutrition (TPN)
Surgical	Gastric electrical stimulation Gastric bypass surgery Subtotal colectomy

G. Triadafilopoulos (✉)
Department of Gastroenterology, Hepatology and Nutrition, UT MD Anderson Cancer Center, Houston, TX, USA
e-mail: gtriadafilopoulo@mdanderson.org

G. Triadafilopoulos (ed.), *Onco-Neurogastroenterology*,
https://doi.org/10.1007/978-3-031-98848-6_19

19.1 Endoscopic Therapies

19.1.1 Endoscopic Stricture Dilation

Endoscopic stricture dilation in patients with chronic dysmotility may be beneficial at multiple levels along the GI tract to mitigate the likelihood of progressive luminal dilation proximal to the stricture. Depending on the underlying etiology for stricture formation (i.e., malignant, benign peptic, postoperative), the response to initial dilation, or the frequency of recurrences, additional measures may need to be undertaken, such as PPI therapy; intralesional steroid injection (ILSI); mitomycin C topical application or injection; repeat procedure to higher levels of luminal dilation; temporary use of self-expanding metal stenting (SEMS), self-expanding plastic stents (SEPS), or lumen-apposing metal stents (LAMS); or incisional therapy, using needle knife, typically for distal esophageal rings or anastomotic strictures [1]. Depending on the location, endoscopic dilation may be performed using bougie (Savary) dilators or, more frequently, through-the-scope (TTS) balloon dilation, available at multiple diameter sizes. Repeat dilation sessions may be necessary. The end goal of managing any stricture is to re-establish an adequate and durable luminal patency that is sufficient to resolve the presenting clinical symptoms. For select patients with head and neck cancer, self-dilations may be needed. Endoscopic management of strictures may be challenging and depends on the type of stricture (malignant vs benign), their complexity and length, and their location and accessibility. Further, malignant strictures are often managed either surgically or with radiation and/or chemotherapy. Endoscopic therapies are typically palliative or used as a bridge therapy to surgery [2].

Endoscopic dilation therapy for benign esophageal strictures has success rates ranging from 70% to 90%, but up to 40% of patients require more than three dilation sessions. Gastric outlet obstruction may be benign, caused by chronic peptic ulcer or caustic ingestion or following gastrectomy or gastrojejunostomy, or malignant. TTS balloon dilation is the first-line treatment for benign gastric outlet obstruction followed by enteral stenting, if multiple dilation sessions fail [3].

Small bowel strictures, typically a result of previous abdominal surgery, radiation, or ischemia, may cause obstruction, perforation, and fistula formation [4]. Recurrent diverticulitis, inflammatory bowel disease, colonic ischemia, pelvic radiation, or prior endoscopic submucosal dissection and colonic resection may cause benign colonic strictures and proximal colonic dilation. TTS balloon dilation causes symptomatic relief of obstruction, but repeat dilation is usually needed [5].

19.2 Botulinum Toxin Injection

Achalasia and spastic esophageal dysmotility As an acetylcholine inhibitor, Botox injection of the EGJ decreases LES pressure and improves esophageal clearance in patients with achalasia. Injections may be repeated as needed to sustain symptomatic response over months or years.

Gastroparesis Since prolonged pyloric tonic elevations and increases in phasic contractions are found in some patients with gastroparesis, endoscopic intra-pyloric BoTox injection may accelerate gastric emptying and improve symptoms for 1–6 months after injection. Clinical responses are dose-dependent and are better in women; those under 50 years old; patients with non-diabetic, non-postsurgical gastroparesis; and possibly individuals without retained food, long-standing opiate use, or with severely delayed gastric emptying. Repeat injections, performed even years after initial therapy, do not affect the reinjection interval but may require higher dosage per session.

Sphincter of Oddi dysfunction Intra-sphincteric injection of BoTox reduces sphincter of Oddi pressure in patients with both biliary and pancreatic SOD. Because of the high risk of post-procedural pancreatitis in patients with SOD undergoing ERCP and SO manometry with or without sphincterotomy, the less invasive option of BoTox injection is not only attractive but also it may predict successive outcome of sphincterotomy and could be useful in patient selection and management. Easy to administer using the duodenoscope without cannulation of the ampulla and free of side effects, intra-sphincteric injection of BoTox has a durability of <12 months, but it can be repeated as needed [6].

Pelvic floor dysfunction and anismus BoTox selectively weakens the external anal sphincter if injected anally and the puborectalis muscle when injected preferably under transrectal ultrasound and may increase anorectal angle during straining and decrease anismus, thereby facilitating evacuation, symptomatic relief, and manometric and defecographic improvement. Although simple, safe, and effective in such patients with obstructed defecation, it may require repeated injections to maintain efficacy [7].

19.3 Pneumatic Balloon Dilation

Pneumatic dilation (PD) for achalasia is performed using large-diameter (30–40 mm) balloons that are passed over a guidewire and positioned under fluoroscopic guidance to straddle the EGJ visualized endoscopically and fluoroscopically, and it has a success rate of 70–80%. The decision between PD and surgical or endoscopic myotomy as initial therapy for achalasia should be based upon patient's preferences, clinical status, and available expertise. While evidence suggests that peroral endoscopic myotomy (POEM) may be preferred for type III achalasia, PD remains a valuable alternative for patients with a straight, non-dilated esophagus, who prioritize the preservation of anatomical integrity and a lower risk of post-procedural gastroesophageal reflux disease (GERD). While PD carries a non-negligible risk of perforation, it has an excellent safety profile and minimal likelihood of post-procedural GERD causing permanent esophageal mucosal damage and scarring [8].

Pneumatic dilation of the pylorus, using through-the-scope (TTS) balloons (20 mm), may benefit a subset of patients with gastroparesis who have normal gastric myoelectrical activity (GMA) and pyloric dysfunction with an effect lasting for up to 12 months [9].

Peroral endoscopic myotomy (POEM) (gastric, G-POEM) Third-space endoscopy (TSE) allows for peroral endoscopic myotomy (POEM) or gastric (G-POEM) endoscopic pyloromyotomy. Under upper endoscopy using a standard endoscope, an access to the LES muscle fibers is attained by submucosal saline lifting and balloon orifice dilation, a few centimeters above the LES, followed by the introduction of the scope through the new interlayer's space and advancing it toward the visible fibers of the LES. Once incision of the circular muscle is made by electrocautery knife, the scope is withdrawn back into the lumen, and the mucosal defect is closed with endoscopically applied clips. The procedure is safe and effective in patients with achalasia [10].

Endoscopic therapies for GERD Endoscopic therapies for GERD are minimally invasive outpatient alternatives to medical or surgical treatments. Many GERD patients require a life-long therapy with PPIs, with associated poor compliance, high costs, and possible intolerance and side effects. Antireflux surgery carries surgical risks and side effects, particularly gas-bloat and dysphagia. The Stretta device delivers computer-regulated radiofrequency energy to the gastroesophageal junction causing shrinkage and cellular response in the submucosal tissue decreasing the frequency of transient LES relaxations reducing acid reflux through a less compliant gastroesophageal junction [11]. Transoral incisionless fundoplication (TIF) endoscopically delivers multiple T-fasteners, which pleat the fundus to the esophageal wall, in turn restoring the angle of His and creating serosa-to-serosa fusions. Although successful against GERD symptoms, these procedures have not been shown to protect against GERD-related Barrett's dysplasia and its progression to esophageal adenocarcinoma [12].

Endoscopic food disimpaction Distinct from foreign body impaction, esophageal food bolus impaction (EFBI) is the third most common non-biliary emergency in gastroenterology with an annual incidence rate of 13 episodes per 100,000 person-years and 1500 deaths/year. Esophageal motility disorders are associated with poor esophageal clearance and may promote food impaction, especially of meat, chicken, or other dry foods. Patients who are unable to swallow oral secretions require endoscopic disimpaction using baskets, forceps, snares, or nets, with vigilant push technique alone or in combination with extraction [13]. Most patients have underlying esophageal pathology, such as esophageal rings, peptic or radiation-induced stricture, or cancer. More than 30% of patients resolve spontaneously. The treatment of choice, endoscopic disimpaction typically performed in the emergency department in patients with acute dysphagia, is safe and effective, even if it is performed within a median of 10 h. Endoscopic interventions include endoscope-guided push, extraction by Roth net and/or rat tooth forceps, and, infrequently, TTS balloon dilation. Overall, EFBI is not an emergency, since endoscopy with disimpaction can be done safely with less time constraints and cost savings [14]. Gastric bezoars, often associated with gastroparesis, may also call for endoscopic fragmentation of the bezoar, followed by extraction using snares and nets [15]. Figure 19.1 outlines the three key reasons for esophageal food bolus—as well as foreign body—impaction in patients across the cancer spectrum and highlights other associated symptoms and the steps to be considered for the correct diagnosis in order to prevent recurrences.

Foreign body extraction Foreign body ingestion is a common emergency in cancer patients with cognitive impairment, usually a result of significant fluid and electrolyte disturbances or central nervous system (CNS) involvement by metastatic disease or other age-related neurodegenerative conditions. Although over 80% of foreign bodies pass spontaneously without intervention, 10–20% of them need to be removed urgently by endoscopy (i.e., batteries, partial dentures) and less than 1% surgically [16]. Foreign body impaction should be an important medico-surgical consideration in patients with previously known underlying cancer-related dysmotility, prior surgery, or radiation affecting the gastrointestinal tract that would compromise spontaneous passage of the foreign body in the stool.

Endoscopic gastric electrical stimulation (GES) The placement of temporary GES electrodes endoscopically or through a percutaneous endoscopic gastrostomy could be a predictor of subsequent success of permanent surgical GES placement [17]. Currently, endoscopic placement of temporary GES is not widely used.

Endoscopic sphincterotomy for SOD For patients with SOD, sphincterotomy is challenging, invasive, and associated with increased risk of pancreatitis, bleeding, and perforation. Patients with high probability for biliary or pancreatic SOD (type I), liver or pancreatic enzyme increases, and ductal dilation usually respond to sphincterotomy, which can be performed without prior manometry. In patients with intermediate probability (type II), sphincterotomy is generally being considered after finding high SO pressures or abnormal response to CCK analogues. Low probability patients (type III) should not have sphincterotomy since their symptoms may be attributable to functional bowel disease [18]. Because of the associated risks of post-ERCP complications and the lack of demonstrable clinical benefits, this approach is rarely used [19].

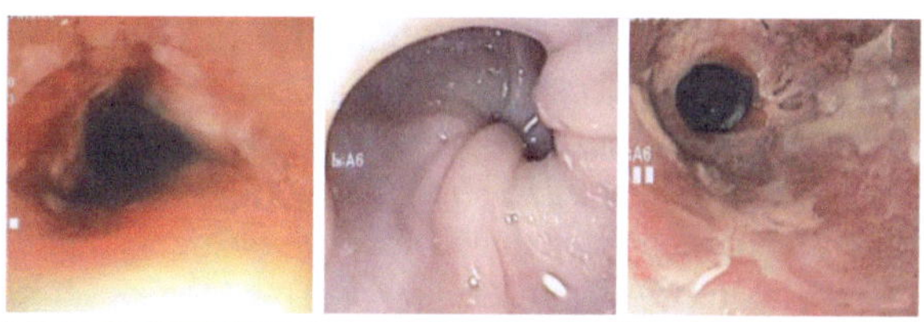

Cancer	Dysmotility	Peptic stricture
Recent onset dysphagia & weight loss	Longstanding, intermittent dysphagia	Heartburn and acid regurgitation
Biopsy	Motility study	pH study

Fig. 19.1 Key reasons for esophageal food bolus impaction in patients with cancer

Endoscopic colonic decompression Acute colonic pseudo-obstruction (ACPO, Ogilvie's syndrome) may require endoscopic decompression to prevent colonic ischemia and perforation. Colonic decompression should be performed without preceding oral preparation, using cautious CO_2 insufflation and continuous aspiration while the colonoscope is inserted and withdrawn. Since one-third of patients may require repeat decompression because of recurrent colonic distention, insertion of a long, fenestrated decompression tube over a guidewire upon completion of the decompression decreases relapses. Adequate decompression may be obtained if at least the hepatic flexure is intubated. Post-procedure oral administration of polyethylene glycol is recommended to prevent relapse. Colonoscopy-guided percutaneous cecostomy may be suggested to patients with recurrent colonic pseudo-obstruction as a potentially attractive alternative to surgical or fluoroscopic placement [20].

Celiac plexus block and neurolysis EUS-guided celiac plexus block and celiac plexus neurolysis are safe and effective modalities used to alleviate pain. Celiac plexus block is a transient interruption of the plexus by local anesthetic, while celiac plexus neurolysis is prolonged interruption of the transmission of pain from the celiac plexus using chemical ablation. Celiac plexus block is generally performed in the unilateral position, while celiac plexus neurolysis is performed in the unilateral or bilateral position [21]. Careful consideration and thoughtful exchange among the onco-neurogastroenterologist, the endoscopic ultrasonographer, and the pain management specialist is needed on every patient requiring such approach.

19.4 Feeding G and J Tube Placement

Generally, naso-enteral tubes are used if tube feeding is expected to be less than 30 days long. Gastrostomy or jejunostomy tubes are ideal for patients needing enteral nutrition for more than 30 days [22]. The percutaneous endoscopic gastrostomy (PEG) technique is an effective, safe, and reliable source of enteral nutrition for both home-based and hospitalized patients. PEG tubes are increasingly used in patients with terminal cancer, for improvement of quality of life in patients with prolonged irreversible conditions and morbidity benefits for patients undergoing radiation therapy for head and neck cancer and for patients with malnutrition. However, a PEG does not reduce the risk of aspiration pneumonia or mortality (Fig. 19.2) [23]. Percutaneous endoscopic jejunostomy (PEJ) is widely used as an alternative when PEG is contraindicated in general or if gastric feedings are not tolerated [24].

Enteral feeding intolerance (EFI) is the development of nausea, vomiting, abdominal cramps, bloating/distension, constipation, and diarrhea that require a change in the protocol and/or introduction of a specific treatment, such as antiemetics or prokinetics. Such intolerance is common in patients with gastrointestinal dysmotility [25]. The resulting delay in administering enteral feeds results in suboptimal nutrition, longer hospitalization, and increased mortality [26]. The utilization of gastric residual volumes (GRVs) to determine feed intolerance is questionable due to the lack of a reliable threshold (range from 50 mL to 500 mL) [27].

Fig. 19.2 Abdominal CT imaging revealing a PEG tube (white half ring) in the stomach

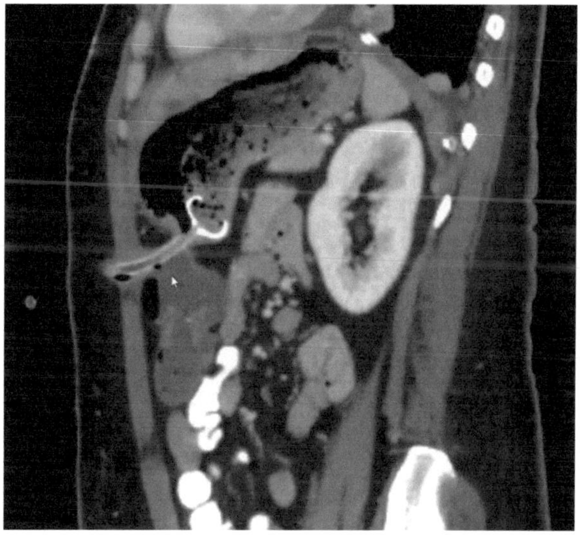

19.5 Venting Tube Placement

In contrast to a conventional venting trans-nasal small intestinal tube that is invasive and painful, percutaneous endoscopic gastro-jejunostomy is a noninvasive, novel decompression therapy available at home and can improve abdominal symptoms and nutritional status in CIPO patients [28]. This approach is also frequently used for malignant obstructions in patients who are not surgical candidates due to widely metastatic disease, multilevel obstructions, or peritoneal carcinomatosis, and it typically employs 24 Fr tubes to allow better venting.

19.5.1 Radiologic Interventions

Many feeding and venting tubes are placed radiologically, particularly if malignant ascites or peritoneal carcinomatosis is present. Similarly, in patients with severe CIPO, who are poor surgical candidates for any surgical treatment, percutaneous endoscopic colostomy by placing a 20 Fr tube in the cecum with the introducer method may lead to durable symptom relief without complications [29].

19.5.2 Nutritional Considerations

Enteral feedings Enteral nutrition (EN) therapy can provide vital nutrition support for patients with various medical conditions, and it is the preferred method for providing nutrition to patients who cannot meet their recommended caloric intake per day through oral intake while maintaining a functional and intact gastrointestinal system. If tolerated in patients with dysmotility, EN is preferable, but it frequently poses challenges because of early satiety, nausea, vomiting, and postprandial bloating. Depending on the formula administered, EN may cause fecal urgency and diarrhea leading to poor compliance and failure to reach the desirable caloric and protein intake and subsequent need for total parenteral nutrition (TPN).

Total parenteral nutrition (TPN) Total parenteral nutrition (TPN) is a life-saving intervention for patients in whom enteral nutrition (EN) cannot be achieved. TPN contains the essential components, such as carbohydrates, lipids, amino acids, vitamins, trace elements, electrolytes, and water, and it has to be administered through a central line because of its hypertonicity. For shorter term, peripheral parenteral nutrition (PPN), which has lower nutrient content and larger volume, can be administered through a non-central line. Parenteral nutrition is costly and associated with metabolic complications related to macro- and micronutrient disturbances, such as hyperglycemia, hypertriglyceridemia, and electrolyte imbalance, as well as infectious complications, mostly related to venous access. In patients with chronic gastrointestinal dysmotility, where weaning from the parenteral approach is frequent, long-term complications, such as hepatobiliary and metabolic bone disease, are often encountered. To prevent and mitigate such potential complications, optimal monitoring and early management of metabolic imbalances are needed [30].

19.6 Surgical Interventions in Onco-neurogastroenterology

Gastric electrical stimulation Gastric electrical stimulation (GES) is an accepted therapy for gastroparesis and the compassionate management of patients with refractory nausea and vomiting [31]. High-frequency gastric electrical stimulation (Enterra, Medtronic Inc., Minneapolis, MN), using pacing electrodes implanted to the proximal gastric muscle layer, reduces nausea and vomiting, improves nutrition and quality of life, but does not always normalize gastric emptying. The device is implanted subcutaneously during laparoscopic surgery assisted by endoscopy, since it is essential that the electrode wires do not penetrate the gastric mucosa during placement [32]. The procedure has low morbidity, but bleeding, infection, and lead migration may occur. The efficacy of the procedure may last for up to 10 years.

Gastric bypass surgery Management of refractory gastroparesis may be challenging after diet, prokinetics, G-POEM, and long-term nutritional support have failed, and surgical interventions (sleeve gastrectomy and Roux-en-Y gastric bypass surgery) may be considered. In such patients, all studies report improvement of nausea and vomiting postoperatively, while gastric emptying improves postoperatively in 45–67% for sleeve gastrectomy and 87% for Roux-en-Y gastric bypass [33].

Subtotal colectomy Surgery can be successful in alleviating chronic constipation, but the decision to proceed with surgical treatment is complex and will require multimodality testing (Fig. 19.3) and medico-surgical input as well as patient understanding of its long-term implications.

Subtotal colectomy with ileo-rectal anastomosis improves health-related quality of life (HRQoL) in most patients with slow-transit constipation. However, symptoms of bloating and abdominal pain may persist following surgery, probably a result of undetected concomitant small bowel or gastric dysmotility (Fig. 19.4).

Approximately 5–15% of patients may experience diarrhea and fecal incontinence for the first few months following colectomy, while ongoing constipation may be experienced by 10–30% of patients [34]. Perioperative complications may be seen in 20–30% of patients and may require re-hospitalization and re-laparotomy [35].

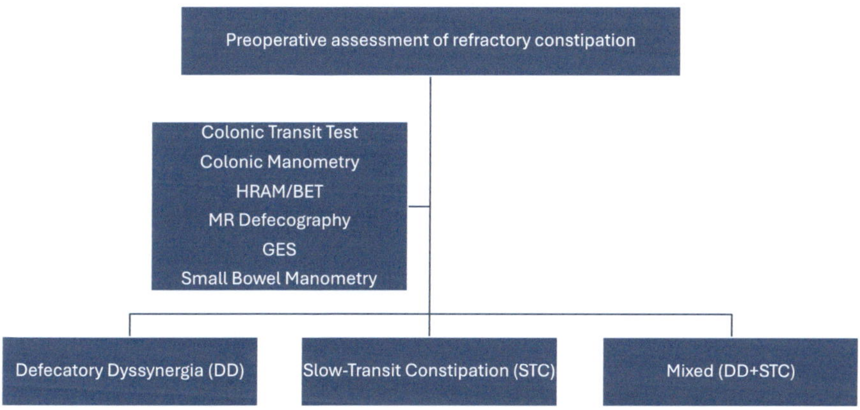

Fig. 19.3 Outline of the multimodality testing prior to a decision for colectomy in refractory constipation. Colonic transit time (CTT) is often assessed using Sitzmarks. If available, colonic manometry substantiates slow-transit constipation (STC). HRAM/BET and MR defecography are useful in excluding dyssynergic defecation (DD). Gastric emptying scan (GES) assesses for concomitant gastroparesis, and small bowel manometry evaluates for concomitant small intestinal dysmotility, typically in the context of chronic intestinal pseudo-obstruction (CIPO)

Fig. 19.4 Key determinants of clinical outcomes after colectomy for refractory constipation, based on multimodality preoperative testing. Best outcomes after surgery are accomplished in patients with pure STC, without significant DD or gastric/small bowel dysmotility

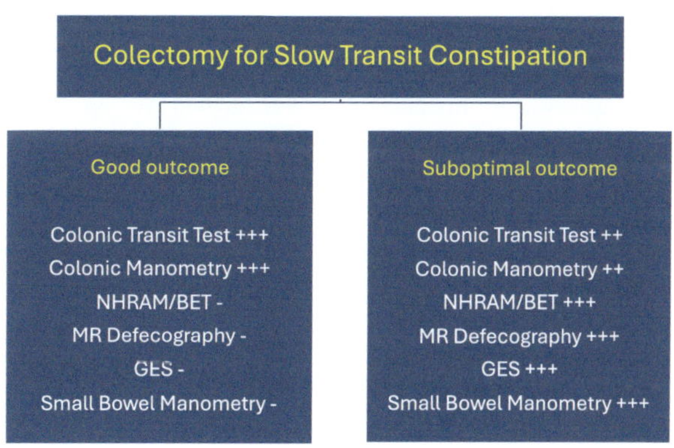

References

1. Siersema PD. How to approach a patient with refractory or recurrent benign esophageal stricture. Gastroenterology. 2019;156(1):7–10. https://doi.org/10.1053/j.gastro.2018.11.040. Epub 2018 Nov 22. PMID: 30472230.
2. Daoud ND, Ghoz H, Mzaik O, Zaver HB, McKinney M, Brahmbhatt B, Woodward T. Endoscopic management of luminal strictures: beyond dilation. Dig Dis Sci. 2022;67(5):1480–99. https://doi.org/10.1007/s10620-022-07396-w. Epub 2022 Feb 25. PMID: 35212884.
3. Lau JY, Chung SC, Sung JJ, Chan AC, Ng EK, Suen RC, Li AK. Through-the-scope balloon dilation for pyloric stenosis: long-term results. Gastrointest Endosc. 1996;43(2 Pt 1):98–101. https://doi.org/10.1016/s0016-5107(06)80107-0. PMID: 8635729.
4. Durmush D, Kaffes AJ. Small bowel strictures. Curr Opin Gastroenterol. 2019;35(3):235–42. https://doi.org/10.1097/MOG.0000000000000531. PMID: 30865041.
5. Adler DG. Colonic strictures: dilation and stents. Gastrointest Endosc Clin N Am. 2015;25(2):359–71. https://doi.org/10.1016/j.giec.2014.11.001. Epub 2014 Dec 30. PMID: 25839690.
6. Friedenberg F, Gollamudi S, Parkman HP. The use of botulinum toxin for the treatment of gastrointestinal motility disorders. Dig Dis Sci. 2004;49:165–75.
7. Maria G, Cadeddu F, Brandara F, Marniga G, Brisinda G. Experience with type a botulinum toxin for treatment of outlet-type constipation. Am J Gastroenterol. 2006;101:2570–5.
8. Vespa E, Barchi A, Passaretti S, Danese S, Savarino EV. Pneumatic dilation for achalasia in the "POEM era": still a valuable ally. Dig Liver Dis. 2024;56(5):778–85. https://doi.org/10.1016/j.dld.2023.10.019. Epub 2023 Nov 4. PMID: 37932169.
9. Noar M, Khan S. Gastric myoelectrical activity-based AI-derived threshold predicts resolution of gastroparesis post-pyloric balloon dilation. Surg Endosc. 2023;37(3):1789–98. https://doi.org/10.1007/s00464-022-09642-8. Epub 2022 Oct 13. PMID: 36229558.
10. North A, Tewari N. Peroral endoscopic myotomy compared to laparoscopic Heller myotomy and pneumatic dilation in the treatment of achalasia: a systematic review. Dis Esophagus. 2024;37(1):doad055. https://doi.org/10.1093/dote/doad055. PMID: 37539633; PMCID: PMC10762503.
11. Triadafilopoulos G. Endoscopic non-ablative radiofrequency treatment (Stretta) for gastroesophageal reflux disease (GERD). Curr Gastroenterol Rep. 2024;26(4):93–8. https://doi.org/10.1007/s11894-024-00917-9. Epub 2024 Feb 23. PMID: 38393432.
12. Triadafilopoulos G. Endoscopic options for gastroesophageal reflux: where are we now and what does the future hold? Curr Gastroenterol Rep. 2016;18(9):47. https://doi.org/10.1007/s11894-016-0521-1. PMID: 27424219.
13. Krill T, Samuel R, Vela A, Marcondes F, Zaibaq J, Guturu P, Parupudi S. Outcomes of delayed endoscopic management for esophageal soft food impactions. Gastrointest Endosc. 2020;91(4):806–12. https://doi.org/10.1016/j.gie.2019.12.020. Epub 2019 Dec 24. PMID: 31874159.
14. Triadafilopoulos G, Gardner JD. Timing and outcomes of endoscopy for esophageal food bolus impaction. Foregut. 2023;3(2):149–54.
15. Katsinelos P, Kountouras J, Paroutoglou G, Zavos C, Mimidis K, Chatzimavroudis G. Endoscopic techniques and management of foreign body ingestion and food bolus impaction in the upper gastrointestinal tract: a retrospective analysis of 139 cases. J Clin Gastroenterol. 2006;40:784–9.
16. Wang X, Zhao J, Jiao Y, Wang X, Jiang D. Upper gastrointestinal foreign bodies in adults: a systematic review. Am J Emerg Med. 2021;50:136–41. https://doi.org/10.1016/j.ajem.2021.07.048. Epub 2021 Jul 29. PMID: 34365062.
17. Ayinala S, Batista O, Goyal A, Al-Juburi A, Abidi N, Familoni B, Abell T. Temporary gastric electrical stimulation with orally or PEG-placed electrodes in patients with drug refractory gastroparesis. Gastrointest Endosc. 2005;61(3):455–61. https://doi.org/10.1016/s0016-5107(05)00076-3. PMID: 15758925.

18. Villavicencio Kim J, Wu GY. Update on Sphincter of Oddi dysfunction: a review. J Clin Transl Hepatol. 2022;10(3):515–21. https://doi.org/10.14218/JCTH.2021.00167. Epub 2022 Jan 11. PMID: 35836767; PMCID: PMC9240241.
19. Cotton PB, Durkalski V, Romagnuolo J, Pauls Q, Fogel E, Tarnasky P, Aliperti G, Freeman M, Kozarek R, Jamidar P, Wilcox M, Serrano J, Brawman-Mintzer O, Elta G, Mauldin P, Thornhill A, Hawes R, Wood-Williams A, Orrell K, Drossman D, Robuck P. Effect of endoscopic sphincterotomy for suspected sphincter of Oddi dysfunction on pain-related disability following cholecystectomy: the EPISOD randomized clinical trial. JAMA. 2014;311(20):2101–9. https://doi.org/10.1001/jama.2014.5220. PMID: 24867013; PMCID: PMC4428324.
20. Mankaney GN, Sarvepalli S, Arora Z, Kamal A, Lopez R, Vargo JJ, Burke CA. Colonic decompression reduces proximal acute colonic pseudo-obstruction and related symptoms. Dis Colon Rectum. 2020;63(1):60–7. https://doi.org/10.1097/DCR.0000000000001492. PMID: 31567918.
21. Sachdev AH, Gress FG. Celiac plexus block and neurolysis: a review. Gastrointest Endosc Clin N Am. 2018;28(4):579–86. https://doi.org/10.1016/j.giec.2018.06.004. Epub 2018 Aug 3. PMID: 30241645.
22. ASGE Standards of Practice CommitteeJain R, Maple JT, Anderson MA, Appalaneni V, Ben-Menachem T, et al. The role of endoscopy in enteral feeding. Gastrointest Endosc. 2011;74(1):7–12.
23. Onur OE, Onur E, Guneysel O, Akoglu H, Denizbasi A, Demir H. Endoscopic gastrostomy, nasojejunal and oral feeding comparison in aspiration pneumonia patients. J Res Med Sci. 2013;18(12):1097–102.
24. Ponsky JL, Aszodi A. Percutaneous endoscopic jejunostomy. Am J Gastroenterol. 1984;79(2):113–6. PMID: 6421149.
25. Wang K, McIlroy K, Plank LD, Petrov MS, Windsor JA. Prevalence, outcomes, and management of enteral tube feeding intolerance: a retrospective cohort study in a tertiary center. J Parenter Enter Nutr. 2017;41(6):959–67.
26. Gungabissoon U, Hacquoil K, Bains C, Irizarry M, Dukes G, Williamson R, et al. Prevalence, risk factors, clinical consequences, and treatment of enteral feed intolerance during critical illness. J Parenter Enter Nutr. 2015;39(4):441–8.
27. McClave SA, Lukan JK, Stefater JA, Lowen CC, Looney SW, Matheson PJ, et al. Poor validity of residual volumes as a marker for risk of aspiration in critically ill patients. Crit Care Med. 2005;33(2):324–30.
28. Ohkubo H, Fuyuki A, Arimoto J, Higurashi T, Nonaka T, Inoh Y, Iida H, Inamori M, Kaneda T, Nakajima A. Efficacy of percutaneous endoscopic gastro-jejunostomy (PEG-J) decompression therapy for patients with chronic intestinal pseudo-obstruction (CIPO). Neurogastroenterol Motil. 2017;29(12). https://doi.org/10.1111/nmo.13127. Epub 2017 Jun 20. PMID: 28631871.
29. Küllmer A, Schmidt A, Caca K. Percutaneous endoscopic cecostomy (introducer method) in chronic intestinal pseudo-obstruction: report of two cases and literature review. Dig Endosc. 2016;28(2):210–5. https://doi.org/10.1111/den.12561. Epub 2016 Feb 4. PMID: 26493622.
30. Berlana D. Parenteral nutrition overview. Nutrients. 2022;14(21):4480. https://doi.org/10.3390/nu14214480. PMID: 36364743; PMCID: PMC9659055.
31. Camilleri M, Parkman HP, Shafi MA, et al. For the American College of Gastroenterology. Clinical guideline: management of gastroparesis. Am J Gastroenterol. 2013;108:18–37.
32. Wendorf G, Lahr C, Tang SJ, Shah A, Islam S, Abell T. Importance of endoscopy during permanent gastric stimulator placement. VideoGIE. 2020;5(7):289–91. https://doi.org/10.1016/j.vgie.2020.03.003. PMID: 32642614; PMCID: PMC7332708.
33. Masclee GMC, Keszthelyi D, Conchillo JM, Kruimel JW, Bouvy ND, Masclee AAM. Systematic review on sleeve gastrectomy or Roux-en-Y gastric bypass surgery for refractory gastroparesis. Surg Obes Relat Dis. 2023;19(3):253–64. https://doi.org/10.1016/j.soard.2022.09.009. Epub 2022 Sep 16. PMID: 36274017.

34. Corsetti M, Brown S, Chiarioni G, Dimidi E, Dudding T, Emmanuel A, Fox M, Ford AC, Giordano P, Grossi U, Henderson M, Knowles CH, O'Connell PR, Quigley EMM, Simren M, Spiller R, Whelan K, Whitehead WE, Williams AB, Scott SM. Chronic constipation in adults: contemporary perspectives and clinical challenges. 2: conservative, behavioural, medical and surgical treatment. Neurogastroenterol Motil. 2021;33(7):e14070. https://doi.org/10.1111/nmo.14070. Epub 2021 Feb 1. PMID: 33522079.
35. Pluta H, Bowes KL, Jewell LD. Long-term results of total abdominal colectomy for chronic idiopathic constipation. Value of preoperative assessment. Dis Colon Rectum. 1996;39(2):160–6. https://doi.org/10.1007/BF02068070. PMID: 8620782.

Emergencies in Onco-neurogastroenterology

20

George Triadafilopoulos

Most patients with gut motor or sensory dysfunction have a subacute or chronic presentation. However, there are rare instances of gastrointestinal emergencies that must not be ignored, particularly in patients with active cancer under treatment who are immunocompromised. This chapter highlights important emergencies to be always considered in these patients that will require an urgent evaluation by a gastroenterologist in consideration of endoscopic intervention and a surgeon, in case surgery is required. In cases of emergency surgery for non-intestinal issues, the surgeon also needs to consider any possible risks that the underlying gut dysmotility poses in the perioperative period, such as pulmonary aspiration.

20.1 Acute Dysphagia

Difficulty swallowing (dysphagia) is quite prevalent in onco-neurogastroenterology. Although usually of gradual onset and intermittent over months or years, dysphagia may present acutely, typically in the form of complete inability to swallow (aphagia). Food bolus (such as dry meat) impaction should be always considered, particularly if the patient suddenly cannot handle their own saliva with ensuing need to constantly spit. Drug- or radiation-induced esophageal injury leading to obstruction needs to be considered [1]. Urgent endoscopy should be undertaken particularly if associated with acute onset of painful swallowing (odynophagia) especially if the patient is unable to handle oropharyngeal secretions and is at risk for pulmonary aspiration.

G. Triadafilopoulos (✉)
Department of Gastroenterology, Hepatology and Nutrition, UT MD Anderson Cancer Center, Houston, TX, USA
e-mail: gtriadafilopoulo@mdanderson.org

G. Triadafilopoulos (ed.), *Onco-Neurogastroenterology*,
https://doi.org/10.1007/978-3-031-98848-6_20

20.2 Esophageal Perforation

Esophageal perforation is rare but potentially fatal, and it requires prompt diagnosis and treatment. In patients with chronically abnormal motility and sensation, esophageal perforation may be iatrogenic, typically in the context of food bolus impaction, and efforts toward endoscopic disimpaction, or spontaneously, resulting from retching (Boerhaave's syndrome) and underlying severe gastroparesis. The clinical presentation depends on the cause and location of the perforation, as well as the length of time since its occurrence. Cervical perforation can present with neck pain, erythema, and edema, whereas thoracic perforations can present with chest pain; gastroesophageal junction perforations can present with either chest or abdominal pain or both. Subcutaneous emphysema and signs of sepsis and multiorgan failure may be seen. A high index of suspicion, a complete history, and physical examination are key. Imaging involves a computed tomography scan of the neck and chest with oral contrast. The gold standard is a fluoroscopic contrast esophagram using gastrografin, followed by thin barium if the diagnosis is not confirmed.

Surgery has traditionally been required for treatment, but endoscopic stenting, over-the-scope clipping, and endoscopic vacuum therapy are increasingly used therapies that are safe and effective in many patients [2]. Primary surgical repair may be possible but is contraindicated in diffuse mediastinal necrosis or a large perforation, preexisting severe benign esophageal disease, and clinical instability. All patients suspected of esophageal perforation should be fasted and started on appropriate intravenous antimicrobial therapy. For those who are hemodynamically unstable or show signs of clinical deterioration, operative debridement and control of contamination is recommended [3].

20.3 Acute Gastric Volvulus

Gastric volvulus is a life-threatening condition, requiring prompt diagnosis and treatment. The condition is characterized by abnormal rotation of the stomach by more than 180°. As such, it carries the risk of strangulation, resulting in necrosis, perforation, hypovolemic shock, and a mortality of 30–50% [4]. The clinical presentation may be acute or chronic and depends upon the speed of onset, the type of volvulus, and the degree of obstruction. Those with the acute form present with pain in the upper abdomen or lower chest, associated with severe retching and inability to pass a nasogastric tube.

Acutely, open surgical reduction with or without gastropexy is most frequently performed. However, several other operative approaches may be used, including diaphragmatic hernia repair, gastropexy, partial gastrectomy, or fundo-antral gastrogastrostomy. However, in the elderly population with chronic dysmotility, or those with chronic gastric volvulus, laparoscopic surgery or endoscopic reduction with insertion of a percutaneous gastrostomy tube is used [5].

20.4 Acute Colonic Volvulus

Acute colonic volvulus may occur either in the sigmoid colon or the cecum and causes large bowel obstruction. It presents with acute diffuse abdominal pain and distention, nausea, vomiting, and inability to pass stool or gas through the rectum. If untreated, it can progress to bowel gangrene and frank peritonitis secondary to colonic perforation. Sigmoid volvulus affects older patients who are debilitated by long-standing constipation and colonic dysmotility. Mortality can be quite high, around 10% for uncomplicated cases and up to 60% if bowel gangrene develops [6].

The presentation can be acute or subacute, associated with progressively worsening abdominal pain. A plain abdominal radiograph can be obtained first, but it only establishes the diagnosis in 60% of cases. Oftentimes, an abdominal CT scan is needed, which will also rule out other causes of obstruction. Management is either endoscopic reduction or surgical resection. If bowel necrosis is suspected, emergent surgery is imperative. If bowel necrosis is not suspected, non-surgical reduction with colonoscopy is preferred, being successful in up to 75% of cases. However, recurrence can happen in up to 57% of these patients. Elective resection, after initial endoscopic reduction, may be needed to prevent recurrence [7].

20.5 Acute Fecal Impaction

Acute fecal impaction (FI) is defined by a large mass of stool in the rectum and/or distal colon that cannot be evacuated. FI is more prevalent with increasing age and in patients with chronic constipation, intestinal pseudo-obstruction, or other neurological disorders. A digital rectal examination should be performed on all patients with suspected fecal impaction for both diagnosis and management. However, impaction can also occur in the proximal rectum and sigmoid colon, so an abdominal radiograph should be obtained if digital rectal examination is negative. Management consists of manual disimpaction, liberal enema use, and establishment of an effective long-term maintenance bowel regimen. Abdominal surgery, both for bowel resections for ischemia/necrosis of the small bowel and colon, is associated with very high mortality [8].

Prolonged and inadequately treated constipation in patients with chronic intestinal dysmotility may lead not only to fecal impaction but also, rarely, stercoral colitis, an uncommon but potentially life-threatening condition that can present acutely, and it is characterized by impacted fecal material causing increased colonic intraluminal pressure and inflammation. If not recognized and treated, stercoral colitis may lead to dangerous complications, such as ischemic necrosis, perforation, and/or sepsis, with a mortality rate up to 63% [8–10]. Management consists of manual stool disimpaction, liberal enema use, and establishment of an effective long-term maintenance bowel regimen. If manual disimpaction and enemas fail, colonoscopic disimpaction may be pursued.

20.6 Intestinal Perforation

Elderly patients with long-standing history of constipation inadequately treated with laxatives may develop stercoral ulcer and colonic perforation with peritonitis. If not suspected in a timely fashion, assessed by abdominal imaging, and attended surgically, perforation carries high mortality [11].

20.7 Acute Colonic Pseudo-obstruction (ACPO)

Ogilvie's syndrome or acute colonic pseudo-obstruction (ACPO) manifests with symptoms of obstruction, such as bloating and abdominal distension, but in the absence of any mechanical blockage. Several associated conditions exist, including electrolyte disturbances, infections, major surgeries (particularly orthopedic), and use of narcotics. Diagnosis is made by plain abdominal radiograph or abdominal CT, which is necessary to rule out mechanical obstruction. Management is often conservative at first, with proximal gastrointestinal decompression (fasting, nasogastric suction), placement of a decompressive rectal tube if the distention extends as far as the sigmoid or rectum, intravenous fluid and electrolyte repletion (correction of hypokalemia and hypomagnesemia), and monitoring for life-threatening complications, such as colonic ischemia and perforation. Intravenous neostigmine, 2 mg intravenously over a period of 3–5 min, monitored by telemetry and quick access to atropine, is the next option if conservative measures fail [12]. If narcotics are being used, peripheral opioid antagonists, such as intravenous methylnaltrexone, should be considered. If there is still no improvement, colonoscopic decompression should be attempted. Surgical or percutaneous decompression should be reserved only for refractory cases or in emergent situations [13].

20.8 Toxic Megacolon

Toxic megacolon (TM) is a potentially fatal condition that can result from various infectious and inflammatory etiologies. The diagnosis of TM is made clinically (fever >101.5°, tachycardia (>120 beats/min), leukocytosis, and anemia, as well as altered mentation, dehydration, hypotension, or electrolyte abnormalities) together with radiographic evidence of colonic non-obstructive dilation (≥5.5 cm), with abnormal haustral appearance, particularly in the transverse and ascending colon. Inflammatory bowel disease (IBD), particularly ulcerative colitis (UC), remains the most common cause of toxic megacolon, followed by infectious colitis due to *Clostridioides difficile* infection and, rarely, ischemic colitis or ICI colitis in cancer patients. The mortality rate can be as high as 80% [14]. The condition needs to be diagnosed and managed early in an intensive care setting, under continuous vigilance by both gastroenterology and colorectal surgery.

Key in the medical management of acute severe IBD (including ICI colitis) with toxic megacolon is the use of intravenous (IV) methylprednisolone 60 mg/day or hydrocortisone 100 mg three to four times daily to induce remission, together with IV hydration and resuscitation, electrolyte replacement as indicated, deep vein thrombosis (DVT) prophylaxis, blood transfusions as needed, and total parenteral nutrition if the patient is malnourished. Nonsteroidal anti-inflammatory medications, anticholinergic medications, antidiarrheal agents, and opiates should be avoided [15]. In cases of *C. difficile* colitis, the first step in management is to discontinue the inciting antibiotics, followed by oral vancomycin at a dose of 500 mg four times daily by mouth or nasogastric tube to directly target the infection in the colonic lumen. IV metronidazole at a dose of 500 mg every 8 h can also be added in the case of ileus. Rectal or intracolonic vancomycin at a dose of 500 mg in 500 mL normal saline every 6 h can be considered in severe cases, when ileus may slow the delivery of oral medication to the colon [16]. The surgical management for patients with severe, fulminant *C. difficile* infection should be reserved for patients with colonic perforation or severe colitis that is not improving with medical therapy.

The role of cytomegalovirus (CMV) infection in exacerbating the severity of ulcerative colitis, the optimal diagnostic tests for CMV, and the timing of antiviral treatment initiation and its response to treatment remain uncertain. In general, CMV colitis, as defined by the presence of intranuclear or intracellular inclusion bodies on hematoxylin and eosin (H&E) staining and/or positive immunohistochemistry (IHC) assay on histology, is associated with more severe colitis [17]. Patients with CMV infection and acute severe colitis are more resistant to treatment with corticosteroids than non-infected patients. This refractoriness to steroids is related to colonic tissue CMV viral load and number of inclusion bodies—a marker of high-grade CMV infection—which may affect clinical outcomes. There is a significant difference in colectomy rates of patients with high-grade CMV infection who received antiviral therapy compared with those who did not. It was therefore proposed that high-grade CMV disease indicating that the virus can be pathogenic. CMV is common in immunocompromised patients. It is associated with high morbidity and mortality, particularly in patients undergoing allogeneic (allo-) hematopoietic stem cell transplantation (HSCT) [18]. Immune checkpoint inhibitor (ICI) colitis and cytomegalovirus (CMV) colitis share many common symptoms, making the diagnosis difficult to distinguish clinically. Accurately diagnosing a superimposed CMV colitis changes clinical management and in turn can improve patient outcomes [19].

References

1. Abdi S, Masbough F, Nazari M, Abbasinazari M. Drug-induced esophagitis and helpful management for healthcare providers. Gastroenterol Hepatol Bed Bench. 2022;15(3):219–24. https://doi.org/10.22037/ghfbb.v15i3.2591. PMID: 36311965; PMCID: PMC9589134.
2. Barakat MT, Girotra M, Banerjee S. (Re)building the wall: recurrent Boerhaave syndrome managed by over-the-scope clip and covered metallic stent placement. Dig Dis Sci. 2018;63(5):1139–42. https://doi.org/10.1007/s10620-017-4756-y. Epub 2017 Sep 25. PMID: 28948439; PMCID: PMC5867198.

3. Fairbairn K, Worrell SG. Esophageal perforation: is surgery still necessary? Thorac Surg Clin. 2023;33(2):117–23. https://doi.org/10.1016/j.thorsurg.2023.01.005. Epub 2023 Feb 26. PMID: 37045480.
4. Chau B, Dufel S. Gastric volvulus. Emerg Med J. 2007;24(6):446–7. https://doi.org/10.1136/emj.2006.041947. PMID: 17513555; PMCID: PMC2658296.
5. Eckhauser ML, Ferron JP. The use of dual percutaneous endoscopic gastrostomy (DPEG) in the management of chronic intermittent gastric volvulus. Gastrointest Endosc. 1985;31(5):340–2. https://doi.org/10.1016/s0016-5107(85)72221-3. PMID: 4043688.
6. Aboelezz AF, Othman MO. Endoscopic management of colonic obstruction. Gastrointest Endosc Clin N Am. 2024;34(1):141–53. https://doi.org/10.1016/j.giec.2023.09.011. Epub 2023 Oct 13. PMID: 37973225.
7. Tian BWCA, Vigutto G, Tan E, van Goor H, Bendinelli C, Abu-Zidan F, Ivatury R, Sakakushev B, Di Carlo I, Sganga G, Maier RV, Coimbra R, Leppäniemi A, Litvin A, Damaskos D, Broek RT, Biffl W, Di Saverio S, De Simone B, Ceresoli M, Picetti E, Galante J, Tebala GD, Beka SG, Bonavina L, Cui Y, Khan J, Cicuttin E, Amico F, Kenji I, Hecker A, Ansaloni L, Sartelli M, Moore EE, Kluger Y, Testini M, Weber D, Agnoletti V, Angelis ND, Coccolini F, Sall I, Catena F. WSES consensus guidelines on sigmoid volvulus management. World J Emerg Surg. 2023;18(1):34. https://doi.org/10.1186/s13017-023-00502-x. PMID: 37189134; PMCID: PMC10186802.
8. Sommers T, Petersen T, Singh P, Rangan V, Hirsch W, Katon J, Ballou S, Cheng V, Friedlander D, Nee J, Lembo A, Iturrino J. Significant morbidity and mortality associated with fecal impaction in patients who present to the emergency department. Dig Dis Sci. 2019;64(5):1320–7. https://doi.org/10.1007/s10620-018-5394-8. Epub 2018 Dec 8. PMID: 30535766; PMCID: PMC6499648.
9. Bae E, Tran J, Shah K. Stercoral colitis in the emergency department: a review of the literature. Int J Emerg Med. 2024;17(1):3. https://doi.org/10.1186/s12245-023-00578-x. PMID: 38166616; PMCID: PMC10759528.
10. Corban C, Sommers T, Sengupta N, Jones M, Cheng V, Friedlander E, Bollom A, Lembo A. Fecal impaction in the emergency department: an analysis of frequency and associated charges in 2011. J Clin Gastroenterol. 2016;50(7):572–7. https://doi.org/10.1097/MCG.0000000000000458. PMID: 26669560.
11. Alburakan A, Alshunaifi A, AlRabah R, Alshammari S, Alnasser S, Nouh T. Chronic constipation that resulted in fecal impaction and colon perforation: a case report. Medicine (Baltimore). 2022;101(34):e30206. https://doi.org/10.1097/MD.0000000000030206. PMID: 36042637; PMCID: PMC9410610.
12. Pereira P, Djeudji F, Leduc P, Fanget F, Barth X. Ogilvie's syndrome-acute colonic pseudo-obstruction. J Visc Surg. 2015;152(2):99–105. https://doi.org/10.1016/j.jviscsurg.2015.02.004. Epub 2015 Mar 11. PMID: 25770746.
13. Khan Z, Challand CP, Lee MJ. Management of acute colonic pseudo-obstruction: opportunities to improve care? Ann R Coll Surg Engl. 2024;107:106. https://doi.org/10.1308/rcsann.2024.0017. Epub ahead of print. PMID: 38445579.
14. Liggett MR, Alam HB. Management of severe colitis and toxic megacolon. Clin Colon Rectal Surg. 2023;37(6):404–10. https://doi.org/10.1055/s-0043-1777665. PMID: 39399135; PMCID: PMC11466533.
15. Rubin DT, Ananthakrishnan AN, Siegel CA, Sauer BG, Long MD. ACG clinical guideline: ulcerative colitis in adults. Am J Gastroenterol. 2019;114(3):384–413. https://doi.org/10.14309/ajg.0000000000000152. PMID: 30840605.
16. Shetler K, Nieuwenhuis R, Wren SM, Triadafilopoulos G. Decompressive colonoscopy with intracolonic vancomycin administration for the treatment of severe pseudomembranous colitis. Surg Endosc. 2001;15(7):653–9. https://doi.org/10.1007/s004640080104. Epub 2001 May 7. PMID: 11591962.
17. Mourad FH, Hashash JG, Kariyawasam VC, Leong RW. Ulcerative colitis and cytomegalovirus infection: from A to Z. J Crohns Colitis. 2020;14(8):1162–71. https://doi.org/10.1093/ecco-jcc/jjaa036. PMID: 32103246.

18. Allaw F, Haddad SF, Zakhour J, Kanj SS. Management of cytomegalovirus infection in allogeneic hematopoietic stem cell transplants. Int J Antimicrob Agents. 2023;62(2):106860. https://doi.org/10.1016/j.ijantimicag.2023.106860. Epub 2023 May 21. PMID: 37220849.
19. Harris KB, Funchain P, Baggott BB. CMV coinfection in treatment refractory immune checkpoint inhibitor colitis. BMJ Case Rep. 2020;13(5):e233519. https://doi.org/10.1136/bcr-2019-233519. PMID: 32434876; PMCID: PMC7244273.

21 Nutritional Issues

George Triadafilopoulos, David M. Richards, and Mehnaz A. Shafi

21.1 Malnutrition

Because sensory and motor dysfunction of the digestive tract compromises the key role of the gut in handling and efficiently processing nutrients, the onco-neurogastroenterologist is often confronted with chronically malnourished patients. Figure 21.1 outlines the sequence followed in the evaluation of malnutrition, starting from screening and complete assessment of possible etiologies to diagnosis and severity assessment, ultimately defining the magnitude of the problem and the need for urgent intervention, either enterally or parenterally.

Malnutrition is a key factor for general health and well-being, particularly in the elderly. Functional and mobility limitations, due to weakness and muscle atrophy (sarcopenia), reduce quality of life and overall survival. Aging increases nutritional risk because of diminished organ system reserves. Up to 70% of older adults are malnourished, which in turn is associated with increased mortality. The nutritional needs of older adults depend on multiple factors, most importantly disease-related organ dysfunction, and the person's energy expenditures, as well as the ability to access, prepare, ingest, and digest food. The diagnosis requires the combination of at least one phenotypic (involuntary weight loss, low body mass index (BMI), or reduced muscle mass) and one etiologic criterion, such as reduced food intake or absorption, or underlying inflammation, due to acute disease/injury, or chronic disease (Fig. 21.2). Malnutrition can be seen across the cancer spectrum with impacts on treatments and survival [1].

G. Triadafilopoulos (✉) · D. M. Richards · M. A. Shafi
Department of Gastroenterology, Hepatology and Nutrition, UT MD Anderson Cancer Center, Houston, TX, USA
e-mail: GTriadafilopoulo@mdanderson.org; DMRichards@mdanderson.org; mashafi@mdanderson.org

G. Triadafilopoulos (ed.), *Onco-Neurogastroenterology*,
https://doi.org/10.1007/978-3-031-98848-6_21

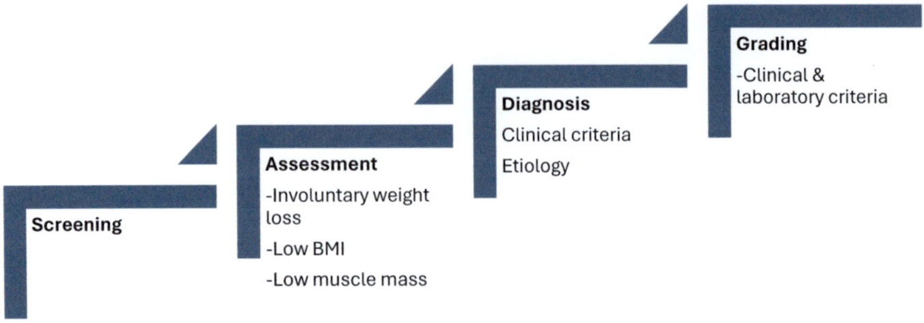

Fig. 21.1 Sequence of steps in the evaluation of malnutrition

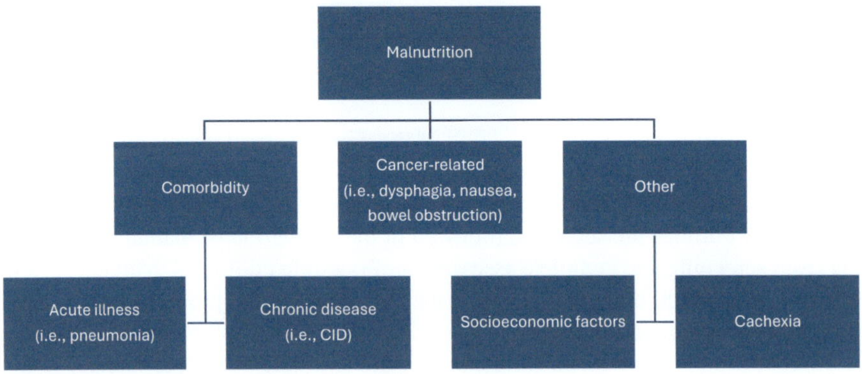

Fig. 21.2 Important elements for consideration when managing a patient with malnutrition

Involuntary weight loss in patients with motor and/or sensory dysfunction may be driven by a variety of factors, such as inadequate dietary intake, loss of appetite, muscle atrophy (sarcopenia), inflammatory effects of disease (cachexia), or a combination of these factors. Associated medical and psychiatric issues, such as malignancy and depression, play a key role. Additional contributors may include loss of smell and taste, dysphagia, fasting associated with drug administration, chemotherapy-induced nausea and/or vomiting, and poor appetite, all of which can affect food intake and absorption. Female sex, old age, depression, cognitive decline, and depression may also contribute (Fig. 21.3).

Often resistant to nutritional intervention, cachexia is a complex metabolic syndrome associated with underlying illness, characterized by loss of muscle, with or without loss of fat mass, anorexia, inflammation, insulin resistance, and increased muscle protein breakdown. Sarcopenia, a syndrome characterized by the loss of muscle mass, strength, and function without underlying illness, is associated with increased rates of functional impairment, disability, falls, and mortality. Sarcopenia often occurs in people with cancer [2].

To evaluate weight loss and malnutrition, one should start by performing a complete history and physical examination, followed by laboratory evaluation for

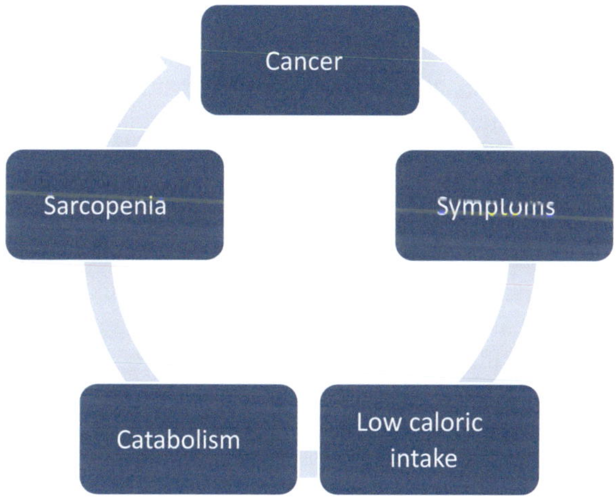

Fig. 21.3 Cycle of events relating cancer to malnutrition

evidence of metabolic or inflammatory disease, such as comprehensive chemistry profile, thyroid-stimulating hormone (TSH), complete blood count (CBC), and C-reactive protein (CRP). Screening involves the serial measurements of weight, calculating the percentage weight loss, and utilizing screening tools, such as the Mini Nutritional Assessment (MNA). Weight loss is significant if it exceeds 5% in 3 months or more than 10% in 6 months [3]. A dietician or nutritionist should assess if calorie and protein requirements are met and, together with clinical criteria, grade the severity of malnutrition.

In resistant cases where symptom-focused simple modalities and behavioral changes have failed, the use of appetite stimulants could be cautiously considered. Megestrol acetate may lead to weight gain in patients with anorexia and cachexia. Several studies have shown appetite improvement in advanced cancer, and a meta-analysis showed 1 in 4 patients will improve their appetite and 1 in 12 will improve their weight [4]. But megestrol use is risky, particularly in elderly patients. Notable side effects include risks of thrombophlebitis, adrenal insufficiency with abrupt withdrawal, impotence in males, and menstrual bleeding with drug withdrawal in women [4]. Dronabinol may be useful for anorexia, weight gain, and behavior problems in patients with advanced cancer who are refusing food but has significant central nervous system side effects, limiting its use. Mirtazapine, an antidepressant that leads to more weight gain than selective serotonin reuptake inhibitor (SSRI) antidepressants, is commonly used for management of depression and weight loss [5]. It is important to remember that while appetite stimulants may improve appetite, they do not appear to improve global quality of life or survival [4]. It is important to clearly define the goal of using an appetite stimulant and to inform patients of expected side effects prior to use.

21.2 Obesity

Many patients across the cancer spectrum have obesity. Hence, it is essential to consider the impact of obesity and its various medical and surgical therapies on gastrointestinal motility and sensation and their potential role in symptom induction. Obesity has been traditionally defined as a body mass index (BMI) of at least 30 kg/m^2. It is further categorized into class I obesity (BMI 30–34.9 kg/m^2), class II obesity (BMI 35–39.9 kg/m^2), and class III obesity (BMI $\geq$40 kg/m^2) [6]. Obesity increases the risk of gastroesophageal reflux disease, erosive esophagitis, and esophageal adenocarcinoma by 2-, 1.8-, and 2.8-fold, respectively [7]. Obesity increases the risk for gastric cancer (OR, 1.55), colon polyps (OR, 1.44) and colorectal cancer (RR, 1.3), dyssynergic defecation (OR, 1.64), and diarrhea (OR, 2.7) [8].

The management of both type 2 diabetes and obesity has dramatically changed with the availability of glucagon-like peptide-1 (GLP-1) receptor agonists (RAs), such as liraglutide or semaglutide, and tirzepatide, a GLP-1 and glucose-dependent insulinotropic polypeptide co-agonist. However, both long-acting and short-acting GLP-1RAs delay gastric emptying with a consequent increased risk of aspiration at the time of surgery or upper gastrointestinal endoscopy, and special precautions are needed [9].

Significant changes in gastrointestinal motility, mostly in the stomach, occur after metabolic and bariatric surgery (MBS) [10]. Esophageal dysmotility after MBS may include esophagogastric junction outflow obstruction (EGJOO), absent contractility, and secondary achalasia-like pattern called post-obesity surgery esophageal dysfunction (POSED), contributing to postoperative dysphagia and/or gastroesophageal reflux disease. Altered postsurgical anatomy after MBS contributes to changes in gastric motility. After laparoscopic sleeve gastrectomy (LSG), the creation of the sleeve decreases the gastric reservoir, while the removal of the gastric fundus leads to reduced distensibility and loss of the gastric pacemaker, all leading to accelerated gastric emptying, at times dumping syndrome. The consequent rapid emptying of undigested nutrients leads to elevated levels of GLP-1 and PYY leading to improved satiation and weight loss [11]. Dumping syndrome has been described in patients after LSG, and the underlying pathophysiology lies in such rapid gastric emptying.

Similarly, in cases of Roux-en-Y gastric bypass (RYGB), the creation of the gastric pouch leads to rapid gastric emptying variably depending on the dimensions of the pouch and the width of the gastrojejunal anastomosis. High-resolution manometry has shown that the Roux limb exhibits regular migrating motility complexes, suggesting that the gastric pouch and the Roux limb behave as a common cavity during food ingestion [12]. Since they improve symptoms and gastric emptying in patients with severe gastroparesis and obesity, both LSG and RYGB are good treatment options in patients with refractory disease. RYGB is the preferred therapy in patients with obesity and severe GERD since the creation of a pouch compared to a sleeve causes lower increases in intragastric pressure and is less likely to provoke reflux. After LSG and RYGB, accelerated gastric emptying and subsequent premature arrival of contents into the small intestine lead to acceleration of small intestinal transit, but we have less data about ileocecal and colonic transit in patients after MBS.

References

1. Jensen GL, Cederholm T, Correia MITID, Gonzalez MC, Fukushima R, Higashiguchi T, de Baptista GA, Barazzoni R, Blaauw R, Coats AJS, Crivelli A, Evans DC, Gramlich L, Fuchs-Tarlovsky V, Keller H, Llido L, Malone A, Mogensen KM, Morley JE, Muscaritoli M, Nyulasi I, Pirlich M, Pisprasert V, de van der Schueren M, Siltharm S, Singer P, Tappenden KA, Velasco N, Waitzberg DL, Yamwong P, Yu J, Compher C, Van Gossum A. GLIM criteria for the diagnosis of malnutrition: a consensus report from the global clinical nutrition community. J Parenter Enteral Nutr. 2019;43(1):32–40. https://doi.org/10.1002/jpen.1440. Epub 2018 Sep 2. PMID: 30175461.
2. Evans WJ, Morley JE, Argilés J, Bales C, Baracos V, Guttridge D, Jatoi A, Kalantar-Zadeh K, Lochs H, Mantovani G, Marks D, Mitch WE, Muscaritoli M, Najand A, Ponikowski P, Rossi Fanelli F, Schambelan M, Schols A, Schuster M, Thomas D, Wolfe R, Anker SD. Cachexia: a new definition. Clin Nutr. 2008;27(6):793–9. https://doi.org/10.1016/j.clnu.2008.06.013. Epub 2008 Aug 21. PMID: 18718696.
3. Zawada ET Jr. Malnutrition in the elderly. Is it simply a matter of not eating enough? Postgrad Med. 1996;100(1):207–8, 211–4, 220–2. https://doi.org/10.3810/pgm.1996.07.17.
4. Childs DS, Jatoi A. A hunger for hunger: a review of palliative therapies for cancer-associated anorexia. Ann Palliat Med. 2019;8(1):50–8. https://doi.org/10.21037/apm.2018.05.08. Epub 2018 May 24. PMID: 29860861; PMCID: PMC6252156.
5. Chowdhury IH, Rahman S, Afroze YJ, Shovah ST. IUPHAR ECR review: cancer-related anorexia-cachexia in cancer patients: pathophysiology and treatment. Pharmacol Res. 2024;203:107129. https://doi.org/10.1016/j.phrs.2024.107129. Epub 2024 Mar 9. PMID: 38461961.
6. Jirapinyo P, Thompson CC. Obesity primer for the practicing gastroenterologist. Am J Gastroenterol. 2021;116(5):918–34. https://doi.org/10.14309/ajg.0000000000001200.
7. El-Serag H. The association between obesity and GERD: a review of the epidemiological evidence. Dig Dis Sci. 2008;53(9):2307–12. https://doi.org/10.1007/s10620-008-0413-9. Epub 2008 Jul 24. PMID: 18651221; PMCID: PMC2827866.
8. Camilleri M, Malhi H, Acosta A. Gastrointestinal complications of obesity. Gastroenterology. 2017;152(7):1656–70. https://doi.org/10.1053/j.gastro.2016.12.052. Epub 2017 Feb 10. PMID: 28192107; PMCID: PMC5609829
9. Jalleh RJ, Rayner CK, Hausken T, Jones KL, Camilleri M, Horowitz M. Gastrointestinal effects of GLP-1 receptor agonists: mechanisms, management, and future directions. Lancet Gastroenterol Hepatol. 2024;9(10):957–64. https://doi.org/10.1016/S2468-1253(24)00188-2. Epub 2024 Aug 1. PMID: 39096914.
10. Gala K, Ghusn W, Abu Dayyeh BK. Gut motility and hormone changes after bariatric procedures. Curr Opin Endocrinol Diabetes Obes. 2024;31(3):131–7. https://doi.org/10.1097/MED.0000000000000860. Epub 2024 Mar 27. PMID: 38533785.
11. Sioka E, Tzovaras G, Perivoliotis K, et al. Impact of laparoscopic sleeve gastrectomy on gastrointestinal motility. Gastroenterol Res Pract. 2018;2018:4135813.
12. Bjorklund P, Lonroth H, Fandriks L. Manometry of the upper gut following Roux-en-Y gastric bypass indicates that the gastric pouch and roux limb act as a common cavity. Obes Surg. 2015;25:1833–41.

22 Care Coordination in Onco-neurogastroenterology

George Triadafilopoulos

Onco-neurogastroenterology is multidimensional, with both structural and functional elements (both gastrointestinal and neurological) that frequently interact and complicate both diagnosis and management. It is important for the physician to be fully informed about the severity, acuity, and, to a degree possible, disease prognosis, both acutely and long term, before spending time informing the patient and their family of their findings and outlining a therapeutic plan. Table 22.1 highlights the essential elements of the first interaction between the onco-neurogastroenterologist and the patient, particularly if the clinical issues are chronic and relapsing in nature (as they frequently are). During this pivotal visit, there is no room for diagnostic uncertainty; it is a time for building trust in the therapeutic relationship, which will only remain effective in the long term if it is based on transparency and perpetual open-mindedness from either side.

As with any chronic illness, effective and encouraging patient-physician interaction remains paramount for all patients. Such interaction needs to come from multiple directions (i.e., oncology, endoscopy, surgery) emphasizing the positives while acknowledging any challenges. Table 22.2 provides a list of issues in onco-neurogastroenterology that require regular consideration when managing such patients who, during their illness, may experience a physical, emotional, or cognitive decline. During follow-up, it is often useful to first privately interact with the escorting family member or caretaker to be kept abreast of recent changes in the patient's clinical and psychological performance. This information facilitates the subsequent interview and decision-making that ultimately will remain patient-centered and direct.

G. Triadafilopoulos (✉)
Department of Gastroenterology, Hepatology and Nutrition, UT MD Anderson Cancer Center, Houston, TX, USA
e-mail: gtriadafilopoulo@mdanderson.org

G. Triadafilopoulos (ed.), *Onco-Neurogastroenterology*,
https://doi.org/10.1007/978-3-031-98848-6_22

Table 22.1 Essential elements of the first interaction between the onco-neurogastroenterologist and the patient

Points to be considered when breaking the news about onco-neurogastrointestinal conditions
Prepare fully, checking notes, test results, and time arranged for follow-up tests, or planned admission
Break bad news in a suitable room, perhaps with a nurse present. Ensure privacy, with no interruptions
Allow adequate time
Make sure patients and relatives know who you are and the purpose of the consultation
Remember that what is hopeful news for you might still be bad news for the patient and vice versa
Do not assume that someone else has handled important parts of the information giving
Do not be falsely reassuring; provide as much positive practical support and information as possible
Ensure that the patient has enough time to let the news sink in—check understanding before they leave
Offer follow-up appointment, number to call, or addresses or other helpful agencies
Ensure that they understand that you are working closely with others, particularly, their oncology team

Table 22.2 Issues in onco-neurogastroenterology that require regular consideration

Issues to be addressed	Patient-physician exchange examples
Assess patient's awareness of the problem	Tell me what worries you the most
Address understanding of prognosis	We will try to minimize any functional decline
Clarification of natural history	We have several ways to control the disease
Explore patient's emotions toward gut issues	I can imagine that this is hard for you and your family
Engage caretakers in disease understanding	We should engage a partner in our discussions
Examine what matters the most	We can prioritize the control of your constipation

It is often useful to consider the patients' perspectives and concerns about their disease prior to engaging into a dialogue about diagnostic investigations, therapeutic options, and other management decisions. Table 22.3 shows a list of issues of concern for most patients with symptoms stemming from abnormal gastrointestinal sensory or motor function. Although at first glance this list may seem overwhelming, it is time-saving in the long term, since many of these issues can be addressed pre-emptively. This approach also helps patients build trust toward their neurogastroenterologist and the other members of their clinical team.

Table 22.4 is based upon the original concepts of the Kübler-Ross model of the five stages of grief, and physicians caring for patients with incurable chronic or relapsing gastrointestinal sensory and/or motor dysfunction should keep in mind the various stages of dealing with their illness [1].

Table 22.3 Issues of concern for most patients with symptoms stemming from abnormal gastrointestinal sensory or motor function

Key issues that concern patients with chronic gastrointestinal sensory and/or motor dysfunction
Fear of incontinence on public transport, shopping, vacation, and work
Fear of hospitals and treatments
Effects on employment including limitations on types of job and promotion prospects
Effects on holiday and medical and life insurance
Guilt because of the effects the above problems have on family
Overwhelming sense of isolation

Table 22.4 Stages of grief and physicians caring for patients with incurable chronic or relapsing gastrointestinal sensory and/or motor dysfunction

Stages of dealing with incurable chronic or relapsing gastrointestinal sensory and/or motor dysfunction
Initial *shock and denial* of the diagnosis; *anger* for getting the disease
Realization of possible morbidity and mortality
Loss of hope and dreams of future
Anxiety and uncertainty of prognosis and evolution
Need for daily medications, their effect(s), or treatment failures
Fear of possible need for other treatments (endoscopic and surgical)
Depression for living with chronic disease and absence of cure
Limited lifestyle because of illness
Professional and social isolation or rejection
Guilt about being a burden to partner or family

22.1 Optimizing Patient-Centered Care in Onco-neurogastroenterology

The clinical presentation of gastrointestinal sensory and/or motor dysfunction is highly heterogeneous and ranges from silent functional disturbance of propulsion, minimally symptomatic chronic infection by *H. pylori* causing intermittent dyspepsia, to significant—but intermittently recurring—dysphagia, nausea (with or without vomiting), or chronic constipation. This multitude of covert abnormalities and symptoms—that vary in sensitivity and specificity as well as frequency and severity—matched with their underlying multifactorial nature, pose significant challenges in long-term management, need for hospitalization, and prevention of complications, such as malnutrition. Therefore, to optimize a patient-centered, individualized approach, clinicians need to consider several important elements.

22.2 Strategic Management in Onco-neurogastroenterology

Strategic management of patients with gastrointestinal sensory and/or motor dysfunction should aim to maintain the best possible gut-related quality of life (QoL) in the context of an indolent or overt, chronic or relapsing neurologic disease affecting the gut. Together, healthcare providers, patients, supporting family, and caretakers should develop a successful road map by adopting a management strategy that fits their mutually agreed-upon short- and long-term health objectives, based on available resources, given the physical and emotional impact and demands of a potentially chronic illness. Figure 22.1 outlines the key advantages of this approach (Table 22.5).

Clear sense of direction Setting specific, achievable directives helps define the patient's perspective of their gut symptoms and defines a gut-specific mission and value, as compared to their overall active or inactive oncologic disease. For the patient to prosper, everyone must strive toward various multidirectional goals that are well orchestrated, non-contradictory, and thereby ultimately effective.

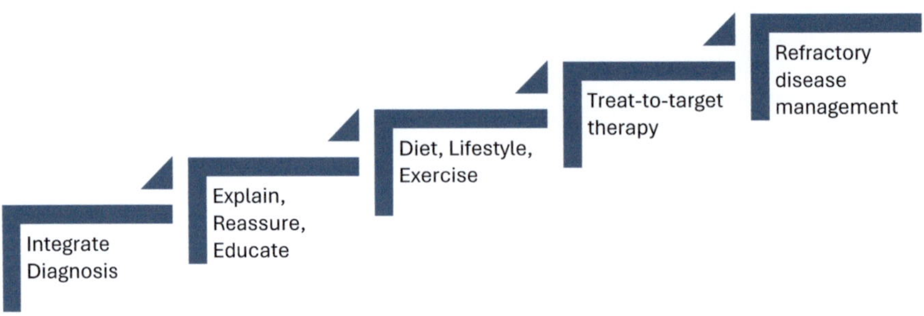

Fig. 22.1 Long-term cohesive approach to management of patients with gastrointestinal sensory and/or motor dysfunction

Table 22.5 Strategic management of patients with chronic gastrointestinal sensory and/or motor dysfunction

Strategic management of patients with chronic gastrointestinal sensory and/or motor dysfunction
Clear sense of direction (ideally patient-driven)
Enhanced decision-making (based on multifaceted information)
Improved resource allocation
Increased tolerance, adaptability, and long-term adherence to therapy
Enhanced physical and psychological performance
Facilitation of changes in management
Increased use of innovation through up-to-date medical education
Improvement in risk management
Enhanced communication
Buildup of healthcare team culture

Enhanced decision-making Healthcare providers may identify areas for improvement and chances for the patient to seize by regularly examining internal (i.e., gut neurologic function and symptoms) and external elements (i.e., new therapy options). This makes it more likely that decision-making will be informed by facts and analysis, rather than intuition.

Improved resource allocation Under the combined guidance of the healthcare team, patients may distribute their available resources efficiently to get optimal results, by selecting and coordinating their strategies aiming to accomplish an enhanced QoL. This guarantees that efforts (i.e., visits) and resources (i.e., medications, interventions) are utilized effectively.

Increased tolerance, adaptability, and long-term adherence The patient becomes more tolerant and adaptable to challenges that originate from multiple directions (i.e., gut, neuromuscular, psychological). Through efficient communication, the healthcare providers may recognize opportunities and risks and create strategies to capitalize or avoid them. This improves the patient's physical condition, well-being, and long-term adherence and clinical success.

Enhanced physical and psychological performance By setting realistic goals and developing strategies, healthcare providers can ensure that everyone in the team centering upon the patient's QoL is working toward the same aims that are not counterproductive, but synergistic. This boosts firm physical and psychological performance and ensures long-term clinical success.

Facilitation of change in management Physicians and other members of the healthcare team may identify areas of need and strategize to successfully implement changes, by assessing various internal and external variables. This ensures that the patient can adjust to shifting clinical circumstances and maintain their QoL.

Increased use of innovation Against an evolving long-term illness, well-informed healthcare providers may promote innovative approaches by examining possibilities in new research and creating plans to take advantage of them. As a discipline, onco-neurogastroenterology is poised to benefit from innovative diagnostic tools that will better quantify motility, secretion, and sensation, as well as therapeutic devices aimed to mitigating or controlling symptoms (i.e., implantable stimulators, medication-perfusing pumps). This helps the patient to stay ahead of the disease and succeed in either neutralizing its impact or improving their physical, mental, and emotional performance.

Improved risk management Regularly assessing various internal and external factors may help the healthcare team identify and mitigate risks. This reduces the consequences of potential threats while ensuring that the patient is prepared for any unexpected events that would in turn compromise their QoL, potentially leading to significant morbidity and mortality. Examples include monitoring for progressive esophageal atony and dilation in patients with achalasia, placing patients at risk for pulmonary aspiration, or, similarly, progressive colonic atony and dilation in patients with slow-transit constipation at risk for obstipation and fecal impaction.

Enhanced communication Through their individual perspectives and using effective communication, the various healthcare providers ensure that everyone on the team is working toward the same goals by establishing clear, non-competing objectives and creating strategies to attain them. This fosters better patient-centered exchange and teamwork. This is particularly applicable to cancer survivors suffering from early oncologic treatment sequela, where the neurogastroenterologist frequently assumes a dominant long-term role in management.

Buildup of a strong healthcare team culture Through strategic management, a strong healthcare team culture and collaboration can be built, particularly in a specialized onco-neurogastroenterology well-integrated in a multidisciplinary medical and surgical oncology setting. By defining focused goals, healthcare providers can ensure that everyone is working toward well-aligned aims for the patient.

In summary, a strategic management of patients with chronic gastrointestinal sensory and/or motor dysfunction plays an essential role during all stages of their disease. It helps with prevention, recognition, multi-angle initial and longitudinal disease assessment, cooperative setup of direction, decision-making, and resource allocation, thereby boosting patients' QoL, improving physical and mental performance, easing the transition to new ways of doing things, fostering creativity, decreasing anxiety about the unknown, and strengthening team bonding, through open lines of communication. Through such management, patients can avoid and respond to shifting disease conditions or complications, by considering all internal and external factors affecting their disease, designing and implementing strategies to meet goals, and monitoring their success over time. This is an ongoing process that requires leadership, clear direction, open lines of communication among providers, and quick thinking to meet shifting demands of a chronic disease state, ultimately aiming at sustaining long-term success.

Strategic management is an iterative process with multiple interdependent steps that, given the evolving nature of the disease, should be periodically reassessed. The major phases are described in Fig. 22.2. The first phase is the creation of its overall structure, during which a patient and their healthcare team generate a multidisciplinary, thorough, and realistic strategy to seamlessly fulfill all their goals and objectives. After such objectives are established, then strategic options must be identified and assessed for their safety, efficacy, feasibility, and acceptance. Depending on the disease and its clinical evolution, goal adjustments are made at least once yearly. This approach has been successfully implemented in other chronic diseases [2].

There are several key steps in structuring the correct management strategy process, and modifications are frequently needed, given the chronicity and unpredictability of the underlying sensory and motor gut manifestations.

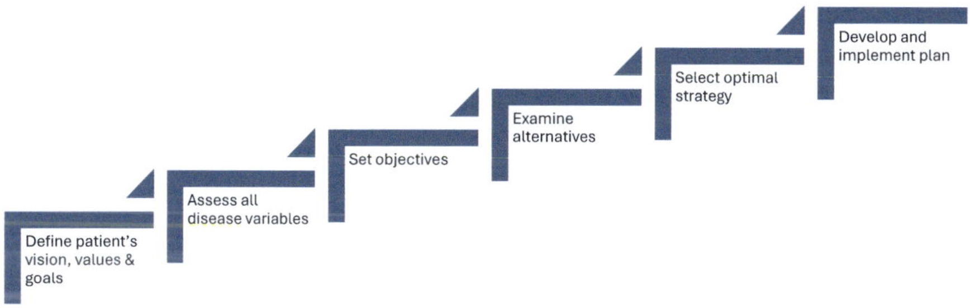

Fig. 22.2 Management strategies in onco-neurogastroenterology

Define the patient's vision, values, and goals The patient's vision, values, and goals provide a key framework for strategic planning. The vision is based on the patient's understanding of the nature, severity, and projected natural history of the disease and its specific manifestations, both neurologic (i.e., pain, dysesthesias) and gut-related (i.e., dysphagia, nausea, constipation), and identifies its long-term objectives. The patient's values help mark the significance and impact of the gut disease beyond that of the neurologic (motor and sensory) manifestations, in turn guiding gut-directed therapy.

Assess all disease variables An assessment of all disease variables involves looking for any external and internal factors to identify therapeutic opportunities and avoid risks. This requires looking at the speed, pattern, and severity of disease, the patients' needs and aspirations, conflicting pre-existing or new therapies (i.e., immunotherapy), disease control at times requiring additional resective surgery, prevailing home and environmental circumstances, home and personal resource availability, physical and emotional strength, mobility, and nutritional status.

Set objectives In setting their objectives based on analysis of all variables, the patient and their care team will also need to consider realistic, organ-focused, and easily quantifiable parameters (i.e., frequency and degree of fecal incontinence) that will need practical periodic reassessment, both clinically and by objective ancillary testing.

Examine alternatives The patient and their healthcare team should periodically identify strategic alternatives (i.e., use of non-pharmacologic alternatives for constipation, such as the vibrating capsule), based on their objectives. This involves generating and evaluating alternative strategies, with their related benefits and risks, which could help the patient achieve their goals. The evaluation and selection of strategic alternatives (i.e., resources, expertise) is always based on their availability, feasibility, suitability, and acceptability and in alignment with the patients' perspectives.

Develop and implement an action plan This is accomplished by allocating resources, outlining roles, establishing deadlines, and setting up feedback loops to track progress. The plan is then communicated to all who are working toward its achievement. SWOT analysis, a management framework widely used in business, can evaluate the patients' strengths, weaknesses, opportunities, and threats, helping to understand the multitude and sometimes conflicting disease variables and build plans to capitalize on opportunities, rectify weaknesses, and mitigate risks (Fig. 22.3).

Using SWOT on every patient with gastrointestinal sensory and/or motor dysfunction, healthcare providers can highlight existing strengths, such as the identification of manageable prodromal or early neuromuscular and sensory compromise, nutritional strength, and preserved physical and mental conditioning; identify weaknesses, such as lack of proper and adequate physical environment, resources, or support, cognitive disabilities, or unwillingness for collaboration with the healthcare team; explore opportunities for new medical (oncologic) therapies and minimally invasive (endoscopic) or surgical interventions, including participation in clinical research trials; and, finally, identify threats, such as risk of pulmonary aspiration, decubitus ulcer formation, and malnutrition. Because of the possibility of neuro-degeneration over time (i.e., after radiation injury) or intervening additional surgical interventions compromising structure and function, SWOT analysis needs to be repeated at least yearly, so relevant adjustments and preventative steps can be timely implemented [3].

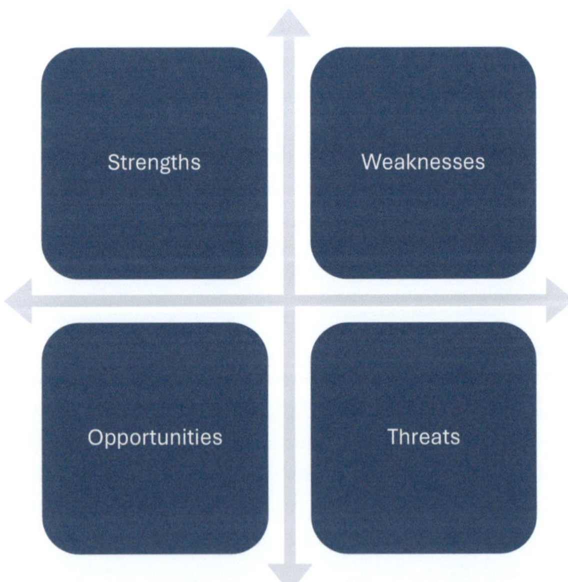

Fig. 22.3 SWOT analysis in onco-neurogastroenterology

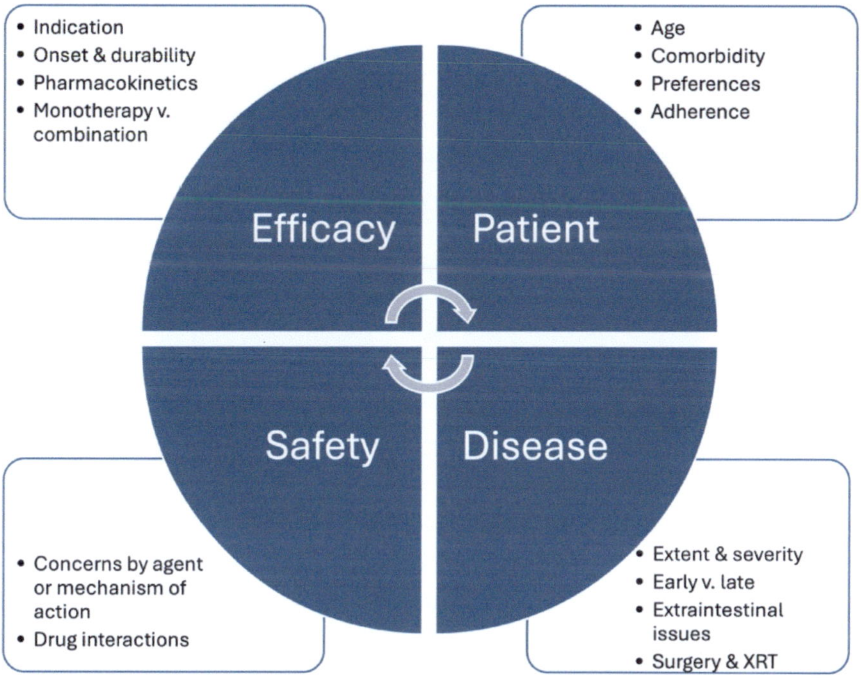

Fig. 22.4 Considerations prior to therapy in patients with symptoms of gastrointestinal sensory and motor dysfunction

22.3 Pieces of the Therapy Choice Puzzle in Onco-neurogastroenterology

Figure 22.4 highlights the various considerations prior to therapy in patients with symptoms of gastrointestinal sensory and motor dysfunction, specifically the patient, disease, safety, and efficacy. Because of the complexities of the patient population, such considerations are important prior to introducing any therapy. Since there is limited outcome data in most instances, and after discussion with patients, carefully designed empirical trials aiming at improving QoL are encouraged.

22.4 Role of Integrated Onco-neurogastroenterology Centers

Integrated Onco-neurogastroenterology Centers (IONCs) An IONC is a multidisciplinary team with expertise, skill, range, and facilities necessary to achieve optimal outcomes in patients with gastrointestinal sensory and motor dysfunction efficiently and expeditiously (Fig. 22.5). Within an IONC, patients presenting with

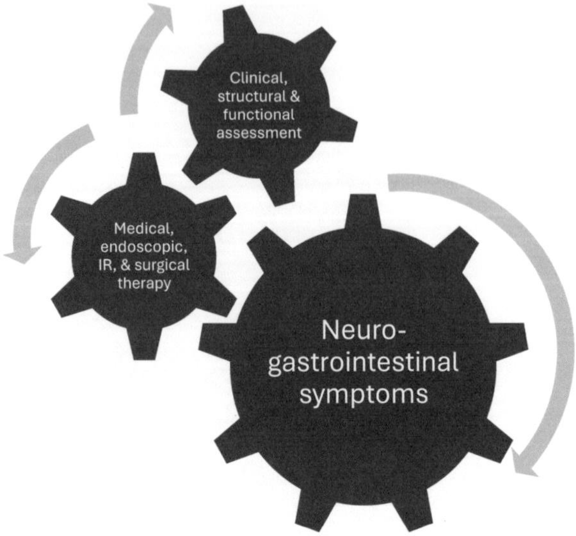

Fig. 22.5 Essential elements of an IONC, incorporating a multidisciplinary team with expertise, skill, range, and facilities necessary to achieve optimal outcomes in patients with gastrointestinal sensory and motor dysfunction

neurogastrointestinal symptoms undergo a detailed clinical, functional, and structural evaluation from mouth to anus, prior to implementation of a properly tailored medical, endoscopic, interventional radiologic, or surgical therapy. Serving as a core, the IONC clinical practice also supports related biotechnological and or pharmacological research and innovation, as well as public and physician education. Referrals to the IONC may be primary, either from primary care or self-initiated, or secondary from other specialty practices, to reassess patients who have previously failed therapies and to manage complex or complicated cases. Such integrated centers are presently at their budding phases of evolution in major cancer centers, but they are expected to grow significantly over the next decade given the increased recognition of patients with gastrointestinal sensory and motor dysfunction and expanding therapeutic options. This multidisciplinary concept has been quite successful in tertiary gastroenterology centers in other areas of the specialty [4].

The IONC bidirectionally interfaces with the referring community, as well as with other disciplines, beyond the relevant medical and surgical oncology services, such as the GI physiology laboratory, therapeutic endoscopy, and interventional radiology, and other supportive services, such as physical and occupational services and pain management. Through ongoing interactions, IONC has the potential to enhance QoL through pharmacologic and biotechnology options emanating from research (Fig. 22.6).

The fundamental goals of the IONC are to provide value for patients with onco-neurogastroenterologic diseases, streamlining complex diagnostic investigations and expediting therapies aiming at reducing costs while improving clinical outcomes, and to accelerate knowledge generation through robust interaction and cross-training across disciplines [5]. The scope is provision of organ-specific care

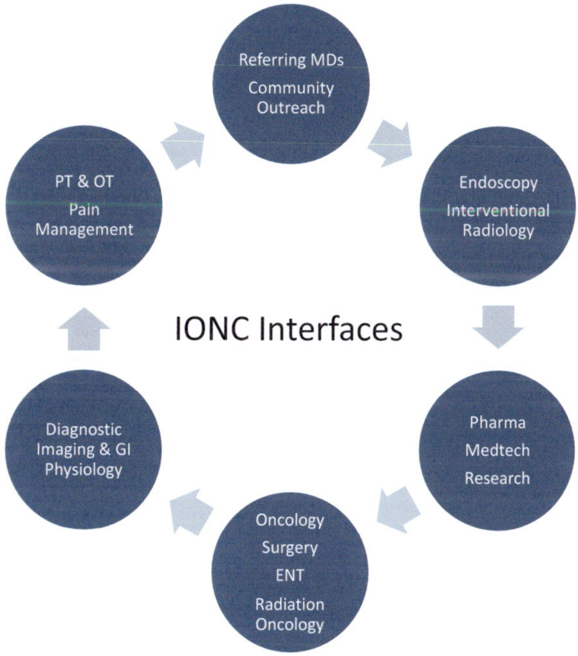

Fig. 22.6 Various disciplines within IONC involved in the care of patients with gastrointestinal sensory and motor dysfunction

through a highly organized team that delivers coordinated care, with lower costs and by negotiating bundled payments with employers and payers. The IONC creates synergies that consolidate volume by condition, coordinating care across sites, thereby allowing value creation, and it can be impactful for large metropolitan areas with adequate geographic population density as well as rural areas by efficiently coordinating a complex visit and evaluation. The core IONC clinical practice manages both primary referrals and secondary/tertiary issues, such as the assessment of medical or surgical failures and the treatment of complications (Fig. 22.7). Ideally, every patient with gastrointestinal sensory and motor dysfunction should be managed by an onco-neurogastroenterologist. Such engagement will allow a more meticulous assessment of underlying gastrointestinal issues and further assessment of the gut physiology using specialty tools, as well as imaging of the gut, as needed. Based on this, diet, special drug therapy, endoscopy, and/or surgery may be needed. Nutrition, pain management, exercise, and physical and occupational therapy are then coordinated under expert guidance. This is particularly true in the pre-cancer and survivorship phases, where acute oncologic and/or surgical care is not a priority.

Advanced (dedicated) fellowship in onco-neurogastroenterology In the setting of an IONC, a third year dedicated fellowship, offering special training in onco-neurogastroenterology, is poised to cross-pollenate clinical and research activities for junior gastroenterologists interested in the field. Such a 1-year program (as part of a subspecialty-focused third year) will comply with ABIM requirement for

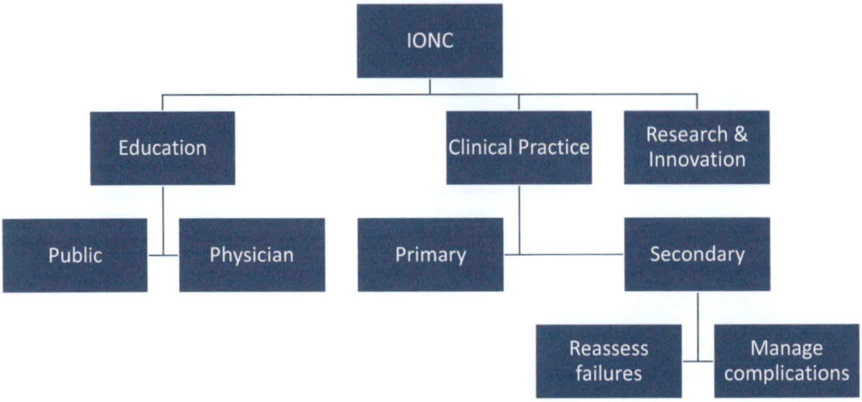

Fig. 22.7 Clinical, educational, and research activities of an integrated onco-neurogastroenterology center (IONC)

Table 22.6 Essential elements of a dedicated fellowship in onco-neurogastroenterology

Therapeutic gastrointestinal endoscopy
Diagnostic imaging
High-resolution esophageal, colonic, and anorectal manometry
Impedance planimetry (EndoFLIP)
Ambulatory esophageal pH monitoring (impedance and wireless)
Clinical trial methodology
General, thoracic, and colorectal surgery
Medical oncology
Radiation oncology
Clinical and translational research in onco-neurogastroenterology
Quality metrics in onco-neurogastroenterology
Basic science in onco-neurogastroenterology

gastroenterology board certification and will be aimed to generate subspecialists in onco-neurogastroenterology who will have a multidisciplinary clinical exposure and education that is based on a diverse curriculum and who will have devoted a minimum of 50% time in basic, clinical, and/or translational research. Institutionally supported and/or sponsored by industry partners, such training can lead to a society-endorsed certification (i.e., American Neurogastroenterology and Motility Society, ANMS). Table 22.6 outlines the various rotations of the fellowship. Broadly described here, the curriculum of such an advanced fellowship in onco-neurogastroenterology has a multidisciplinary content and is based on direct familiarity in both medical, oncologic, and surgical aspects of disease. Fellows rotate in oncology and therapeutic endoscopic settings and also in the operating room and surgical wards.

22.5 Intensive Care

Neurogastrointestinal problems in the intensive care unit (ICU) setting present a unique challenge because critically ill cancer patients often cannot verbalize their symptoms, yet these problems can significantly increase their mortality risk. This increased risk of mortality related to neurogastrointestinal problems is associated with increasing risks of infection, prolonged mechanical ventilation, and an increasing total hospital stay [6]. In critically ill patients, the degree of intestinal dysmotility is directly related to the severity of illness. The most common motility problems encountered in the ICU are gastroesophageal reflux disease (GERD), gastroparesis, ileus, and acute colonic pseudo-obstruction [7].

Figure 22.8 highlights the significant impact of critical illness and mechanical ventilation on the esophageal function and consideration in prevention and management. Similarly, Fig. 22.9 highlights factors contributing to gastric emptying delay in the ventilated ICU patient and steps to be considered.

Adynamic ileus, or gut hypomotility in the absence of mechanical obstruction, is encountered in 50–80% of ICU patients, and it often correlates with the severity of the underlying critical illness. The etiology of ileus in the critical care setting is typically multifactorial, and it involves the activation of inhibitory sympathetic input and the release of inflammatory mediators that inhibit gut motility. The use of narcotics or anticholinergics or metabolic disturbances in such patients may contribute to the severity of ileus and its prolonged natural history leading to longer ICU stays. The use of various pharmacologic agents has been variably successful [8–11].

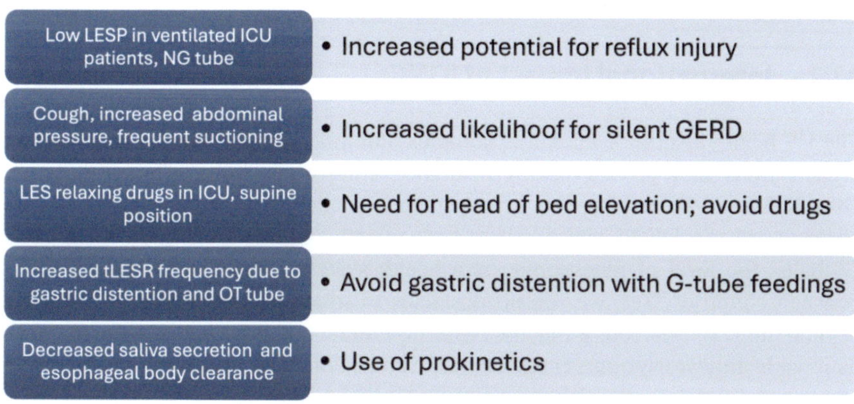

Fig. 22.8 Key considerations on GERD in the ventilated patient

Factor	Intervention
Supine position	Head of bed elevation
Frequent oropharyngeal suctioning	Minimize
Obesity Advanced age	
Severity of critical illness, increase intracranial pressure	Monitor
Ascites, fluid overload	Minimize fluids
Abnormal antropyloric responses to small-volume enteral feeding Increase in pyloric pressure waves	Prokinetcs
Hyperglycemia Electrolyte disturbances	Correct/prevent

Fig. 22.9 Factors contributing to gastric emptying delay in the ventilated ICU patient and interventions to be considered

22.6 Remote Care

Travel may be cumbersome for patients with gastrointestinal sensory and motor dysfunction, and remote clinic-to-clinic telehealth visit to evaluate the multimodal function in such patients is not only feasible but it also helps in improving access to care and research participation, similar to other chronic neurological conditions [12]. However, because functional testing is currently centralized, periodic in-person visits are still needed to monitor for disease evolution and guide therapy.

22.7 International Impact of IONCs

The US health insurance market is complex, comprising many health maintenance organizations and private health insurance companies with different policies. Overall, US physicians have negative perceptions about the effect of managed care on access to specialists, and this may have negative implications for IONCs [13]. Globally, the level of gatekeeping is a health system decision and varies widely between countries. Yet, we see no obstacles in implementing the IONC concept beyond the USA. Indeed, it may be easier to initiate and promote in countries with national healthcare systems (i.e., Canada, Europe) provided that the multiple disciplines involved are available in one geographical area or major cancer center. Outcomes of course will depend on the baseline level of care that is provided before the IONC is formed, which is variable within, as well as across, countries. A balanced assessment that includes the value to patients (e.g., satisfaction, quality of life), the clinical outcomes (e.g., morbidity and mortality reduction, QoL improvement), and the fiscal implications will need to be properly designed and implemented, based on the specifics of geography, disease burden, and overall healthcare delivery models [14]. We anticipate that patients seen in an IONC would have comparable or superior levels of satisfaction, by utilizing less resources and thereby spending less, as compared to those seen outside the center receiving fee-for-service care, akin to the pilot results on accountable care organizations have reported [15].

References

1. Kübler-Ross E. On death and dying. Scribner; 2014.
2. Voigt I, Fischer S, Proschmann U, Konofalska U, Richter P, Schlieter H, Berger T, Meuth SG, Hartung HP, Akgün K, Ziemssen T. Consensus quality indicators for monitoring multiple sclerosis. Lancet Reg Health Eur. 2024;40:100891. https://doi.org/10.1016/j.lanepe.2024.100891. PMID: 38585674; PMCID: PMC10998202.
3. de-Madaria E, Mira JJ, Carrillo I, Afif W, Ang D, Antelo M, Bollipo S, Castells A, Chahal P, Heinrich H, Law JK, van Leerdam ME, Lens S, Pannala R, Park SH, Rabiee A, Savarino EV, Singh VK, Vargo J, Charabaty A, Drenth JPH. The present and future of gastroenterology and hepatology: an international SWOT analysis (the GASTROSWOT project). Lancet Gastroenterol Hepatol. 2022;7(5):485–94. https://doi.org/10.1016/S2468-1253(21)00442-8. Epub 2022 Mar 2. PMID: 35247318.
4. Triadafilopoulos G, Clarke J, Hawn M. Whole greater than the parts: integrated esophageal centers (IEC) and advanced training in esophageal diseases. Dis Esophagus. 2017;30(10):1–9. https://doi.org/10.1093/dote/dox084. PMID: 28859396.
5. Ward L, Powell RE, Scharf ML, Chapman A, Kavuru M. Patient-centered specialty practice: defining the role of specialists in value-based health care. Chest. 2017;151(4):930–5. https://doi.org/10.1016/j.chest.2017.01.006. Epub 2017 Jan 13. PMID: 28089817.
6. Fruhwald S, Kainz J. Effect of ICU interventions on gastrointestinal motility. Curr Opin Crit Care. 2010;16:159–64. Reintam A, Parm P, Redlich U, et al. Gastrointestinal failure in intensive care: a retrospective clinical study in three different intensive care units in Germany and Estonia. BMC Gastroenterol. 2006;6:19.
7. Madl C, Druml W. Gastrointestinal disorders of the critically ill. Systemic consequences of ileus. Best Pract Res Clin Gastroenterol. 2003;17:445–56.
8. van der Spoel JI, Oudemans-van Straaten HM, Kuiper MA, van Roon EN, Zandstra DF, van der Voort PH. Laxation of critically ill patients with lactulose or polyethylene glycol: a two-center randomized, double-blind, placebo-controlled trial. Crit Care Med. 2007;35(12):2726–31. https://doi.org/10.1097/01.CCM.0000287526.08794.29.
9. van Bree SH, Nemethova A, Cailotto C, Gomez-Pinilla PJ, Matteoli G, Boeckxstaens GE. New therapeutic strategies for postoperative ileus. Nat Rev Gastroenterol Hepatol. 2012;9(11):675–83. https://doi.org/10.1038/nrgastro.2012.134. Epub 2012 Jul 17. PMID: 22801725.
10. Bungard TJ, Kale-Pradhan PB. Prokinetic agents for the treatment of postoperative ileus in adults: a review of the literature. Pharmacotherapy. 1999;19(4):416–23. https://doi.org/10.1592/phco.19.6.416.31040. PMID: 10212012.
11. Traut U, Brügger L, Kunz R, Pauli-Magnus C, Haug K, Bucher HC, Koller MT. Systemic prokinetic pharmacologic treatment for postoperative adynamic ileus following abdominal surgery in adults. Cochrane Database Syst Rev. 2008;(1):CD004930. https://doi.org/10.1002/14651858.CD004930.pub3. PMID: 18254064.
12. Virmani T, Pillai L, Smith V, Glover A, Abrams D, Farmer P, Syed S, Spencer HJ, Kemp A, Barron K, Murray T, Morris B, Bowers B, Ward A, Imus T, Larson-Prior LJ, Lotia M, Prior F. Feasibility of regional center telehealth visits utilizing a rural research network in people with Parkinson's disease. J Clin Transl Sci. 2024;8(1):e63. https://doi.org/10.1017/cts.2024.498. PMID: 38655451; PMCID: PMC11036429.

13. Christianson JB, Warrick LH, Wholey DR. Physicians' perceptions of managed care: a review of the literature. Med Care Res Rev. 2005;62(6):635–75. https://doi.org/10.1177/1077558705281060. PMID: 16330819.
14. Vize R. Financial benefits of integration: a case of wishful thinking? BMJ. 2014;348:g3661. https://doi.org/10.1136/bmj.g3661. PMID: 24895204.
15. Nyweide DJ, Lee W, Cuerdon TT, Pham HH, Cox M, Rajkumar R, Conway PH. Association of Pioneer Accountable Care Organizations vs traditional Medicare fee for service with spending, utilization, and patient experience. JAMA. 2015;313(21):2152–61. https://doi.org/10.1001/jama.2015.4930. PMID: 25938875.

Illustrative Cases in Onco-neurogastroenterology

23

George Triadafilopoulos, David M. Richards, Mehnaz A. Shafi, and Lavanya Viswanathan

23.1 Hypopharynx and Esophagus

23.1.1 Oropharyngeal Dysphagia

A 39-year-old woman presented with mostly intermittent solid dysphagia and pill dysphagia after resection of cerebral meningioma. Endoscopy was normal. There is retention of barium tablet in the valleculae, explaining her dysphagia (Fig. 23.1).

23.1.2 Ineffective Esophageal Motility (IEM)

A 35-year-old man, with a personal history of testicular seminoma (s/p orchiectomy and radiation 15 years prior), presented with acid regurgitation and excessive throat clearing. Endoscopy was normal. HREM (Fig. 23.2) showed IEM % failed contractions (70) and mean DCI (411). On esophageal ambulatory pH monitoring (not shown), the % 24-h pH <4 was 3 (normal). There was no need for PPI therapy. Postural and dietary measures were used for symptom relief.

G. Triadafilopoulos (✉) · D. M. Richards · M. A. Shafi · L. Viswanathan
Department of Gastroenterology, Hepatology and Nutrition, UT MD Anderson Cancer Center, Houston, TX, USA
e-mail: gtriadafilopoulo@mdanderson.org

G. Triadafilopoulos (ed.), *Onco-Neurogastroenterology*,
https://doi.org/10.1007/978-3-031-98848-6_23

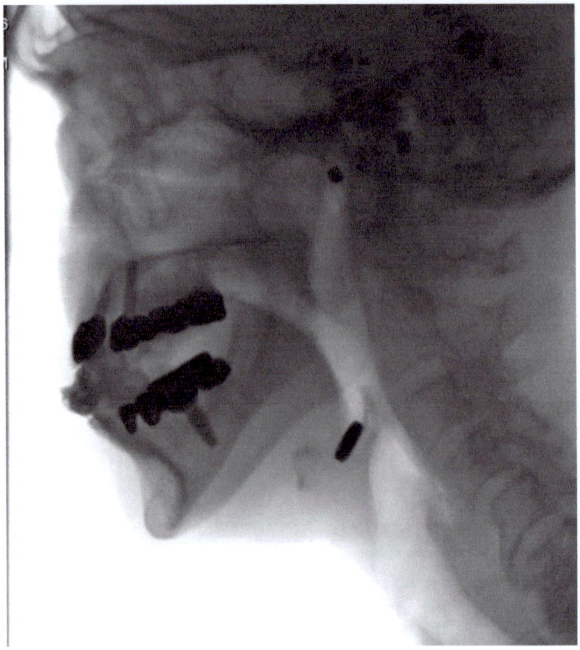

Fig. 23.1 Barium tablet radiography revealing the etiology of oropharyngeal dysphagia. The barium tablet was transiently held up in the valleculae prior to dissolving. She was treated with exercises to improve oropharyngeal clearance, slow and careful mastication, and liquid assistance with meals

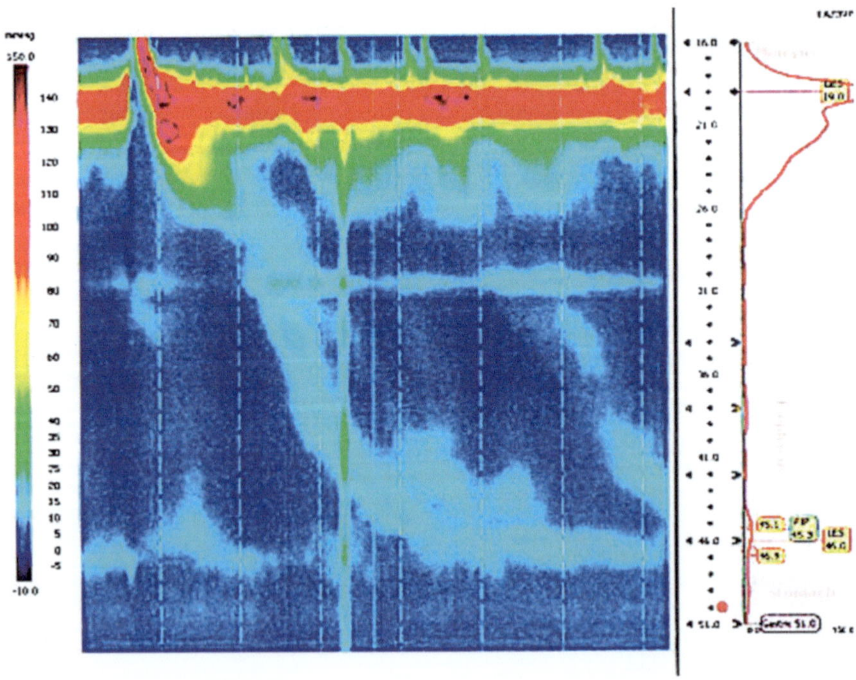

Fig. 23.2 HREM revealing IEM

23.1.3 Ineffective Esophageal Motility (IEM)

A 56-year-old woman presented with intermittent dysphagia to solids and liquids that was progressive over the past 3 years. She also reported mild heartburn and unpleasant regurgitation, particularly nocturnal. She is a breast cancer survivor s/p right mastectomy and radiation that she received 18 years ago. An endoscopy was normal, without evidence of esophagitis or stricture. On the high-resolution esophageal manometry (Fig. 23.3), frequent (>50%) completely failed peristalsis is seen upon swallowing and is associated with lower esophageal sphincter (LES) hypotonicity. IEM appears to be an early, primary event, eventually associated with pathologic acid exposure, particularly supine. In this case, 96-h pH monitoring (not shown) was pathologic (% 24-h pH <4 was 7.6; normal <6%); abnormal impedance (in violet) is also seen, both contributing to positional regurgitation. The patient was treated with aggressive lifestyle and dietary measures and twice daily PPI therapy.

23.1.4 Esophageal Candidiasis

A 51-year-old man presented with acute odynophagia and chest burning several days after initiation of intensive remission induction for recently diagnosed acute myeloblastic leukemia. An endoscopy showed *Candida* esophagitis (Fig. 23.4), a common cause for painful swallowing in this setting. Treatment with fluconazole led to resolution of his symptoms.

23.1.5 Hypercontractile (Corkscrew) Esophagus (HE)

A 46-year-old woman, s/p lumpectomy for breast cancer and without evidence of recurrent disease, presented with difficulty swallowing and retrosternal, noncardiac chest pain. She denied heartburn, regurgitation, or weight loss. Endoscopy was reportedly normal. Simultaneous contractions resulting in a "rosary bead" or

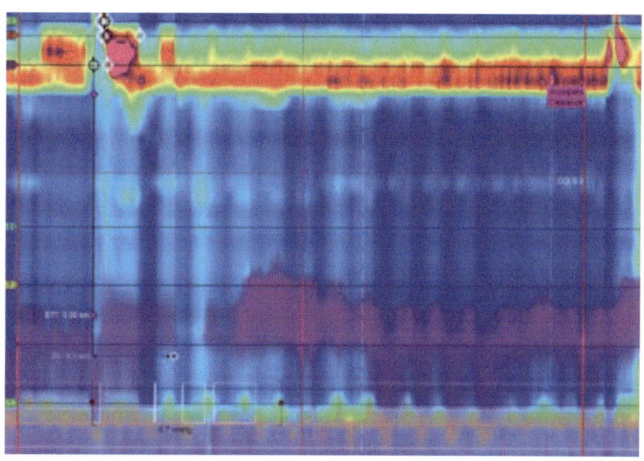

Fig. 23.3 HREM and impedance tracing revealing failed esophageal body peristalsis and LES hypotonicity with retrograde fluid movement upon swallowing

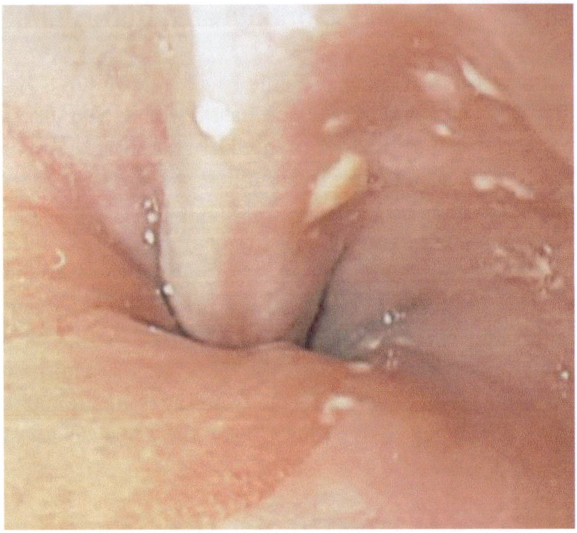

Fig. 23.4 White plaques in the esophagus strongly suggestive of *Candida* infection

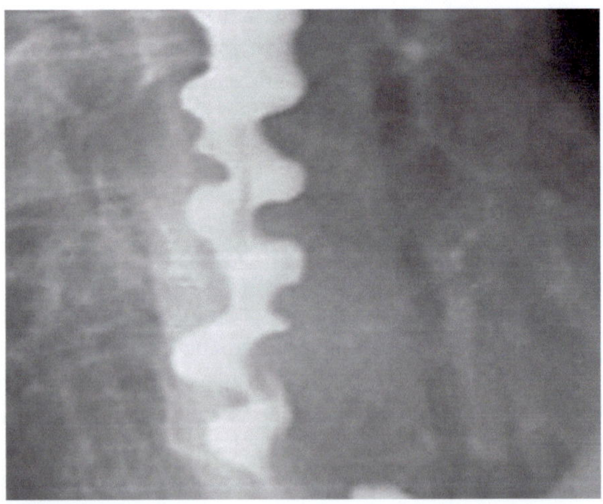

Fig. 23.5 Barium esophagram revealing corkscrew esophagus

"corkscrew" appearance of the esophagus were noted on barium esophagram (Fig. 23.5). She did not respond to calcium channel blockers, and she was treated with endoscopic intramuscular Botox (200 IU) as 25 IU aliquots along the distal esophagus (not the EGJ) in a linear set of injections.

23.1.6 Displaced Nissen Fundoplication Simulating Achalasia

A 79-year-old woman underwent successful endoscopic eradication therapy for stage I esophageal adenocarcinoma 8 years prior, followed by laparoscopic fundoplication for GERD. She now presents with severe regurgitation and intermittent dysphagia without weight loss despite treatment with esomeprazole 40 mg orally twice daily, which effectively controlled her intra-esophageal pH (right panel) (Fig. 23.6). Manometry revealed type II achalasia.

23.1.7 Dislodgement of the Bravo pH

A 36-year-old woman with breast cancer underwent a 96-h ambulatory esophageal pH monitoring because of episodic chest discomfort and non-productive cough suggestive of GERD. Official reading of the study suggested the diagnosis of GERD. However, upon subsequent review, dislodgement of the Bravo pH probe from the esophagus (E) into the stomach (S) and subsequent passage into the duodenum (D) and jejunum (J) was seen (Fig. 23.7).

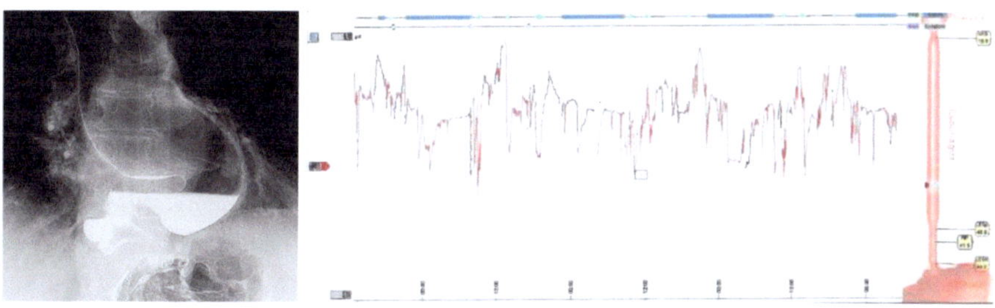

Fig. 23.6 Left panel shows a dilated, sigmoid esophagus, with free barium flow through a displaced fundoplication. Right panel shows a well-controlled distal esophageal pH (% 24-h pH <4.0 of 0%; normal <1.6%) while on esomeprazole 40 mg twice daily

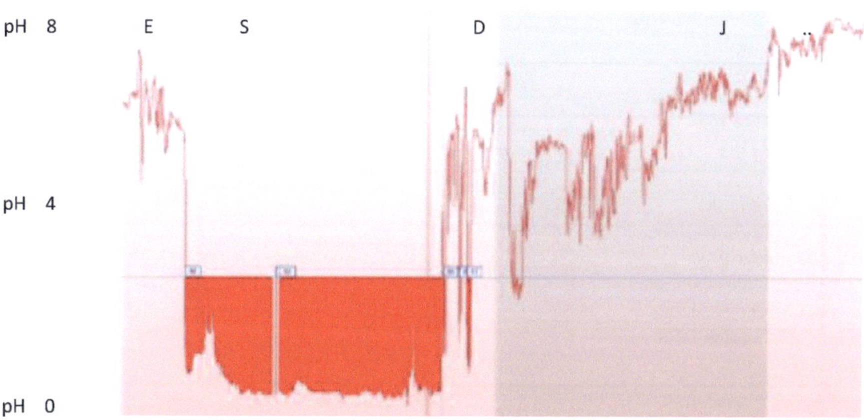

Fig. 23.7 The ongoing ambulatory recording starts with neutral pH (probe in the esophagus), then drops to a persistently acidic one (stomach), and then, suddenly, as it enters the duodenum, becomes alkaline, and increasingly so, as the detached pH capsule enters into the jejunum (J) by the peristaltic wave. It is essential that pH recordings are reviewed prior to reporting, since such occurrence may be misleading and suggestive of esophageal pathologic acid exposure. If this occurs, a repeat study is recommended

23.1.8 Distal Esophageal Spasm (DES)

A 46-year-old woman with prior history of bilateral mastectomy for breast cancer presented with episodic chest pain simulating angina, associated with dysphagia and, at times, odynophagia. Endoscopy showed severe esophageal body spasticity, confirmed manometrically as distal esophageal spasm (DES), without mucosal changes suggestive of acid reflux (Fig. 23.8). She was successfully treated with endoscopic intramuscular Botox (200 IU) as 25 IU aliquots along the distal esophagus (not the EGJ) in a linear set of injections, 2 cm apart from each other.

23.1.9 Distal Esophageal Ring and Hiatal Hernia

A 56-year-old woman with a multifocal T2 N1 M0 invasive ductal carcinoma of the left breast underwent a left mastectomy and axillary lymph node dissection in 2009 and then completed 5 years of aromatase inhibitor therapy. She presented in 2025 with solid food dysphagia and regurgitation. A single- and double-contrast evaluation of the esophagus demonstrates a moderate hiatal hernia. A distal esophageal ring is noted. The barium pill remains trapped at the distal esophagus mucosal ring above the hiatal hernia. The barium pill remained trapped and partially dissolved and required a water bolus to wash it down (Fig. 23.9). She was treated with balloon dilation of the esophagogastric junction (EGJ) to 16 mm diameter with resolution of her symptoms.

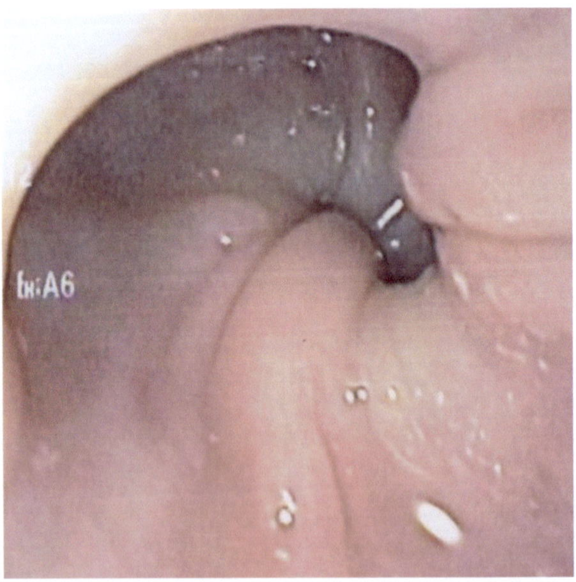

Fig. 23.8 Endoscopic appearance of esophageal spastic dysmotility. High-intensity lumen-obliterating contractions are seen during the inspection of the esophagus, even with the patient being under propofol anesthesia. The mucosal integrity is preserved. Unless assessed by HREM, the clinician cannot distinguish DES from HE

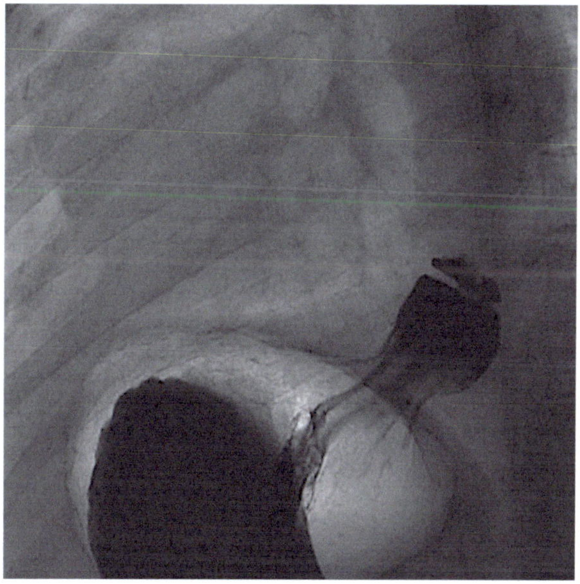

Fig. 23.9 Single barium swallow showing a moderate sliding hiatal hernia, a distal esophageal ring, and a partly dissolving barium tablet just proximal to it

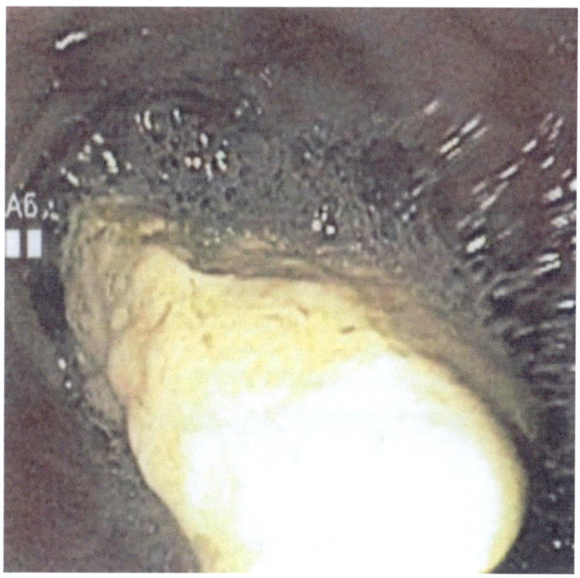

Fig. 23.10 Endoscopic image of complete food impaction. The food bolus and secretions are evident, but the underlying etiology is not shown, and it needs to be entertained prior to intervention

23.1.10 Esophageal Food Bolus Impaction

An 82-year-old man with untreated long-standing dysphagia presented acutely with complete inability to swallow food and oral secretions. A large chicken meat bolus was found on endoscopy (Fig. 23.10), and it was extracted with complete relief. A distal esophageal (Schatzki's) ring and a sliding hiatal hernia were seen distal to the

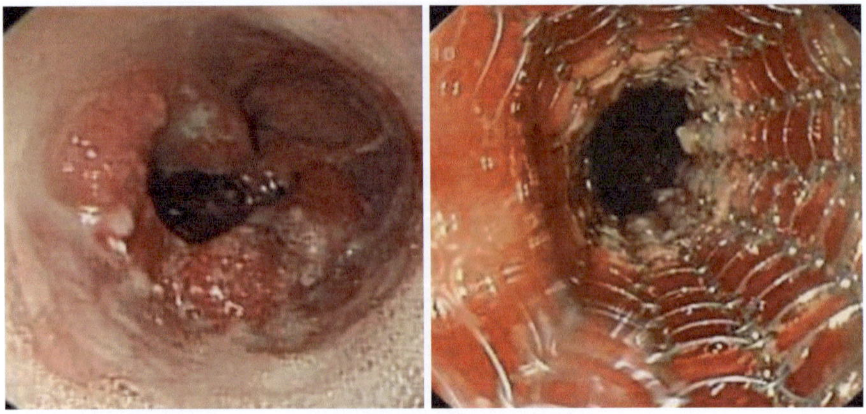

Fig. 23.11 (Left) Endoscopic appearance of EGJ adenocarcinoma compromising the luminal diameter. (Right) Endoscopic appearance of the distal esophagus after placement of a self-expanding metal stent

impaction (not shown). He was eventually treated with endoscopic EGJ balloon dilation to 18 mm diameter, followed by omeprazole 20 mg orally daily with long-term symptom resolution.

23.1.11 Self-Expanding Metal Stenting (SEMS) of the Esophagus

An 84-year-old man presented with solid food dysphagia and weight loss over several months. He has a history of metastatic esophagogastric junction adenocarcinoma. Due to associated comorbidities, it was elected to proceed with self-expanding metal stenting (SEMS) for palliation (Fig. 23.11). The first rule in onco-neurogastroenterology is the assessment for structural mucosal abnormalities causing symptoms. After stent placement, patient experienced resolution of dysphagia, but new onset of mid-chest pain, heartburn, and acid regurgitation, which were treated with twice daily PPI with partial success. Due to the expansion of the stent, some patients may require pain management using narcotics for relief.

23.1.12 Post-esophagectomy Aspiration Pneumonitis

A 53-year-old woman presented with recurrent productive cough and dyspnea secondary to episodic aspiration pneumonitis. Eleven years prior, she had undergone an Ivor Lewis esophagogastrectomy. Surgical pathologic staging was T0N1 adenocarcinoma with 1 of 19 positive lymph nodes positive for metastatic involvement. As part of the evaluation, CT of the chest post-esophagectomy and gastric pull-through

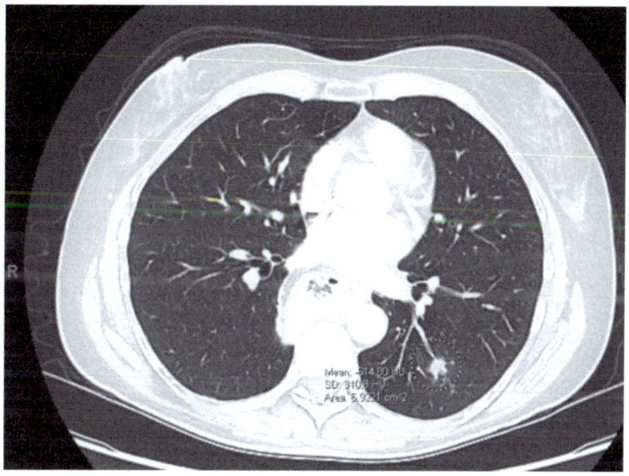

Fig. 23.12 CT of the chest post-esophagectomy and gastric pull-through showing the intrathoracic stomach with opacities in the left lower lobe representing aspiration pneumonitis (circles)

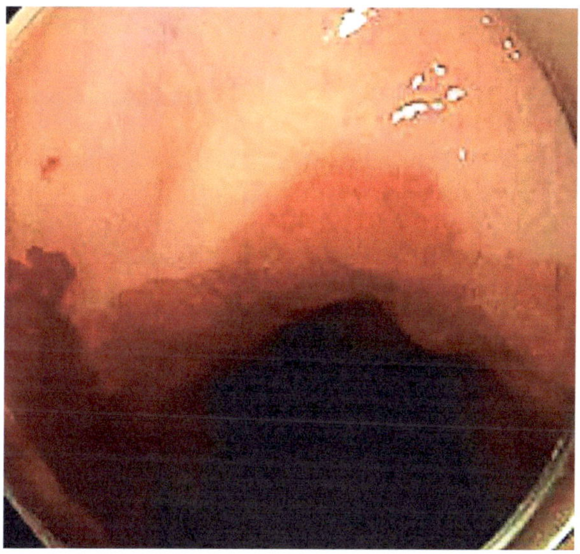

Fig. 23.13 Endoscopic appearance of an intact esophagogastric anastomosis without stricture

with omental flap coverage of the anastomosis showed no evidence of recurrent esophageal adenocarcinoma. There was residual food debris in the intrathoracic stomach with opacities in the left lower lobe representing aspiration pneumonitis (circles, Fig. 23.12). She complained of dysphagia and GERD symptoms despite PPI therapy. On endoscopy, the esophagogastric anastomosis was intact (Fig. 23.13). Dilation was performed in the lower third of the esophagus with a Savary dilator with no resistance felt at 17 mm. Lifestyle (postural) and dietary measures were emphasized, together with continuation of PPI therapy aiming at reducing the volume of gastric acid and fluid secretion.

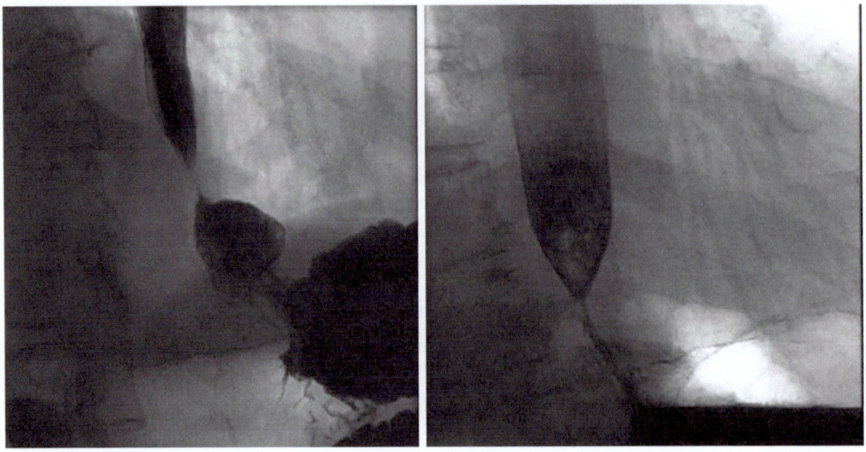

Fig. 23.14 Barium tablet esophagram revealing a sliding hiatal hernia (left) and a stagnating and disintegrating barium tablet (white bubbles) in the distal esophagus above a stricture (right)

23.1.13 Hiatal Hernia and Distal Esophageal Stricture

A 49-year-old man presented with dysphagia and heartburn for several weeks. He had been diagnosed with *H. pylori* infection with gastric intestinal metaplasia 2 years prior and was treated with triple therapy, leading to eradication of the infection. Endoscopy at this time revealed a sliding hiatal hernia and LA grade D esophagitis (not shown). Severe GERD may occur after *H. pylori* eradication, and monitoring is required to avoid complications. Esophagram (Fig. 23.14) with barium tablet confirmed the endoscopic findings of a sliding hiatal hernia (left) and a stagnating and disintegrating barium tablet in the distal esophagus (right). Esophageal through-the-scope (TTS) balloon dilation to 17 mm diameter was successfully performed, and long-term PPI therapy was initiated with rapid symptom relief.

23.1.14 Severe Erosive (Emetogenic) Esophagitis

A 67-year-old woman undergoing chemotherapy for breast cancer developed severe heartburn, lower chest pain, and acid regurgitation after episodes of repetitive severe nausea and vomiting. She denied any prior history of GERD. An endoscopy revealed severe esophagitis (Fig. 23.15). She was treated with antiemetics thrice daily and twice daily proton pump inhibitors with improvement and managed to complete all her chemotherapy cycles.

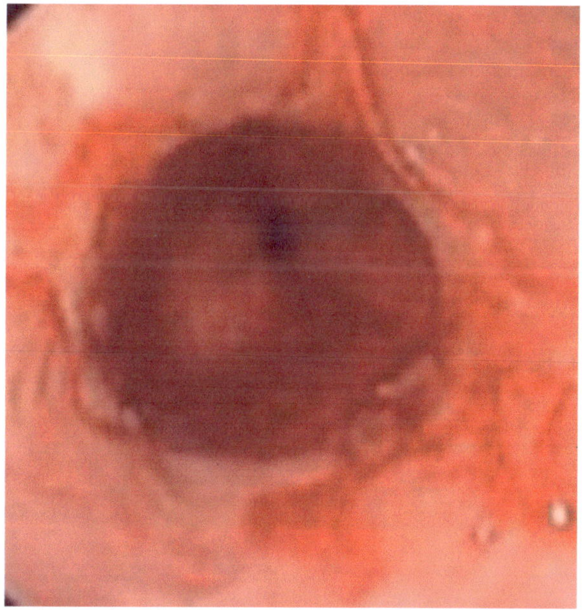

Fig. 23.15 Severe erosive esophagitis in the setting of severe, chemotherapy-induced nausea and vomiting. Linear, confluent, whitish ulcers emanating from the EGJ are noted (LA.C)

23.1.15 GERD with Normal High-Resolution Esophageal Manometry

A 59-year-old woman presented with intermittent dysphagia and heartburn for several years. She is a breast cancer survivor, free of disease after right lumpectomy, lymph node dissection, and chemotherapy without radiation. Endoscopy was normal (not shown). A high-resolution esophageal manometry is an integral part of the evaluation of patients with intermittent dysphagia, and in this case, it was normal. A pH monitoring study however showed moderate acid reflux, with symptom association probability of 96%. Despite her acid reflux severity, the lower esophageal sphincter pressure (LESP) was normal (Fig. 23.16).

23.1.16 A 96-h Ambulatory Esophageal pH Monitoring While on PPI Therapy for GERD

A 53-year-old man presented with long-standing history of heartburn and acid regurgitation that was not responding to acid-suppressive drugs. His father, also with long-standing history of GERD, died of esophageal adenocarcinoma. An endoscopy was normal except for a small sliding hiatal hernia (not shown). Esophageal pH monitoring was performed while the patient was on daily omeprazole 20 mg AC, while the patient was following a liberal diet for the first 48 h, followed by restrictive, anti-reflux diet (Fig. 23.17). Irrespective of the diet, his pH tracing showed no evidence of ongoing pathologic esophageal acid exposure while

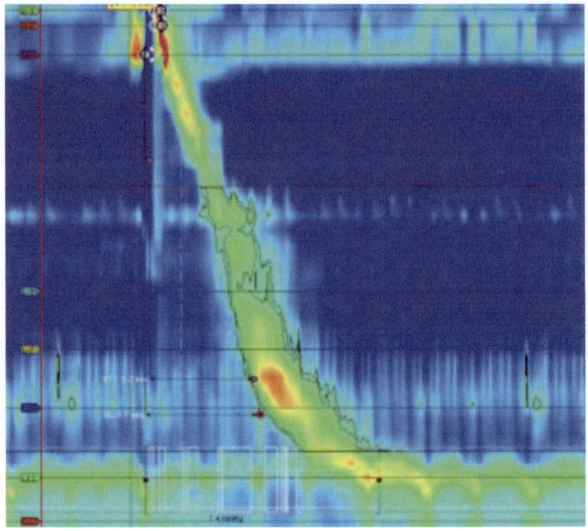

Fig. 23.16 Normal high-resolution esophageal manometry (including LESP) in a patient with GERD symptoms and pathologic acid exposure on pH monitoring

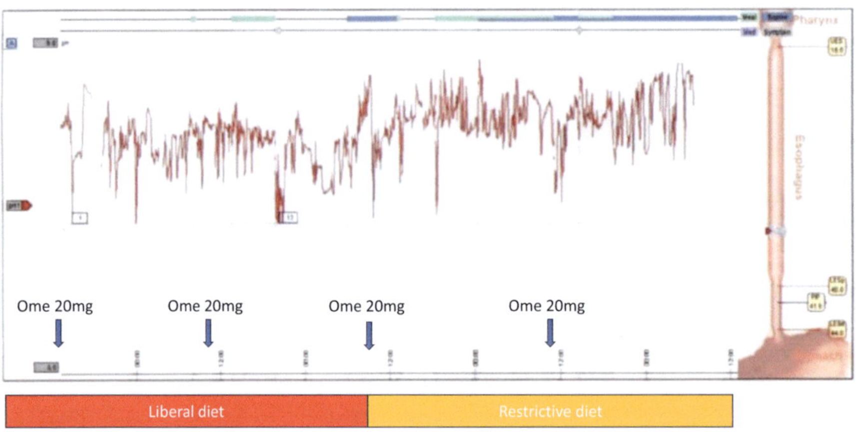

Fig. 23.17 Esophageal pH monitoring performed on daily omeprazole 20 mg AC, while the patient was following a liberal diet for the first 48 h, followed by restrictive, anti-reflux diet

on daily proton pump therapy. The mean % pH <4.0 was 0.4 (normal while on therapy <1.6%). Intraesophageal pH and symptom control are important in protecting patients against Barrett's esophagus and adenocarcinoma.

23.1.17 Hypercontractile Esophagus (HE)

A 76-year-old woman presented with intermittent dysphagia to both solids and liquids and occasional chest pain for the past 2 years. She has no heartburn or regurgitation. She has history of a T-lymphoblastic lymphoma diagnosed in 1995 when she

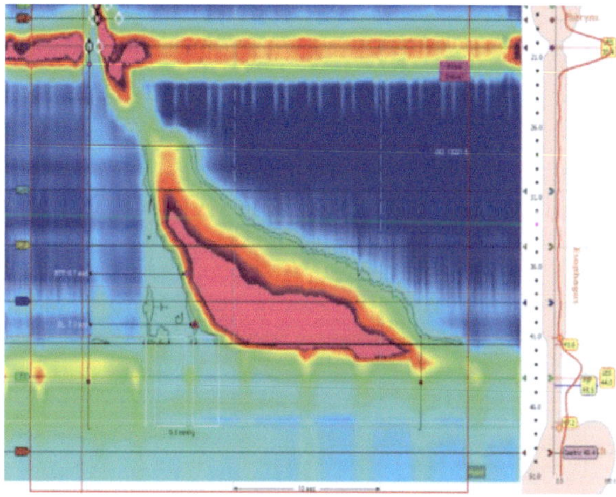

Fig. 23.18 Characteristic HREM tracing of hypercontractile esophagus

received induction therapy with Cytoxan, daunorubicin, prednisone, vincristine, and L-asparaginase and mantle radiation, followed by maintenance protocol with 6-mercaptopurine and methotrexate that was completed in late 1997. At this point, there is no evidence of any disease recurrence (2024). HREM shows characteristic features of hypercontractile esophagus (HE) (Fig. 23.18). HE is a heterogeneous major motility disorder diagnosed when ≥20% hypercontractile peristaltic sequences (distal contractile integral >8000 mmHg·s·cm) are present within the context of normal lower esophageal sphincter (LES) relaxation (integrated relaxation pressure < upper limit of normal) on esophageal high-resolution manometry (HREM). Endoscopy was normal without evidence of esophagitis or stricture. Benign spastic dysmotility, unrelated to cancer, may cause significant decrease in quality of life (QoL). Symptomatically, this patient responded well to intramuscular Botox injection (100 IU) in the distal esophagus.

23.1.18 A 96-h Ambulatory Esophageal pH Monitoring

A 71-year-old man with prostate cancer presented with recent history of heartburn, chest pain, and acid regurgitation that was reportedly not responding to acid-suppressive drugs. An endoscopy showed LA.B esophagitis and a small sliding hiatal hernia (not shown). Esophageal pH monitoring (Fig. 23.19) was performed while the patient was off daily proton pump inhibitor therapy and while the patient was following a liberal diet for the first 48 h, followed by restrictive, anti-reflux diet. His pH tracing showed pathologic esophageal acid exposure (AET 11.2%) only while on liberal diet and normalized to AET 5.2% while on restrictive diet, during the latter part of the study. His symptom association probability (SAP) was 100% for heartburn, chest pain, and acid regurgitation. He was started on omeprazole 20 mg orally daily.

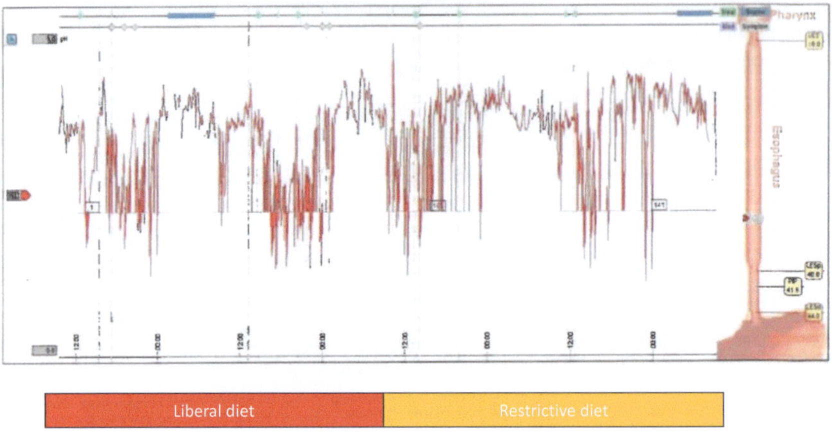

Fig. 23.19 A 96-h ambulatory esophageal pH monitoring showing pathologic esophageal acid exposure only during liberal diet intake

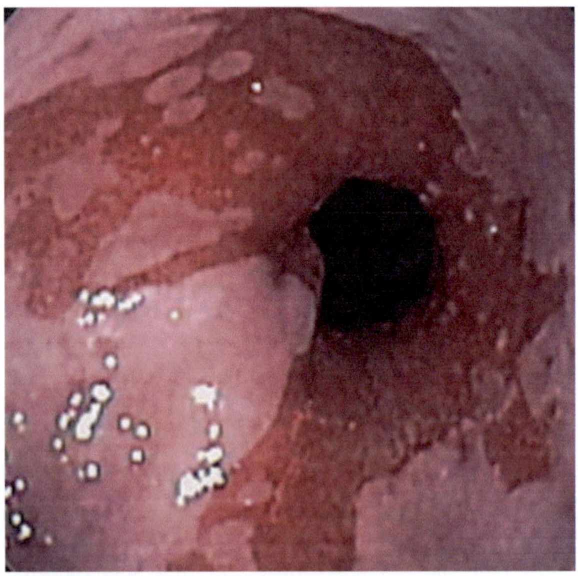

Fig. 23.20 Short-segment (<3 cm) Barrett's esophagus. Using the Prague classification, it was reported as COM2. Several islands of esophageal squamous mucosa appear within the projections of salmon-colored mucosa emanating from a patulous EGJ

23.1.19 Short-Segment Barrett's Esophagus (SSBE)

A 42-year-old obese white man presented with heartburn and acid regurgitation incompletely relieved by using over-the-counter omeprazole 20 mg daily, as needed. Endoscopy (Fig. 23.20) revealed tongues of salmon-colored mucosa. Biopsies were positive for intestinal metaplasia and low-grade dysplasia that was not appreciated endoscopically. He was referred for radiofrequency ablation therapy.

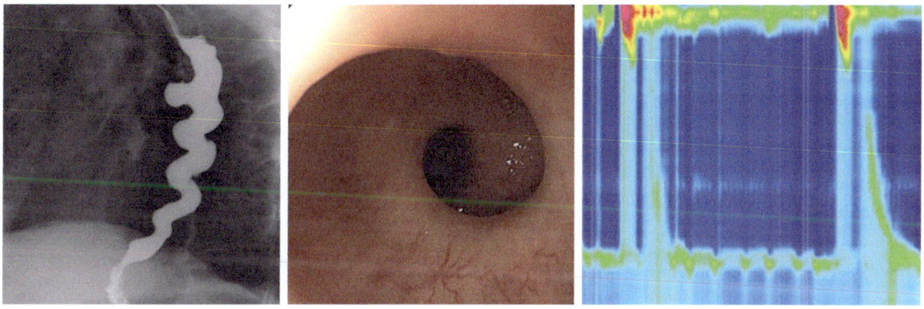

Fig. 23.21 Distal esophageal spasm. (Left) Barium esophagram reveals corkscrew esophagus. (Middle) Endoscopic depiction of esophageal spasticity noted at endoscopy, under propofol anesthesia. (Right) HREM reveals short distal latency (DL) upon water swallowing. Distal latency is measured from the UES swallow-induced relaxation to the contractile deceleration point (CDP). Normal distal latency is greater than 4.5 s, and anything shorter than 4.5 s is considered esophageal spasm

23.1.20 Distal Esophageal Spasm (DES)

A 62-year-old man, prostate cancer survivor, was evaluated for intermittent dysphagia and burning chest pain. He did not respond to PPI therapy. Endoscopy showed spasticity. He switched his diet from solids to minced meals and liquids. He underwent multimodality testing (Fig. 23.21), based on which he was treated successfully using intramuscular Botox injection (100 IU) in the distal esophagus.

23.1.21 GERD with Endoscopically Normal Esophagus

A 59-year-old woman presented with intermittent dysphagia and heartburn for several years. She is a breast cancer survivor, free of disease after right lumpectomy, lymph node dissection, and chemotherapy without radiation. An upper endoscopy was normal (Fig. 23.22). An endoscopy is an essential part of the evaluation of patients with dysphagia. A high-resolution esophageal manometry was normal. A pH monitoring study (not shown) however showed moderate acid reflux, with symptom association probability of 96%. In symptomatic patients, a normal endoscopy should be accompanied by mucosal biopsies to rule out GERD and eosinophilic esophagitis. In this case, long-term PPI therapy was successful in relieving the patient's symptoms.

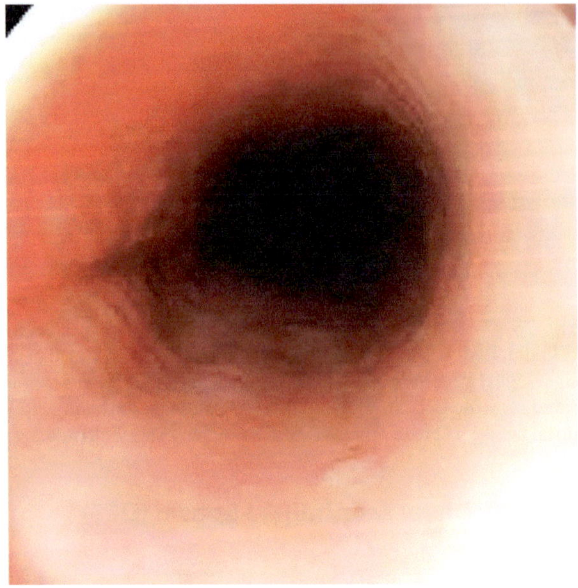

Fig. 23.22 Normal appearance of the esophagus at endoscopy

23.2 Stomach

23.2.1 Atrophic Gastritis

A 49-year-old woman with family history of gastric cancer in her mother presented with troublesome belching, postprandial fullness, and reduced appetite that were not responding to empiric proton pump inhibitors. Endoscopy (Fig. 23.23) showed extensive atrophic gastritis without evidence of *H. pylori* infection or intestinal metaplasia. A 24-h ambulatory gastric pH monitoring (not shown) confirmed achlorhydria, consistent with pernicious anemia. She entered endoscopic surveillance.

23.2.2 Antral Non-erosive Gastritis

A 33-year-old, Mexican-born woman presented with nonspecific but troublesome indigestion for several months that was partially responsive to over-the-counter acid suppressants. She reported history of her mother dying of stomach cancer at age 52. Endoscopy revealed non-erosive gastritis (Fig. 23.24). Biopsies of the antrum revealed *H. pylori* infection and gastric intestinal metaplasia. She was treated successfully with triple anti-*H. pylori* therapy, which expectedly will mitigate the risk for peptic ulcer disease and gastric cancer. Histologic gastric intestinal metaplasia (GIM) typically resolves after *H. pylori* eradication, but endoscopic validation is advised in such cases. She entered endoscopic surveillance.

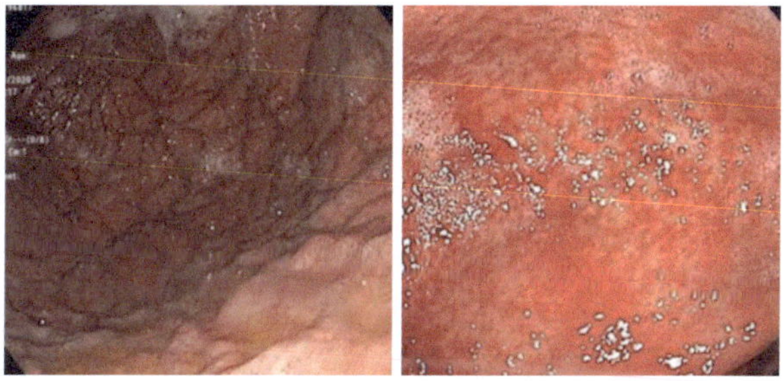

Fig. 23.23 Endoscopic appearance of atrophic gastritis

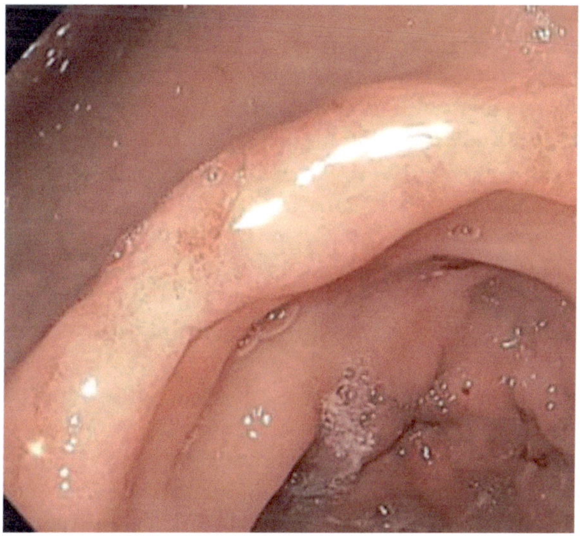

Fig. 23.24 Endoscopic appearance of antral non-erosive gastritis

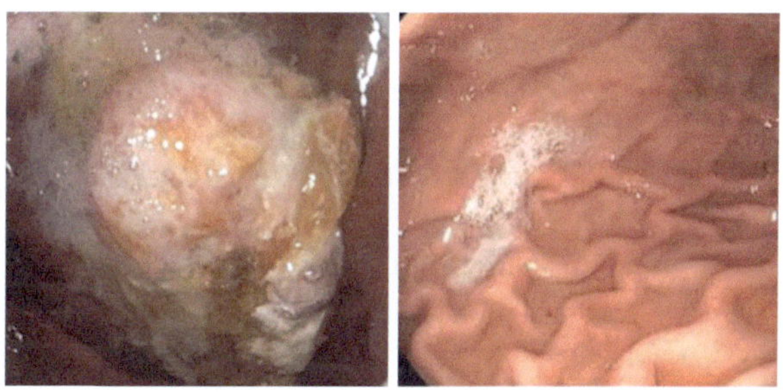

Fig. 23.25 Endoscopy (left) showing a bezoar, suggestive of underlying gastroparesis. After fasting, the gastric mucosa and pylorus were noted intact (right)

23.2.3 Gastroparesis with Food Bezoar

A 51-year-old woman presented with anorexia, postprandial fullness, and early satiety, nausea, vomiting, epigastric abdominal pain, and profound weight loss for several months. An endoscopy (Fig. 23.25) revealed a food bezoar (left), and the procedure was aborted to prevent pulmonary aspiration. Repeat endoscopy

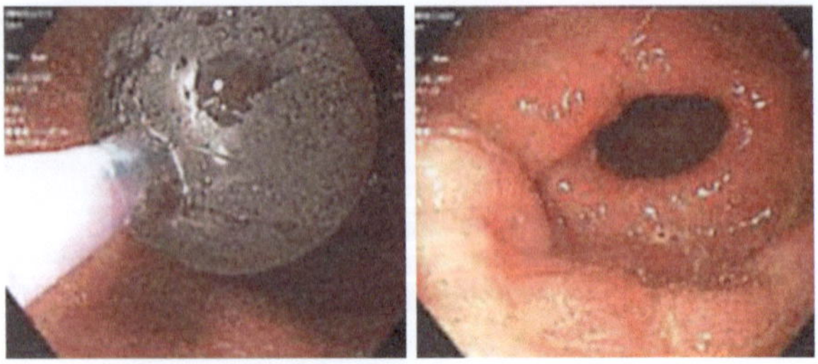

Fig. 23.26 Endoscopic images of a 20 mm TTS balloon dilation during (left) and immediately thereafter (right)

after 5 days of clear liquids (right) revealed normal stomach and pylorus without structural gastric outlet obstruction. She was eventually found to have malignancy-associated gastroparesis (MAG), resulting from paraneoplastic dysmotility with autoantibody-mediated destruction of the ICC or of the myenteric plexus. She was treated with dietary modification and prokinetics. Because of incomplete clinical response, she ultimately received endoscopically a four-quadrant intra-pyloric Botox (100 IU) injection with clinical improvement. The effect of Botox typically lasts 6–12 months, and the procedure typically needs to be repeated, as needed.

23.2.4 Balloon Dilation for Obstructive Gastroparesis

A 55-year-old woman, a breast cancer survivor, presented with early satiety, post-prandial fullness, and reduced appetite. A gastric emptying scan (not shown) revealed evidence of delayed gastric emptying; electrogastrography showed a 3 cpm antral pattern. Figure 23.26 depicts transpyloric dilation using a 20 mm balloon led to symptomatic improvement that lasted for 4 months but had to be repeated for symptom recurrence.

23.3 Small Intestine

23.3.1 Post-bulbar, Radiation-Induced Duodenal Stricture

A 61-year-old woman with renal cell carcinoma presented with right-sided upper back and abdominal pain, prandial fullness, and heartburn, after receiving radiation therapy for painful tumor recurrence in the right renal bed. An endoscopy showed fluid retention in the stomach, but otherwise showed normal mucosa. Barium radiograph (Fig. 23.27) showed a radiation-induced post-bulbar duodenal stricture (arrow). Bowel enteroscopy (not shown) allowed balloon dilation of the stenosis with symptom improvement. Even using endoscopy, subtle structural abnormalities may be missed, and contrast imaging is helpful in providing an explanation for the patient's symptoms.

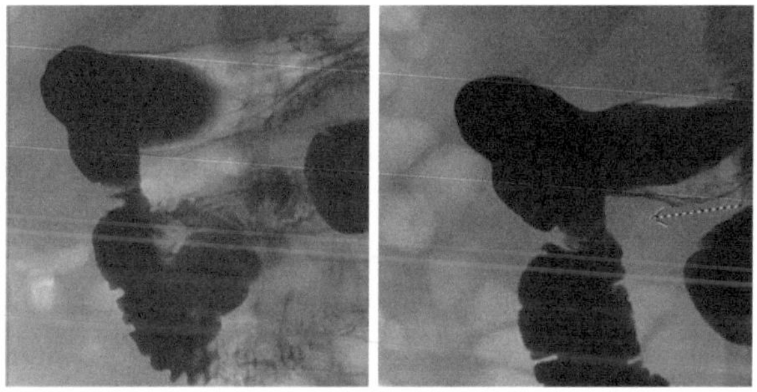

Fig. 23.27 Radiation-induced duodenal stricture

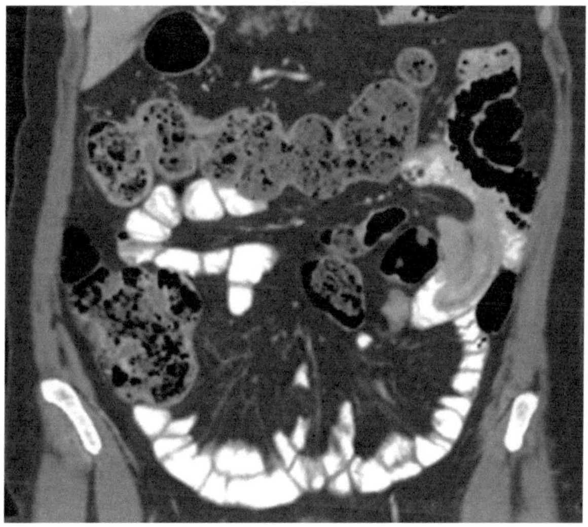

Fig. 23.28 CT appearance of small bowel intussusception. The underlying GIST is not appreciated in this image

23.3.2 Small Bowel Intussusception

A 51-year-old woman presented initially with abdominal bloating and was found to have small intestinal bacterial overgrowth (SIBO), which was treated successfully with rifaximin. However, over the ensuing several months, she had recurrences of symptoms for which she was retreated. One year later, she started experiencing colicky postprandial abdominal discomfort and variable nausea intermittently over several weeks. CT scan of the abdomen and pelvis showed small bowel intussusception (Fig. 23.28) causing intermittent partial small bowel obstruction. The leading point for intussusception was a small gastrointestinal stromal tumor (GIST) (not shown) that was found and resected surgically, leading to clinical resolution.

23.3.3 Small Intestinal Obstruction

A 59-year-old woman with ovarian cancer s/p extensive debulking surgery presented with crampy abdominal pain, abdominal distention, nausea, and vomiting.

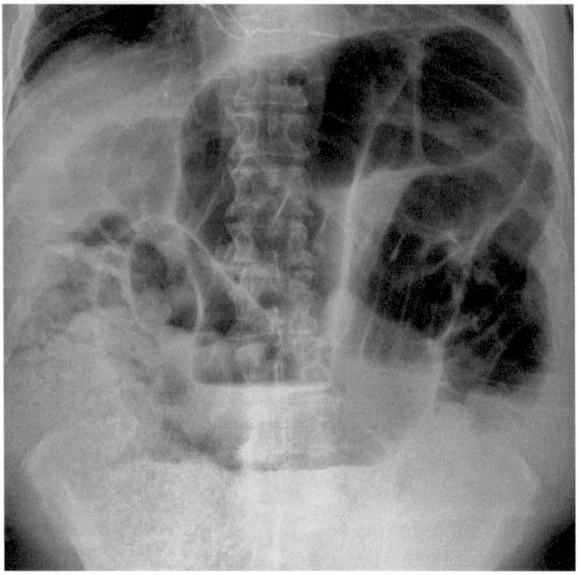

Fig. 23.29 Plain abdominal radiograph revealing dilated loops of bowel, air-fluid levels, and fecal stasis suggestive of obstruction or paralytic ileus. There is no gas within the pelvis to suggest the latter

Abdominal series (Fig. 23.29) revealed air-fluid levels. The clinical distinction is important since treatment may be conservative (medical) or surgical. In the cancer patient population, narcotic use for pain needs to be considered. She was treated with nasogastric decompression. Her small intestinal obstruction was eventually attributed to peritoneal carcinomatosis.

23.3.4 Small Bowel Intussusception

A 65-year-old female with a past history of adenocarcinoma of the lung, s/p right lower lobectomy, Nissen fundoplication, and cholecystectomy, underwent an abdominal CT imaging because of intermittent diffuse, colicky abdominal pain and diarrhea. She had tested positive for SIBO twice and was treated initially with ciprofloxacin plus metronidazole and then with rifaximin, each for 2 weeks with transient improvement. An area of small bowel-to-small bowel intussusception in the left abdomen is present (target sign, circle), with no distinct mass or small bowel obstructive changes (Fig. 23.30). On two prior successive CT studies, months apart, she exhibited small bowel intussusception. During the running of the small bowel at diagnostic laparotomy, no visible masses or other pathology was identified except for segmental jejunal fecalization, suggestive of small bowel dysmotility.

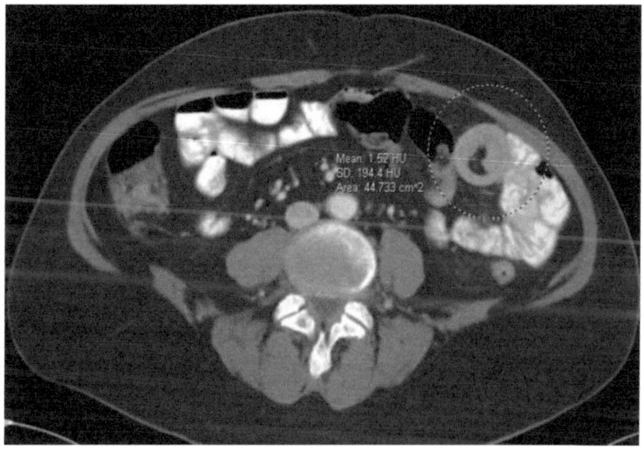

Fig. 23.30 CT image of idiopathic small bowel intussusception revealing a target sign (circle)

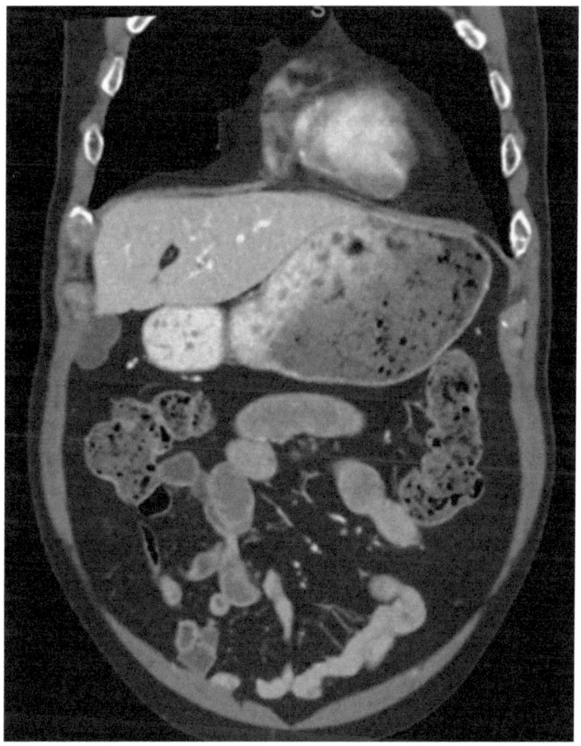

Fig. 23.31 CT image of the abdomen depicting gastric retention and fecalomas, suggestive of CIPO. There was no evidence of dilated small bowel, a key feature in this condition. The constellation of these imaging findings is frequently seen in patients using narcotics

23.3.5 Chronic Intestinal Pseudo-obstruction (CIPO)

A 56-year-old man presented with chronic postprandial abdominal distention and constipation, 7 years after sigmoid resection for colon cancer. He was not receiving any anti-motility agents (i.e., narcotics). CT scan of the abdomen and pelvis (Fig. 23.31) shows gastric retention and fecalomas suggestive of diffuse intestinal dysmotility with stasis.

23.4 Colon and Rectum

23.4.1 Defecatory Dyssynergia

A 63-year-old woman presented with straining and constipation for several weeks. She is 14 years s/p abdominal hysterectomy for uterine leiomyoma. HRAM, RST, and BET are performed to further evaluate the symptoms and guide management. The resting anal pressures are below normal. The squeeze pressure is below normal. The squeeze duration is adequate. During the push maneuver, the residual anal pressure is high (Fig. 23.32), and the percent anal relaxation is only 6% (normal 15–35%); therefore, RAIR is not seen. The sensory pressures are mildly impaired. Balloon expulsion was not achieved. She was referred to pelvic floor physical therapy.

23.4.2 Sigmoid Diverticulitis

A 48-year-old woman underwent colonoscopy because of left lower abdominal pain and recent change in her bowel evacuation pattern, to rule out colonic neoplasia. The colonoscopy showed edema and severe inflammation of the sigmoid colon that

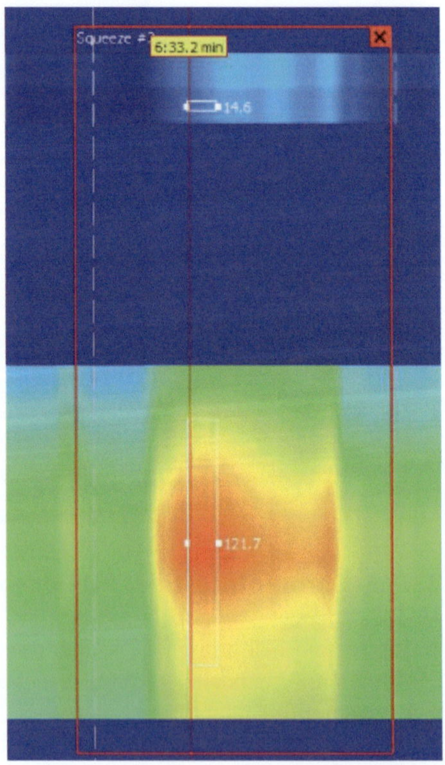

Fig. 23.32 HRAM in defecatory dyssynergia

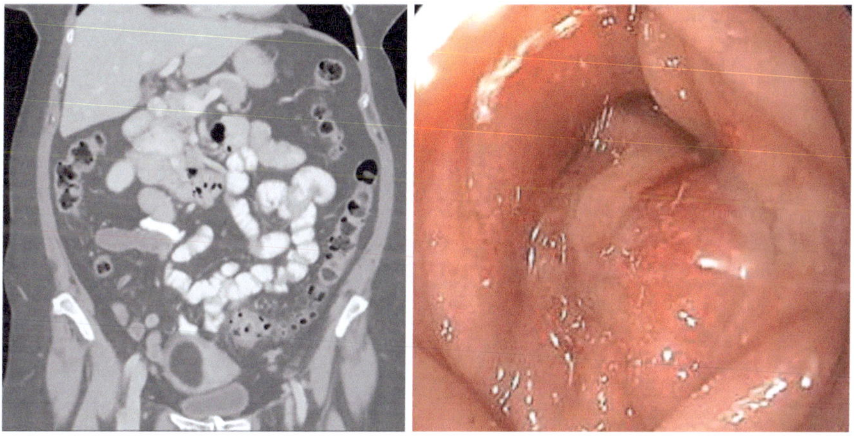

Fig. 23.33 (Left) CT of the abdomen and pelvis revealing colonic diverticulosis, particularly in the sigmoid colon. There is thickening of the sigmoid wall, associated with soft tissue stranding and fluid in the sigmoid mesentery consistent with acute diverticulitis. (Right) Attempted colonoscopy showed edema and severe inflammation of the sigmoid colon that did not allow a safe passage of the colonoscope beyond that point

did not allow a safe passage of the colonoscope beyond that point. CT of the abdomen and pelvis revealed colonic diverticulosis, particularly in the sigmoid colon. There is thickening of the sigmoid wall, associated with soft tissue stranding and fluid in the sigmoid mesentery consistent with acute diverticulitis (Fig. 23.33). Under the circumstances, colonoscopy becomes unsafe.

23.4.3 Low Anterior Resection (LAR) for Rectal Cancer

A 57-year-old man presented with fecal urgency and stool frequency after undergoing LAR for rectal cancer. Surveillance colonoscopy 1 year later did not show cancer recurrence, but transient prolapse at the anastomosis, which was easily crossed with air insufflation (Fig. 23.34). Such structural, postoperative alterations may also be associated with abnormal anorectal function defined by anorectal manometry, rectal sensory testing, and balloon expulsion testing (not shown), which in turn may aid management.

23.4.4 Postoperative Bile Acid Malabsorption (BAM)

A 55-year-old man presented with diarrhea 9–10 times per day after right hemicolectomy with ileocolonic anastomosis for cecal cancer. A colonoscopy revealed a normal right colonic resection with a healthy-appearing ileo-ascending anastomosis (Fig. 23.35). A trial of cholestyramine was successful in slowing the frequency of evacuation, but some fecal urgency persisted, particularly after rich meals.

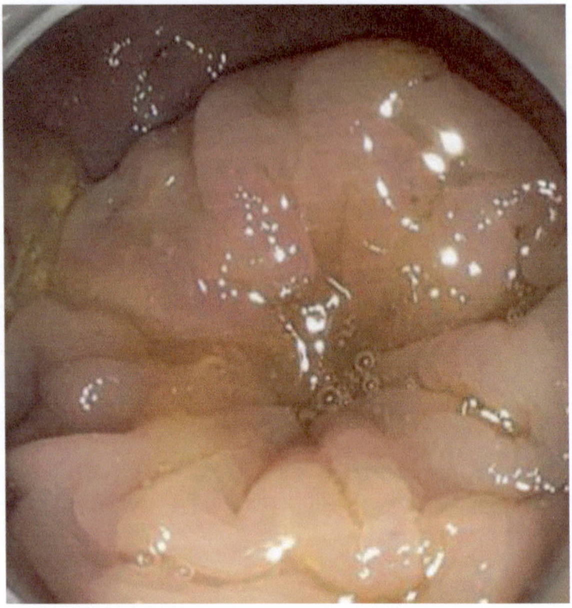

Fig. 23.34 Colonoscopic view of transient prolapse at the colorectal anastomosis, which was easily crossed with air insufflation

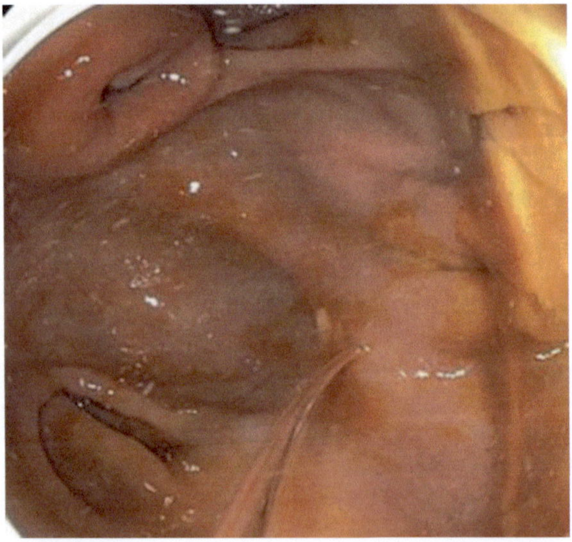

Fig. 23.35 Colonoscopic appearance of a normal ileo-ascending anastomosis. Despite the neovalvular configuration, postoperative bile acid malabsorption (BAM) ensued

23.4.5 Slow-Transit Constipation

A 49-year-old woman, breast cancer survivor on no active oncologic therapy after lumpectomy and breast radiation, presented with severe constipation that had failed osmotic laxatives, prokinetics, stimulant laxatives, and pyridostigmine. On the fifth day after Sitzmarks capsule ingestion, a plain radiography of the abdomen and pelvis shows retention of many radio-opaque markers in the right and left colon,

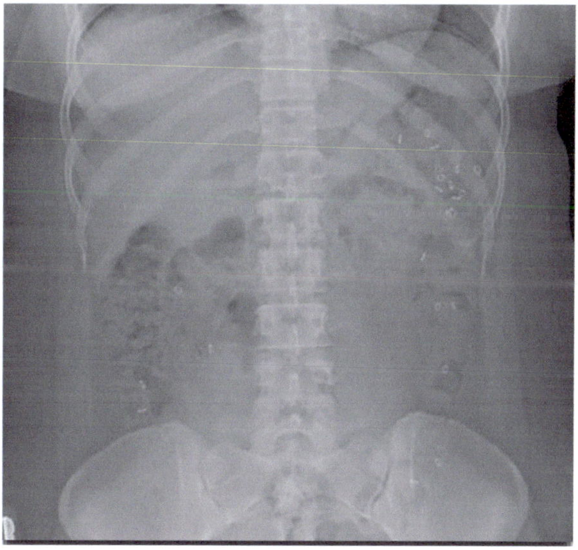

Fig. 23.36 Plain abdominal radiograph showing retained radio-opaque markers in the right and left colon, suggestive of slow-transit constipation

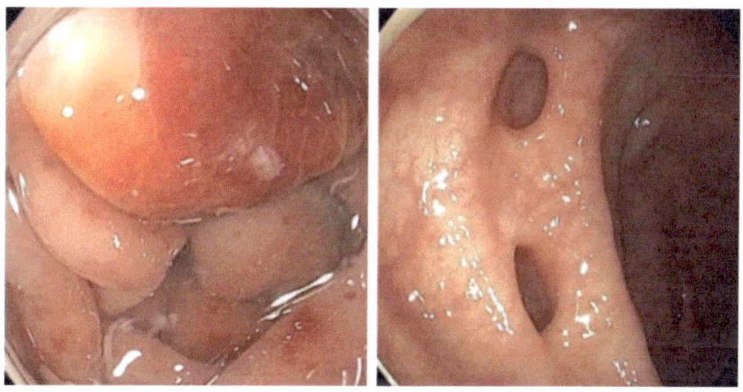

Fig. 23.37 Colonoscopic view of segmental colitis associated with diverticulosis (SCAD)

suggestive of slow-transit constipation (colonic inertia) (Fig. 23.36). Due to the refractoriness of her symptoms to multiple therapies, a subtotal colectomy with ileo-sigmoid anastomosis is planned. This drastic surgical approach can be done minimally invasively, with low probability for temporary colostomy and minimal (if any) impact on genitourinary function postoperatively. The functional outcome ranges from eight to ten bowel evacuations per day over the next 6 months to four to five controlled bowel evacuations per day at 12 months.

23.4.6 Segmental Colitis Associated with Diverticulosis (SCAD)

A 73-year-old obese female developed left lower abdominal pain while receiving R-CHOP chemotherapy for advanced-stage diffuse large B cell lymphoma. A colonoscopy (Fig. 23.37) revealed chronic inflammation and superficial ulcerations (left), involving a segment of the left colon that contains diverticulosis (right).

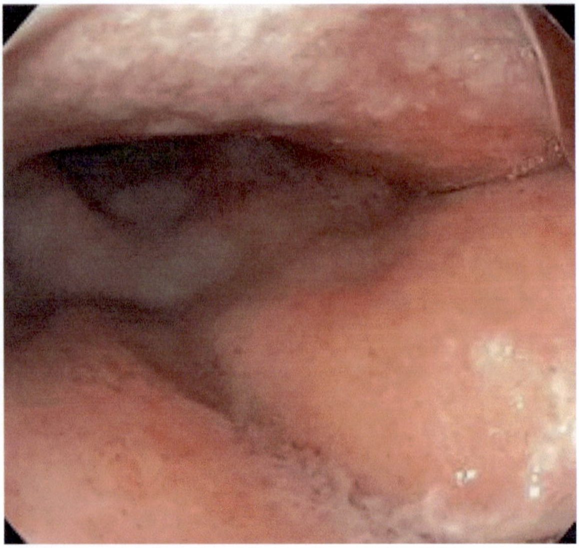

Fig. 23.38 Colonoscopic view of the rectum revealing changes of mucosal prolapse

Patients who are immunocompromised because of corticosteroids or while receiving chemotherapy (or both) are at risk of SCAD complications. 5-ASA agents have been used under the circumstances with success.

23.4.7 Rectal Prolapse and Rectocele

A 59-year-old woman presented with constipation and straining at bowel movements, hard-formed stools, and incomplete emptying of bowels. She is a breast cancer survivor for 11 years s/p lumpectomy. She takes OTC Citrucel once daily. She reports intermittent urgency and diarrhea with loose and watery stools without blood. Patient only noted blood when wiping on toilet paper. Rectal examination and colonoscopy revealed rectal prolapse (Fig. 23.38) and a rectocele. Her symptoms were adequately controlled using a daily osmotic laxative (MiraLAX). MR defecography and high-resolution anorectal manometry (not shown) are useful tool in further assessing such patients, particularly if surgery is considered.

23.4.8 Rectosigmoid Cancer

A 51-year-old man presented for screening colonoscopy. He reported intermittent mild constipation and fecal urgency that was not progressive over the past 2 years. A circumferential exophytic lesion, 2 cm in length (Fig. 23.39), was noted in the rectosigmoid colon; the remaining of the colon was normal, without polyps. Colonoscopy to r/o structural colonic abnormalities is imperative in such cases.

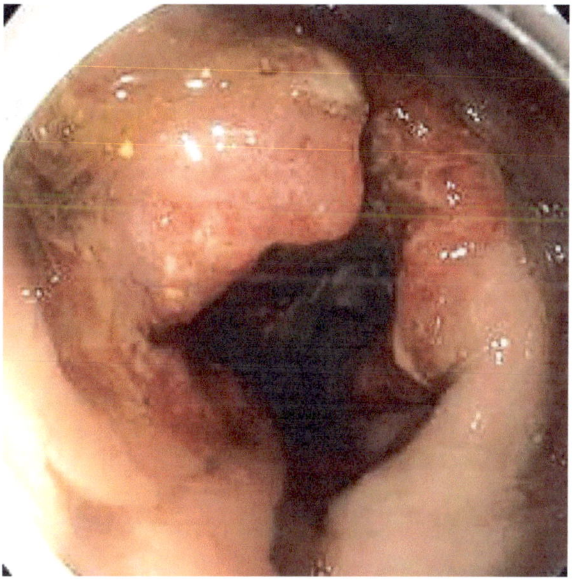

Fig. 23.39 Colonoscopic view of rectosigmoid cancer

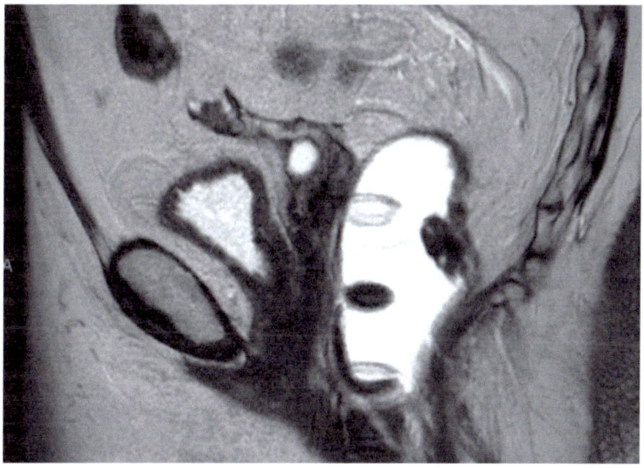

Fig. 23.40 MR defecography revealing mild widening of the pelvic hiatus in resting state with intact squeeze response, consistent with tricompartmental descent, and limited evacuation

Oncologic management and resective surgery were curative in this case. This is a reminder that structural abnormalities need to be fully explored first, before attributing symptoms, such as constipation or fecal urgency, to altered motility of sensation.

23.4.9 MR Defecography

A 72-year-old woman presented with episodes of self-described diarrhea but, upon clinical questioning, more suggestive of fecal incontinence: Defecography (Fig. 23.40) showed widening of pelvic hiatus ("H"-line; normal <=

5 cm)—6.4 cm—and pelvic floor descent ("M"-line; normal <= 2 cm): 2.7. Anorectal angle: 106°. Squeeze: normal pelvic floor ascent, normal appearance of the levators and puborectalis. Evacuation: anterior compartment—the inferior margin of the bladder extends 1 cm below the pubococcygeal line. Middle compartment: greater than expected descent of the vagina. Cul-de-sac: no enterocele or peritoneocele. There was no rectal intussusception. The amount of contrast evacuated was poor (approximately 1/3 of contrast material). Overall, the study showed mild widening of the pelvic hiatus in resting state with intact squeeze response and consistent with tricompartmental descent and limited evacuation. She was referred with pelvic floor physical therapy.

23.4.10 J-Pouch for Familial Adenomatous Polyposis (FAP)

A 69-year-old woman presented with relentless anal pain after J-pouch requiring narcotics for control. Endoscopically (Fig. 23.41), there was no evidence of pouchitis, which, in contrast to the IBD population undergoing similar surgery, is unusual. Suppositories containing anti-inflammatory agents, anesthetics, and corticosteroids were used to partial benefit. Pelvic floor physical therapy was unsuccessful.

23.4.11 Radiation Proctitis

A 52-year-old man s/p external beam radiation for anorectal cancer 12 years ago presented with constipation and intermittent, self-limited rectal bleeding over the

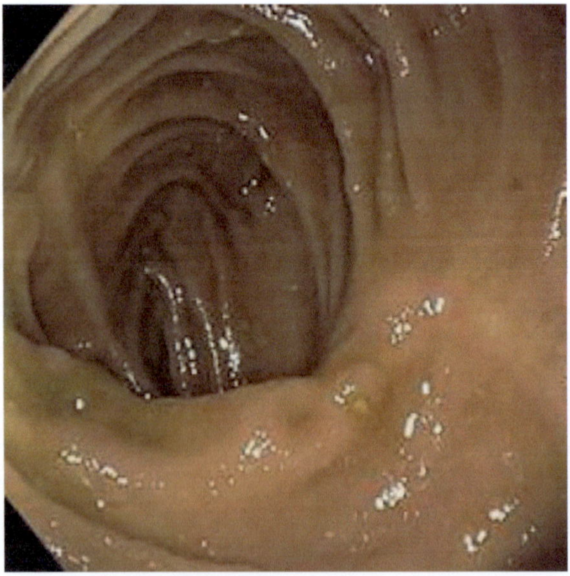

Fig. 23.41 Normal colonoscopic appearance of a J-pouch performed for familial adenomatous polyposis (FAP)

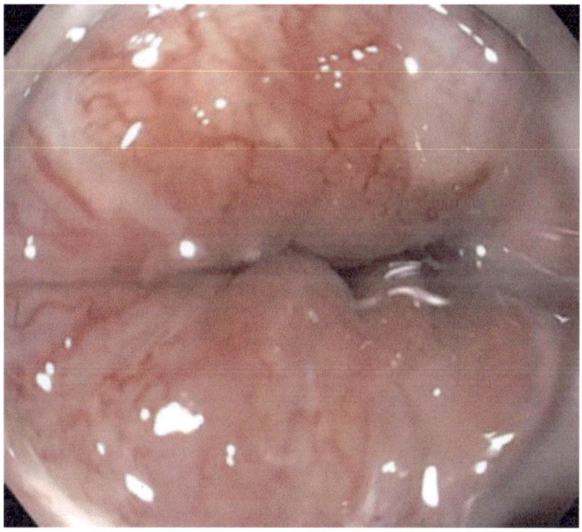

Fig. 23.42 Radiation proctitis at the anorectal junction revealing the characteristic mucosa with sparsity of the blood vessels and telangiectasias

past 2 years. The colonoscopy showed anorectal radiation injury, but it was otherwise normal (Fig. 23.42). High-resolution anorectal manometry (not shown) revealed dyssynergic defecation of questionable clinical significance since the patient passed balloon expulsion test (BET). There was low resting anal sphincter pressure, low maximal squeeze pressure, and minimally abnormal rectal sensation all consistent with radiation injury extending beyond the mucosa to the muscle. Combating constipation using osmotic laxatives is typically effective in managing constipation and mitigating rectal bleeding in such cases.

23.4.12 Sigmoid Diverticulosis

A 63-year-old woman presented for colorectal cancer screening. She reported mild to moderate intermittent constipation and left lower quadrant pain relieved by bowel movements. At the time of colonoscopy, it was impossible to safely traverse the sigmoid colon due to severe fixation of the distal colon impairing scope passage. A CT scan was performed (Fig. 23.43) and revealed severe sigmoid diverticulosis. Although rare, severe diverticulosis with bowel fixation in the pelvis may mitigate successful colorectal cancer screening. In women, this may be aggravated by the presence of pelvic adhesions from prior gynecologic surgery for benign or malignant disease. Under the circumstances, a CT colonography is suggested.

23.4.13 Rectal Intussusception

A 68-year-old woman presented with severe constipation and straining at evacuation. She is a breast cancer survivor. A colonoscopy was performed to rule out

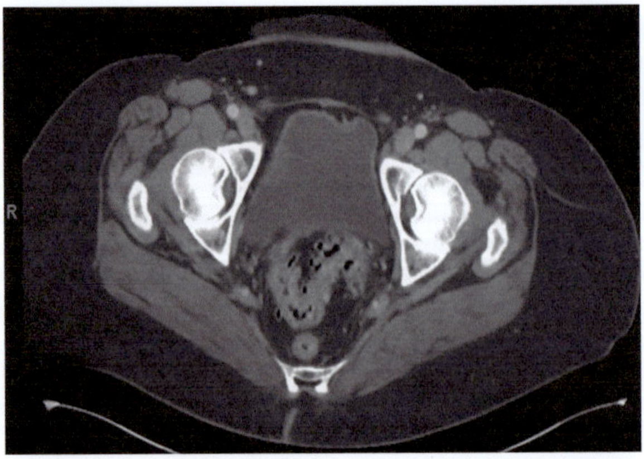

Fig. 23.43 CT of the abdomen and pelvis revealing severe diverticulosis

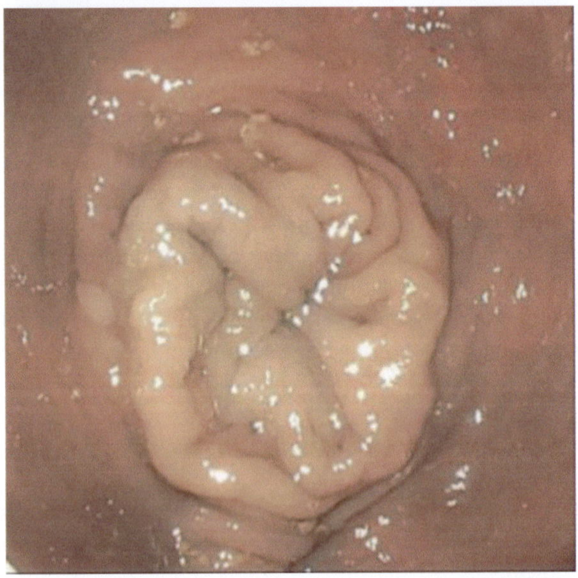

Fig. 23.44 Colonoscopic view of Oxford I rectal intussusception

colon polyps or cancer and to rule out colonic obstruction as a cause of her constipation. This nonspecific endoscopic finding of rectal intussusception (Fig. 23.44) was quite persistent, making colonoscopy a challenge, albeit ultimately successful. No other colonic abnormalities were seen. High-resolution anorectal manometry showed defecatory dyssynergia (not shown). In some cases, stercoral ulcers, resulting from intermittent mucosal ischemia, may be seen endoscopically and proven by biopsies. The diagnosis should be formally made using imaging, preferably MR defecography.

23.4.14 Low Anterior Resection Syndrome (LARS) with Coloanal Anastomosis

A 44-year-old man with history of rectal cancer stage IIIA (pT1, pN1a, cM0) presented with increased frequency of pencil-thin stools every alternate day and mild intermittent urgency without fecal incontinence. One year ago, he had undergone a robotic-assisted low anterior resection (LAR) with coloanal anastomosis and diverting ileostomy that was later reversed. Colonoscopy revealed changes of a healthy coloanal anastomosis (Fig. 23.45). He was treated successfully with fiber supplementation and loperamide 2 mg twice per week. Rectal hypersensitivity is frequently responsible for fecal urgency; it improves over time (years) with diet, antidiarrheals, and pelvic floor physical therapy as needed.

23.4.15 Chronic Constipation

A 72-year-old woman presented with no bowel movements 7 days after undergoing a normal colonoscopy. She has had no urge to defecate for many years and uses senna suppositories to assist with evacuation. Abdominal radiograph (Fig. 23.46) reveals extensive ground-glass appearance of the abdomen, due to fecal accumulation. She was treated with prucalopride 2 mg daily in conjunction with twice daily osmotic laxatives for suspected slow-transit constipation.

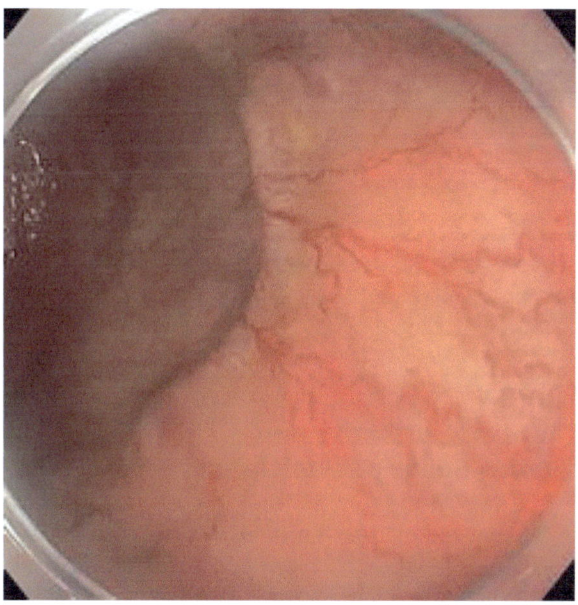

Fig. 23.45 Colonoscopic appearance of an intact coloanal anastomosis

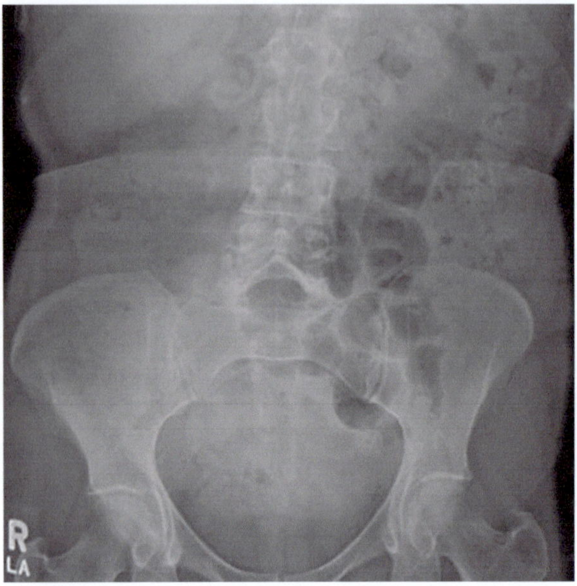

Fig. 23.46 Plain abdominal radiograph revealing changes of constipation, with significant stool burden throughout

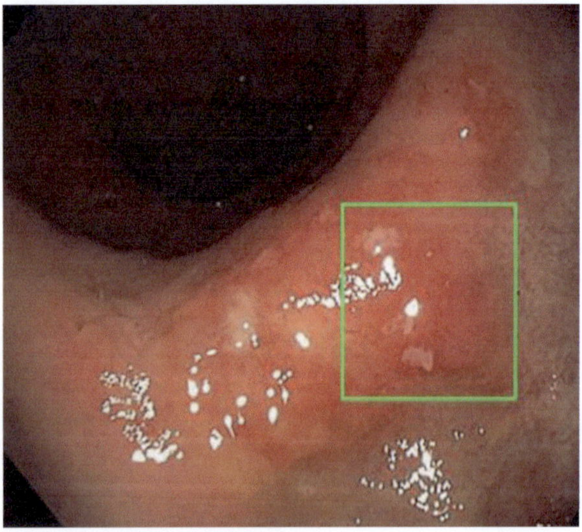

Fig. 23.47 Colonoscopic view of solitary rectal ulcer syndrome (stercoral colitis)

23.4.16 Solitary Rectal Ulcer Syndrome (SRUS)

A 59-year-old man with past history of colon polyps containing high-grade dysplasia presented with severe constipation and straining, with rare episodes of rectal bleeding. Colonoscopy showed stercoral colitis and SRUS (Fig. 23.47) that was confirmed histologically. He was successfully treated with osmotic laxatives.

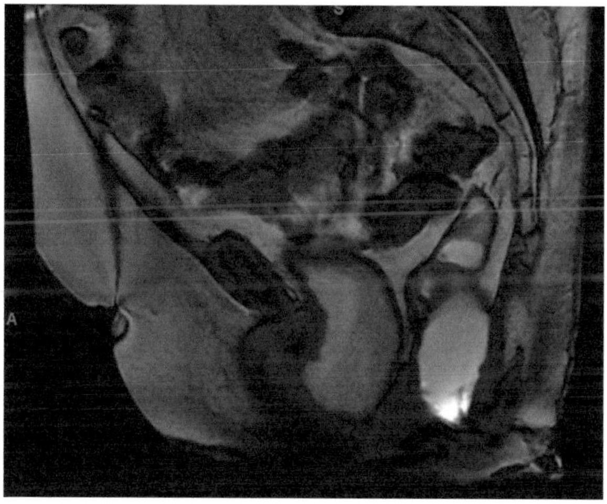

Fig. 23.48 MR defecography revealing several abnormalities of the pelvic floor in a woman after hysterectomy

23.4.17 MR Defecography

A 75-year-old woman presented with constipation and severe defecatory and urinary difficulties after abdominal hysterectomy for uterine cancer. MR defecography (Fig. 23.48) showed the following: anterior compartment, large cystocele measuring 6 cm below the pubococcygeal line with associated urethral hypermobility; middle compartment, moderate to severe vaginal apex prolapse measuring 4.2 cm below the pubococcygeal line; cul-de-sac, small peritoneocele measuring 3.1 cm below the pubococcygeal line; and posterior compartment, tiny anterior rectocele measuring 1 cm. There is exaggerated pelvic floor descent (M-line 6.5 cm at strain) with caudal angulation of the levators. There is no rectal intussusception. The amount of rectal contrast evacuated was poor (approximately 1/3 of contrast material was evacuated). She was referred for pelvic floor physical therapy as a first step, prior to consideration of pelvic reconstructive surgery.

23.4.18 Ogilvie's Syndrome

A 69-year-old man with metastatic prostate cancer underwent left hip replacement after he suffered a fall. On the second postoperative day, he developed severe abdominal distention, bloating, and inability to pass gas and stool. An abdominal radiograph (Fig. 23.49) revealed dilated loops of the small bowel and colon consistent with ileus and Ogilvie's syndrome. He was treated with neostigmine (2 mg) delivered by slow intravenous injection that led to spontaneous bowel evacuation and rapid resolution.

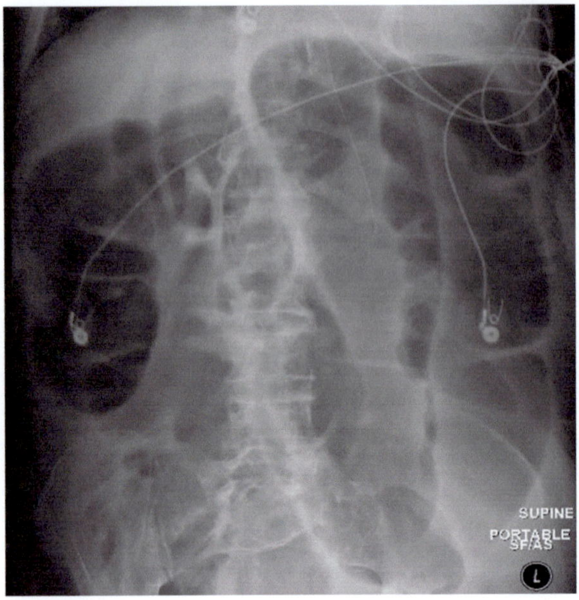

Fig. 23.49 Plain abdominal radiograph in Ogilvie's syndrome

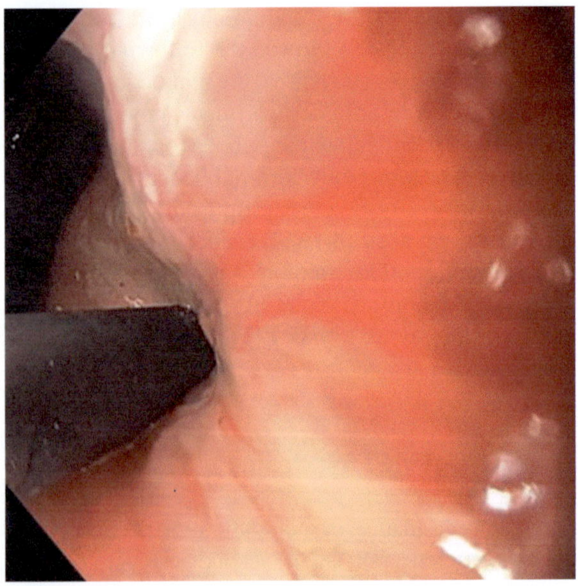

Fig. 23.50 Colonoscopic view of anal Botox injection for outlet constipation (anismus)

23.4.19 Anal Botox Injection

A 36-year-old woman with breast cancer presented with severe outlet constipation and defecatory straining. High-resolution anorectal manometry revealed severe hypertonicity of the anal sphincter (330 mmHg) (not shown). Endoscopic, intramuscular injection of Botox (100 IU) was administered successfully (Fig. 23.50).

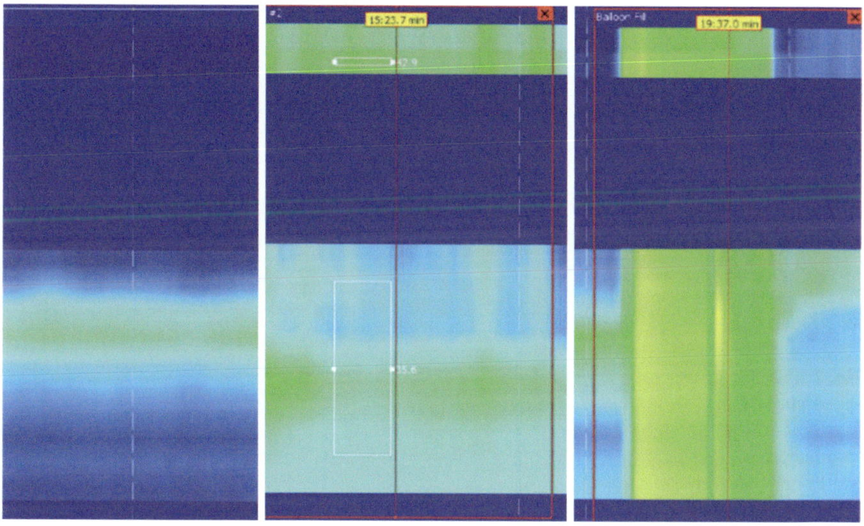

Fig. 23.51 High-resolution anorectal manometry (HR-ARM) in pelvic floor dyssynergia

23.4.20 High-Resolution Anorectal Manometry (HR-ARM) in Pelvic Floor Dyssynergia

A 65-year-old woman presented with chronic diarrhea and fecal incontinence. She has history of uterine cancer, status hysterectomy and post-bilateral salpingo-oophorectomy, chemotherapy, and external beam pelvic radiation 2 years ago. Anorectal manometry (Fig. 23.51) showed a maximum resting pressure of 41.5 mmHg (normal 58–68 mmHg) and high-pressure zone (HPZ) length of 2.6 cm (normal 3.3–3.7 cm) (left); push maneuver showed a residual anal pressure of 40.3 mmHg (normal 27–37 mmHg), normal % anal relaxation of 26% (normal 15–35%) (center), intrarectal pressure of 65 mmHg (normal 27–37 mmHg), and a recto-anal pressure differential of 24.7 mmHg (normal −18.6 to −6.6 mmHg) (right). Balloon expulsion test was normal. She was treated with pelvic floor physical therapy with improvement.

23.4.21 Type II Dyssynergia

A 57-year-old woman presented with severe constipation and defecatory straining. She is s/p 3 vaginal deliveries and ultimately a hysterectomy for an enlarging uterine myoma 3 years ago. A three-dimensional HR-ARM (Fig. 23.52) shows the following: (left) pressure profile during a squeeze effort and maximum sphincter pressure 324 mmHg (normal <247 mmHg) and (right) pressure profile during bear down (simulated attempted defecation) and residual anal pressure 165 mmHg (normal <65 mmHg). Impaired rectal propagation is associated with paradoxical anal contraction (type II dyssynergia). Pelvic floor physical therapy was partly successful, and she is considering anal Botox injection.

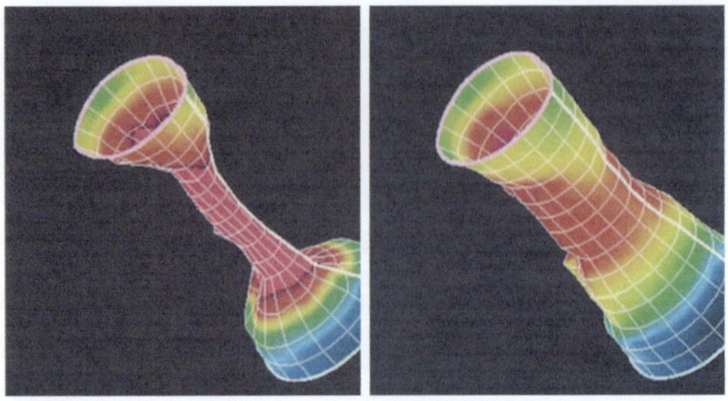

Fig. 23.52 Three-dimensional HR-ARM revealing type II dyssynergia

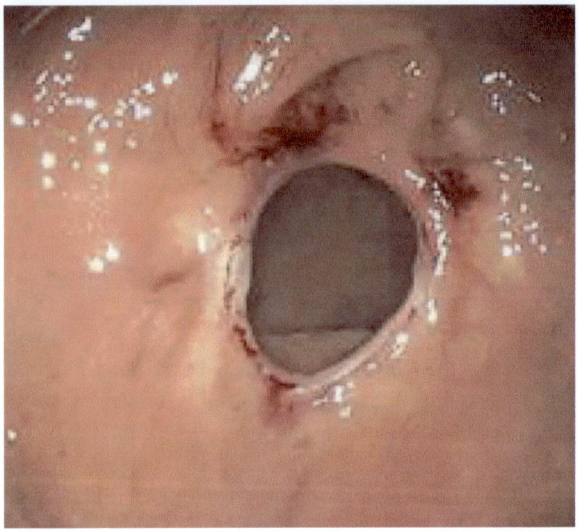

Fig. 23.53 Colonoscopic appearance of an anastomotic stricture after colonic resection and end-to-end anastomosis

23.4.22 Anastomotic Stenosis

A 57-year-old woman presented with progressive constipation and straining almost 1 year after sigmoid resection for colon cancer. A colonoscopy (Fig. 23.53) revealed an anastomotic stricture that was balloon dilated to 18 mm using the colonoscope, followed by daily osmotic laxative use with relief.

23.4.23 Microscopic Colitis

A 76-year-old woman, melanoma survivor but suffering from rheumatoid arthritis, was being treated with non-steroidal anti-inflammatory drugs (NSAIDs) and gastro-protective doses of omeprazole 20 mg daily. She presented with several weeks of watery non-bloody diarrhea, typically explosive, with fecal urgency, and infrequent fecal incontinence. Colonoscopy (Fig. 23.54) showed normal colonic mucosa throughout, but biopsies revealed microscopic colitis. She was treated successfully with budesonide 9 mg daily. Random colonic biopsies should be obtained in all patients presenting with diarrhea.

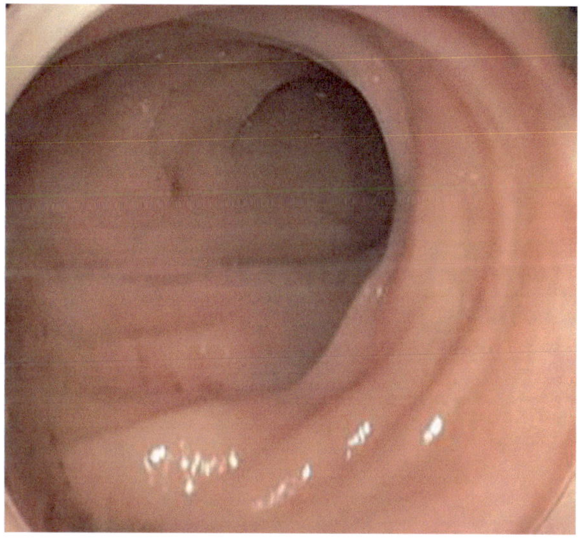

Fig. 23.54 Colonoscopic appearance in microscopic colitis. The mucosa of the colon is normal; the diagnosis is based on random colonic biopsies

23.4.24 Radiation-Induced Pelvic Floor Injury with Dyssynergia and Fecal Incontinence

A 49-year-old woman presented with fecal urgency and straining at evacuation. Fourteen months ago, she was diagnosed with high-intermediate-risk uterine cancer, and she received adjuvant external beam radiation to the pelvis following surgery. A high-resolution anorectal manometry (Fig. 23.55) was performed, revealing type I dyssynergia. She was treated with four-quadrant anal Botox injection (100 IU) with success.

23.4.25 Fecal Impaction

A 53-year-old woman presented with severe constipation and abdominal bloating and nonspecific discomfort without any bowel movements for more than 2 weeks. She had been using hydrocodone regularly for several years for cervical back pain, initially related to a spinal ependymoma that was resected successfully without neurological deficits, or evidence of recurrence thereafter. A plain abdominal radiograph (Fig. 23.56) showed moderate to severe stool burden along the length of the colon due to associated fecal impaction that required manual disimpaction, followed by osmotic laxatives for relief. To avoid recurrences, osmotic laxatives or naloxegol, a peripherally acting mu-opioid receptor antagonist, is used daily, either alone or in combination.

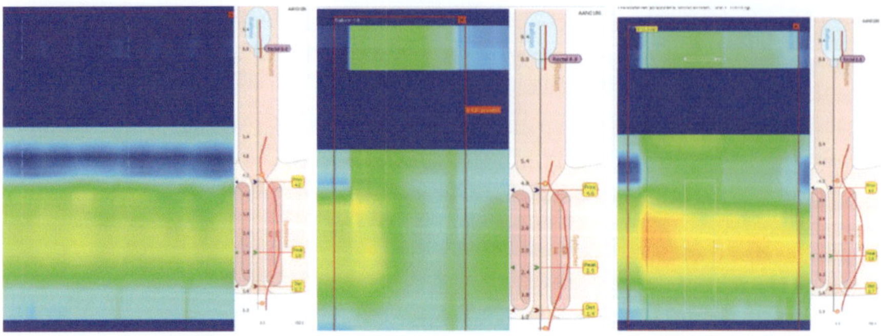

Fig. 23.55 HR-ARM of radiation-induced pelvic floor injury leading to dyssynergia and fecal incontinence. She was diagnosed with type I dyssynergia due to adequate increase in rectal pressure (≥40 mmHg) with paradoxical increase in anal pressure. The tracings show a maximum resting pressure of 76.4 mmHg (normal 83–96 mmHg) (left); the high-pressure zone (HPZ) length was 3.3 cm (normal 4.1–4.5 cm). Upon balloon inflation, the RAIR was present; first sensation was 40 mL (normal 20–25 mL); (center) urge to defecate was 70 mL (normal 140–167 mL) and discomfort 120 mL (normal 192–222 mL). Rectal compliance was poor. Upon pushing, the residual anal pressure was 79.7 mmHg (normal 28–52 mmHg), percent anal relaxation −5%, and recto-anal pressure differential −36.7 mmHg (right)

Fig. 23.56 Plain abdominal radiograph revealing moderate to severe stool burden along the length of the colon and paucity of gas within the pelvis, suggestive of fecal impaction

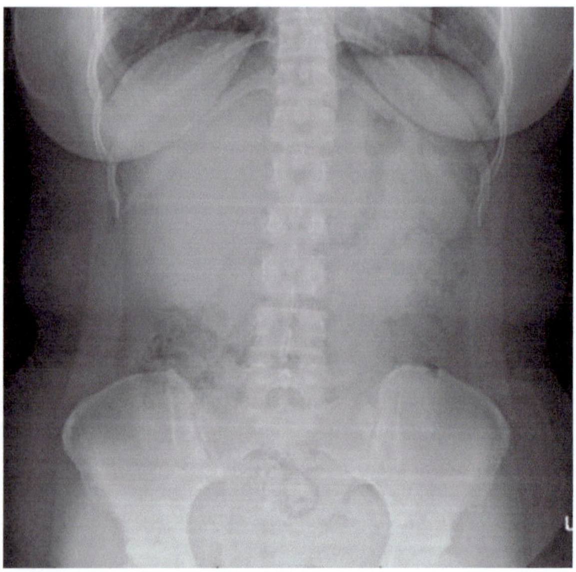

Index

G. Triadafilopoulos (ed.), *Onco-Neurogastroenterology*,
https://doi.org/10.1007/978-3-031-98848-6

N

O

P

MIX
Papier aus verantwortungsvollen Quellen
Paper from responsible sources
FSC® C105338

If you have any concerns about our products,
you can contact us on
ProductSafety@springernature.com

In case Publisher is established outside the EU,
the EU authorized representative is:
Springer Nature Customer Service Center GmbH
Europaplatz 3, 69115 Heidelberg, Germany

Printed by Libri Plureos GmbH
in Hamburg, Germany